Hypoglycaemia in Clinical Diabetes

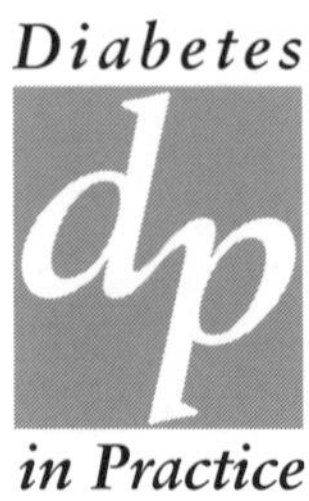

Other titles in the Wiley *Diabetes in Practice Series*

Diabetes in Old Age
Paul Finucane and Alan J. Sinclair (Editors)

Prediction, Prevention and Genetic Counseling in IDDM
Jerry P. Palmer (Editor)

Diabetes and Pregnancy:
An International Approach to Diagnosis and Management
Anne Dornhorst and David R. Hadden (Editors)

Diabetic Complications
Ken M. Shaw (Editor)

Childhood and Adolescent Diabetes
Simon Court and Bill Lamb (Editors)

Exercise and Sport in Diabetes
Bill Burr and Dinesh Nagi (Editors)

Hypoglycaemia in Clinical Diabetes

Edited by

Brian M. Frier

The Royal Infirmary of Edinburgh, Scotland, UK

and

B. Miles Fisher

Royal Alexandra Hospital, Paisley, Scotland, UK

JOHN WILEY & SONS, LTD

Chichester • New York • Weinheim • Brisbane • Singapore • Toronto

Baffins Lane, Chichester,
West Sussex PO19 1UD, England
National 01243 779777
International (+44) 1243 779777
e-mail (for orders and customer service enquiries): cs-books@wiley.co.uk
Visit our Home Page on http://www.wiley.co.uk
or http://www.wiley.com

Reprinted 2000

Other Wiley Editorial Offices

John Wiley & Sons, Inc., 605 Third Avenue,
New York, NY 10158-0012, USA

WILEY-VCH Verlag GmbH, Pappelallee 3,
D-69469 Weinheim, Germany

Jacaranda Wiley Ltd, 33 Park Road, Milton,
Queensland 4064, Australia

John Wiley & Sons (Asia) Pte Ltd, 2 Clementi Loop #02-01,
Jin Xing Distripark, Singapore 129809

John Wiley & Sons (Canada) Ltd, 22 Worcester Road,
Rexdale, Ontario M9W 1L1, Canada

Library of Congress Cataloging-in-Publication Data
Hypoglycaemia in clinical diabetes / edited by Brian M. Frier and B. Miles Fisher.
p. cm. — (Diabetes in practice)
Includes bibliographical references and index.
ISBN 0-471-98264-4 (cased : alk. paper)
1. Hypoglycemia. 2. Diabetes—Treatment—Complications.
3. Hypoglycemic agents—Side effects. I. Frier, Brian M. II. Fisher, B. Miles. III. Series.
[DNLM: 1. Diabetes Mellitus—complications. 2. Hypoglycemia—physiopathology.
3. Insulin—adverse effects. WK 880 H9963 1999]
RC662.2.H965 1999
616.4′66—dc21
DNLM/DLC
for Library of Congress 99-26598
CIP

British Library Cataloguing in Publication Data

A catalogue record for this book is available from the British Library

ISBN 0-471-98264-4

Typeset in 10/12pt Palatino from the author's disks by Keytec Typesetting Ltd., Bridport, Dorset.
Printed and bound in Great Britain by Biddles Ltd, Guildford and King's Lynn
This book is printed on acid-free paper responsibly manufactured from sustainable forestry, in which at least two trees are planted for each one used for paper production.

To
Emily, Ben and Marc

Contents

Contributors

Professor Stephanie A. Amiel *R. D. Lawrence Professor of Diabetes, King's College School of Medicine and Dentistry, Bessemer Road, London SE5 9PJ, UK*

Professor Ian J. Deary *Professor of Differential Psychology, Department of Psychology, University of Edinburgh, 7 George Square, Edinburgh, EH8 9JZ, UK*

Dr B. Miles Fisher *Consultant Physician, Royal Alexandra Hospital, Paisley PA2 9PL, UK*

Dr Brian M. Frier *Consultant Physician, Department of Diabetes, Royal Infirmary, Edinburgh EH3 9YW, UK*

Dr Simon R. Heller *Senior Lecturer in Medicine, Department of Medicine, University of Sheffield, Northern General Hospital, Herries Road, Sheffield S5 7AU, UK*

Dr David Kerr *Consultant Physician, Diabetes & Endocrine Centre, The Royal Bournemouth Hospital, Castle Lane East, Bournemouth, BH7 7DW, UK*

Dr Paromita King *Senior Medical Registrar, Queen's Medical Centre, Nottingham NG7 2UH, UK*

Professor Ian A. Macdonald *Professor of Metabolic Physiology, Department of Physiology and Pharmacology, Medical School, Queen's Medical Centre, Nottingham, NG7 2UH, UK*

Dr Petros Perros *Consultant Physician, Freeman Hospital, Newcastle upon Tyne, NE7 7DN, UK*

Dr Peter G. F. Swift *Consultant Paediatrician, Children's Hospital, Leicester Royal Infirmary, Leicester, LE1 5WW, UK*

Professor Robert B. Tattersall *Curzon House, Curzon Street, Gotham, Nottingham NG11 0HQ, UK*

Preface

Hypoglycaemia is one of the commonest metabolic emergencies encountered in modern clinical practice. Because it is so common, and the outcome generally satisfactory, some clinicians have tended to minimise its importance. Until relatively recently it had not received much detailed scientific analysis or research in comparison to the investigation of the pathogenesis and the complications of diabetes.

The results of the Diabetes Control and Complications Trial in type 1 diabetes, and the UK Prospective Diabetes Study in type 2 diabetes clearly show that strict glycaemic control can reduce the frequency and severity of the complications of diabetes, but intensive insulin therapy incurs the risk of a greater frequency of hypoglycaemia. Clinical staff who look after people with diabetes are often surprised that they are unwilling to accept the risk of hypoglycaemia, and are prepared to risk the development of diabetic complications. This is rarely a surprise to people with diabetes, who live under the shadow of hypoglycaemia on a daily basis. The fear of hypoglycaemia, a recurring theme in this book, is the most common reason why patients are unable to achieve the targets of glycated haemoglobin desired by their medical carers.

Although most people with diabetes know that on most occasions hypoglycaemia does not have any lasting consequences, they are often aware of anecdotal accounts of patients who have suffered mishaps during hypoglycaemia, and of highly publicised sudden and unexpected deaths associated with hypoglycaemia of people with diabetes. This has left an indelible mark on the consciousness of many people with diabetes and their families.

This book on hypoglycaemia and diabetes is one of a series on diabetes in practice, and, as such, attempts to highlight the problems of hypoglycaemia which occur in the daily life of people with diabetes and are common in clinical practice. The contents of this book should be of interest to all members of the diabetes team, from general practitioners to diabetologists and clinical biochemists, from practice nurses to diabetes nurse specialists and dietitians. This text does not attempt to provide a fully comprehensive account of every nuance of hypoglycaemia as it relates to diabetes, and readers who seek further information may find this in other referenced reviews, and in our previous book, *Hypoglycaemia and Diabetes: Clinical and Physiological Aspects*, published in 1993. Instead, we have highlighted common clinical problems, and areas where recent research developments of clinical importance have been reported.

The metabolic and physiological consequences of hypoglycaemia are examined along with the abnormal counterregulatory and symptomatic responses which develop in people with diabetes. The physical consequences of hypoglycaemia are discussed in chapters addressing how hypoglycaemia affects the functioning of the brain and the cardiovascular system.

Hypoglycaemia is of particular importance to certain groups of patients, and a detailed discussion of hypoglycaemia in children and during pregnancy has been provided. This does not diminish the importance of hypoglycaemia to other groups, but simply acknowledges that hypoglycaemia is very common, and has potentially serious consequences, in these two groups. The problems of hypoglycaemia in the elderly and in patients with type 2 diabetes receiving treatment with insulin are two areas where more clinical research is urgently needed, and these areas are discussed briefly in different chapters. These are important topics of increasing relevance to clinical diabetes that will attract greater attention in the future. Finally, but possibly most importantly, the section on living with hypoglycaemia will be of interest not only to clinical staff but also to anyone who has regular contact with people with diabetes, including patients themselves, their relatives and spouses. Medical science progresses rapidly, and there are several potential important developments over the hypoglycaemic horizon, including new non-invasive glucose sensors, and a greater range of insulin analogues which may help to reduce the frequency of hypoglycaemia.

For two busy clinicians it has been difficult to balance the demands of a heavy clinical schedule with the timetable necessary to produce a book of this type. We have been greatly assisted by our fellow contributors who have written their texts with authority and expertise. Inevitably, much of the work on the book has been done out of hours and at home, and we are grateful for the forbearance of our long-suffering families. Finally, we are grateful to our patients who have taught us so much about the real problems of hypoglycaemia.

Brian M. Frier
B. Miles Fisher

1

Normal Glucose Metabolism and Responses to Hypoglycaemia

PAROMITA KING and IAN A. MACDONALD*
Queen's Medical Centre, Nottingham and *University of Nottingham Medical School

INTRODUCTION

Control of blood glucose is a fundamental feature of homeostasis, i.e. the process by which the internal environment of the body is maintained stable allowing optimal function. Blood glucose concentrations are regulated within a narrow range (which in humans is known as *normoglycaemia* or *euglycaemia*) despite wide variability in carbohydrate intake and physical activity. Teleologically, the upper limit is defended because high glucose concentrations cause microvascular disease, and the lower limit, because the brain cannot function without an adequate supply of glucose. In this chapter these mechanisms are described and how hypoglycaemia is avoided in healthy individuals is discussed. The physiological consequences of hypoglycaemia are described.

NORMAL GLUCOSE HOMEOSTASIS

Humans evolved as hunter-gatherers and, unlike people today, did not consume regular meals. Mechanisms therefore evolved for the body to

Hypoglycaemia in Clinical Diabetes. Edited by B. M. Frier and B. M. Fisher.

store food when it was in abundance, and to use these stores to provide an adequate supply of energy, in particular in the form of glucose, when food was scarce. Cahill (1971) originally described the "rules of the metabolic game" which man had to follow to ensure his survival. These have been modified by Tattersall (personal communication) and are:

1. Maintain blood glucose within a very narrow range.
2. Maintain an emergency energy source (glycogen) which can be tapped quickly for fleeing or fighting.
3. Waste not want not, i.e. store fuel (fat and protein) in times of plenty.
4. Use every trick in the book to maintain protein reserves.

To enable the above "rules" to be followed requires various control mechanisms. Insulin and glucagon are the two hormones controlling glucose homeostasis, and the most important processes governed by these hormones are:

- *Glycogen synthesis and breakdown (glycogenolysis): Glycogen*, a carbohydrate, is an energy source stored in the liver and skeletal muscle. Liver glycogen is broken down to provide glucose for all tissues, whereas the breakdown of muscle glycogen results in *lactate* formation (Figure 1.1a).
- *Gluconeogenesis:* This is the production of glucose in the liver from precursors *glycerol, lactate* and *amino acids* (in particular alanine) (Figure 1.1b). The process can also occur in the kidneys but this site is not important under physiological conditions.
- *Glucose uptake and metabolism (glycolysis)* by skeletal muscle and adipose tissue.

The actions of insulin and glucagon are summarised in Boxes 1.1 and 1.2. Insulin is an anabolic hormone, reducing glucose output by the liver (hepatic glucose output), increasing the uptake of glucose by muscle and adipose tissue (increasing peripheral uptake) and increasing protein and fat formation. Glucagon opposes the actions of insulin in the liver. Thus insulin tends to reduce, and glucagon increase blood glucose concentrations.

The metabolic effects of insulin and glucagon and their relationship to glucose homeostasis are best considered in relationship to fasting and the postprandial state (Siegal and Kreisberg, 1975). In both these situations it is the relative and not the absolute concentrations of these hormones that are important.

Fasting (Figure 1.2, left)

During fasting, insulin concentrations are reduced and glucagon increased, which maintains blood glucose concentrations in accordance

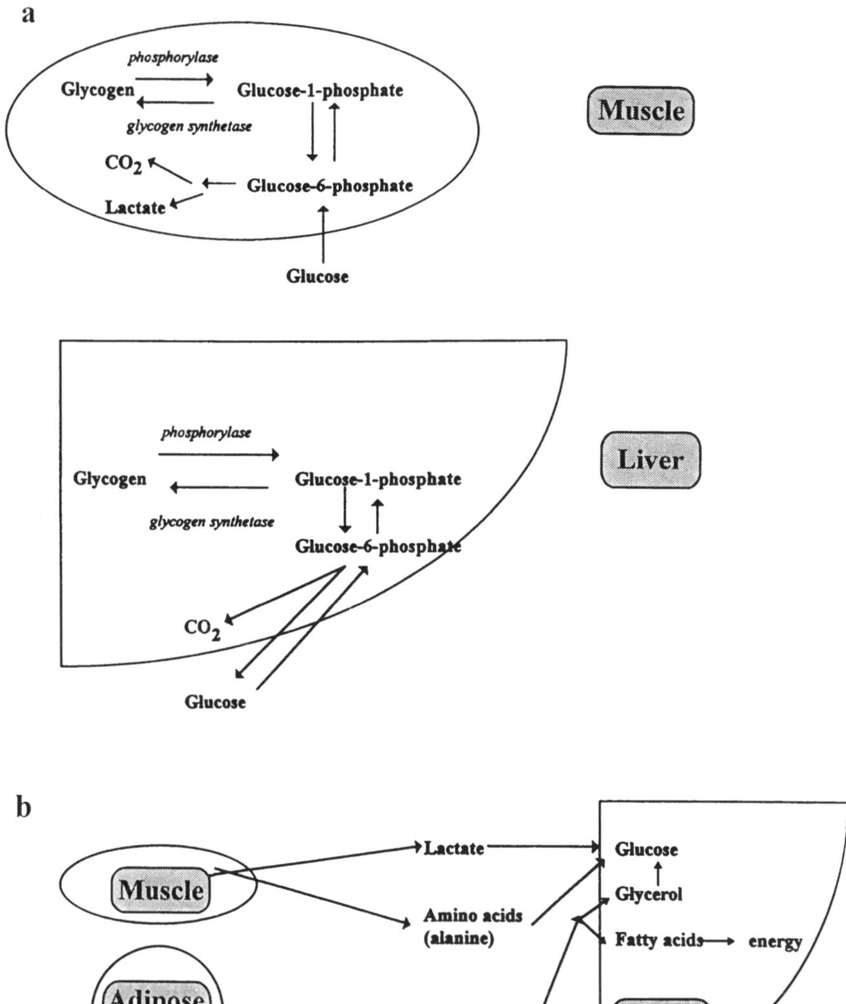

Figure 1.1 (a) Glycogen metabolism; (b) Gluconeogenesis

with rule 1 above. The net effect is to reduce peripheral glucose utilisation, to increase hepatic glucose production and to provide non-glucose fuels for tissues not entirely dependent on glucose. After a short (for example overnight) fast, glucose production needs to be 5–6 g/h to maintain blood glucose concentrations, with the brain using 80% of this. Glycogenolysis provides 60–80% and gluconeogenesis 20–40% of the

Box 1.1 Actions of insulin

Liver
↑ Glycogen synthesis (↑ glycogen synthetase activity)
↑ Glycolysis
↑ Lipid formation
↑ Protein formation
↓ Glycogenolysis (↓ phosphorylase activity)
↓ Gluconeogenesis
↓ Ketone formation

Muscle
↑ Uptake of glucose
amino acids
ketones
potassium
↑ Glycolysis
↑ Synthesis of glycogen
protein
↓ Protein catabolism
↓ Release of amino acids

Adipose tissue
↑ Uptake of glucose
potassium
Storage of triglyceride

Box 1.2 Actions of glucagon

Liver
↑ Glycogenolysis
↑ Gluconeogenesis
↑ Extraction of alanine
↑ Ketogenesis
No significant peripheral action

required glucose. In prolonged fasts, glycogen becomes depleted and glucose production is primarily from gluconeogenesis, with an increasing proportion from the kidney as opposed to the liver. In extreme situations renal gluconeogenesis can contribute as much as 45% of glucose production. Thus glycogen is the short-term or "emergency" fuel source (rule 2), with gluconeogenesis predominating in more prolonged fasts. The fol-

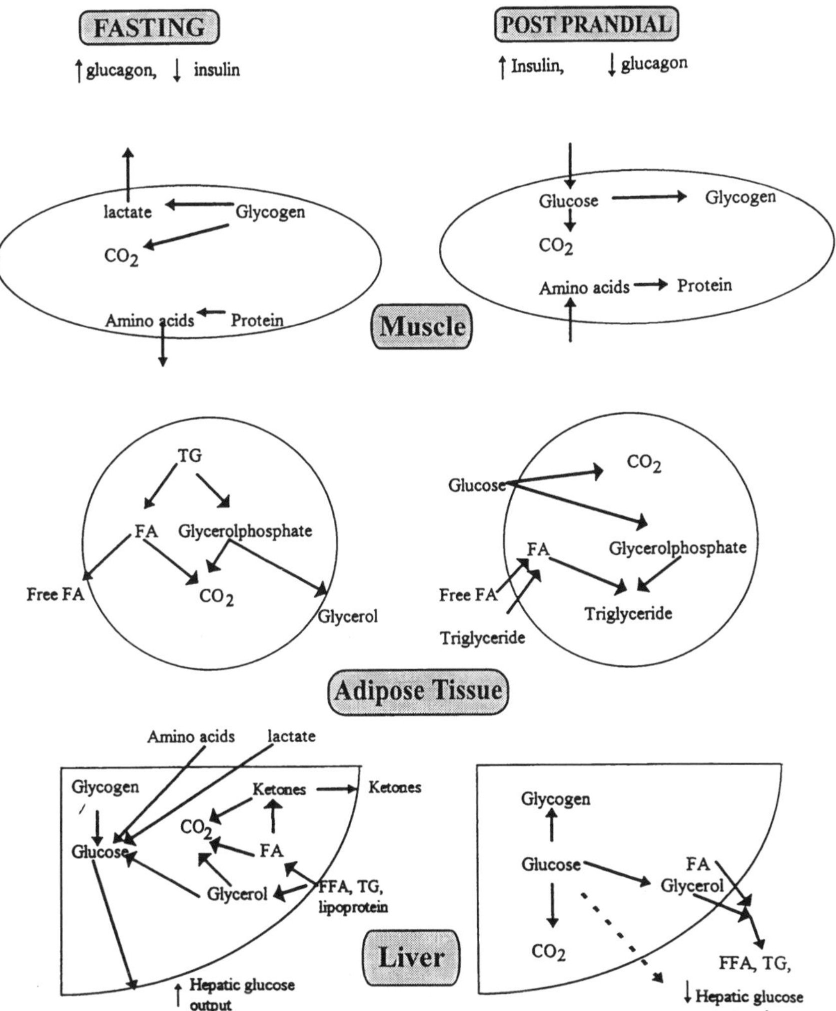

Figure 1.2 Metabolic pathways for glucose homeostasis in muscle, adipose tissue and liver during fasting (left) and postprandially (right). FA = fatty acids; TG = triglycerides

lowing metabolic alterations enable this increase in glucose production to occur.

- *Muscle:* Glucose uptake and oxidative metabolism are reduced and fatty acid oxidation increased. Amino acids are released.

- *Adipose tissue:* There are reductions in glucose uptake and triglyceride storage. The increase in the activity of the enzyme hormone-sensitive lipase, results in hydrolysis of triglyceride to glycerol (a gluconeogenic precursor) and fatty acids, which can be metabolised.
- *Liver:* Increased cAMP concentrations result in increased glycogenolysis and gluconeogenesis, thus increasing hepatic glucose output. The uptake of gluconeogenic precursors (i.e. amino acids, glycerol, lactate and pyruvate) is also increased. Ketone bodies are produced in the liver from fatty acids. This process is normally inhibited by insulin and stimulated by glucagon, thus the hormonal changes during fasting lead to an increase in ketone production. Fatty acids are also a metabolic fuel used by the liver as a source of energy needed for the biochemical reactions involved in gluconeogenesis.

The reduced insulin : glucagon ratio favours a catabolic state, but the effect on fat metabolism is greater than on protein metabolism, and thus muscle is relatively preserved (rule 4). These adaptations meant that not only did the hunter-gatherer have sufficient muscle power to pursue his next meal, but that the function of the brain was optimally maintained to help him do this.

Fed State (Figure 1.2, right)

In the fed state, in accordance with the rules of the metabolic game, the calories from excess food are stored as glycogen, protein and fat (rule 3). The rise in blood glucose concentration results in an increase in insulin and a reduction in glucagon secretion. This balance favours utilisation of glucose, reduction of glucose production and increased formation of glycogen, triglyceride and protein. The following changes enable these processes to occur:

- *Muscle:* Insulin increases glucose transport, oxidative metabolism and glycogen synthesis. Amino acid release is inhibited and protein synthesis is increased.
- *Adipose tissue:* In the fat cells, glucose transport is increased, while lipolysis is inhibited. At the same time the enzyme lipoprotein lipase, located in the capillaries, is activated and causes triglyceride to be broken down to fatty acids and glycerol. The fatty acids are taken up into the fat cells and re-esterified to triglyceride (using glycerol phosphate derived from glucose) before being stored.
- *Liver:* Glucose uptake is increased proportional to blood glucose,

a process which does not need insulin. However, insulin does decrease cAMP concentrations, which causes an increase in glycogen synthesis and the inhibition of glycogenolysis and gluconeogenesis. These effects "retain" glucose in the liver and reduce hepatic glucose output.

This complex interplay between insulin and glucagon maintains euglycaemia and enables the rules of the metabolic game to be followed. This ensures not only the survival of the hunter-gatherer, but also of modern humans.

EFFECTS OF GLUCOSE DEPRIVATION ON CENTRAL NERVOUS SYSTEM METABOLISM

The brain constitutes only 2% of body weight, but consumes 20% of the body's oxygen and receives 15% of its cardiac output (Sokaloff, 1989). It is almost totally dependent on carbohydrate as a fuel and, since it cannot store or synthesise glucose, depends on a continuous supply from the blood. The brain contains the enzymes needed to metabolise fuels other than glucose such as lactate, ketones and amino acids, but under physiological conditions their use is limited by insufficient quantities in the blood or slow rates of transport across the blood–brain barrier. When arterial blood glucose falls below 3.0 mmol/l, cerebral metabolism and function decline. Metabolism of glucose by the brain releases energy, and also generates neurotransmitters such as gamma amino butyric acid (GABA) and acetylcholine, together with phospholipids needed for cell membrane synthesis. When blood glucose concentration falls, changes in the synthesis of these products may occur within minutes because of reduced glucose metabolism, which can alter cerebral function. This is likely to be a factor in producing the subtle changes in cerebral function detectable at blood glucose concentrations as high as 3.0 mmol/l, which is not sufficiently low to cause a major depletion in ATP or creatine phosphate, the brain's two main sources of energy (McCall, 1993).

Isotope techniques and Positron Emission Tomography (PET) allow the study of metabolism in different parts of the brain and show regional variations in metabolism during hypoglycaemia. The neocortex, hippocampus, hypothalamus and cerebellum are most sensitive to hypoglycaemia, whereas metabolism is relatively preserved in the thalamus and brainstem. Changes in cerebral function are initially reversible, but during prolonged severe hypoglycaemia, general energy failure (due to the depletion of ATP and creatine phosphate) can cause permanent cerebral damage. Pathologically, this is caused by selective neuronal necrosis most likely due to "excitotoxin" damage. Local energy failure induces the intrasynaptic release of glutamate or aspartate, and failure of reuptake of the neurotransmitters increases their concentrations. This leads to the activation of N-methyl-D-aspartate (NMDA) receptors causing cerebral damage. One study in rats has shown that an experimental compound called AP7, which blocks the NMDA receptor, can prevent 90% of the cerebral damage associated with severe hypoglycaemia (Wieloch, 1985). In humans with fatal hypoglycaemia, protracted neuroglycopenia causes laminar necrosis in the cerebral cortex and diffuse demyelination. Regional differences in neuronal necrosis are seen, with the basal ganglia and hippocampus being sensitive, but hypothalamus and cerebellum relatively spared (Auer and Siesjö, 1988; Sieber and Traysman, 1992).

The brain is very sensitive to acute hypoglycaemia, but can adapt to chronic fuel deprivation. For example, during starvation, it can metabolise ketones for up to 60% of its energy requirements (Owen et al, 1967). Glucose transport can also be increased in the face of hypoglycaemia. Normally, glucose is transported into tissues using proteins called glucose transporters (GLUT) (Bell et al, 1990). This transport occurs down a concentration gradient faster than it would by simple diffusion and does not require energy (facilitated diffusion). There are several of these transporters, with GLUT 1 being responsible for transporting glucose across the blood–brain barrier and GLUT 3 for transporting glucose into neurones (Figure 1.3). Chronic hypoglycaemia in animals (McCall et al, 1986) and in humans (Boyle et al, 1995) increases cerebral glucose uptake, which is thought to be secondary to an increase in the production and action of GLUT 1 protein. It has not been established whether this adaptation is of major benefit in protecting brain function during hypoglycaemia.

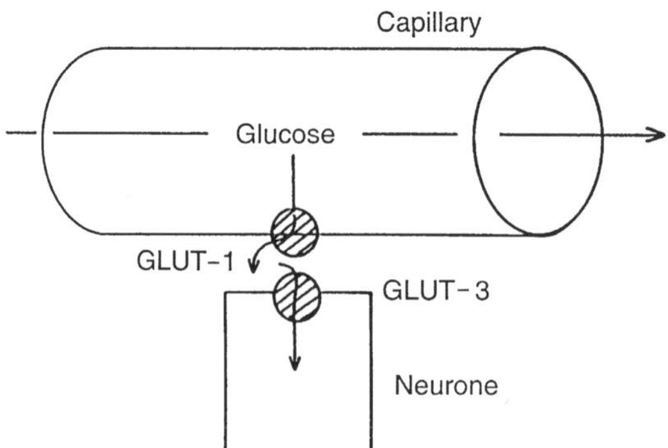

Figure 1.3 Transport of glucose across blood–brain barrier

COUNTERREGULATION DURING HYPOGLYCAEMIA

The potential serious effects of hypoglycaemia on cerebral function mean that not only are stable blood glucose concentrations maintained under physiological conditions, but if hypoglycaemia occurs, mechanisms have developed to combat it. In clinical practice, the principal causes for hypoglycaemia are iatrogenic (as side-effects of insulin and sulphonylureas used to treat diabetes) and excessive alcohol consumption. Insulin-secreting tumours (such as insulinoma) are rare. The mechanisms which correct hypoglycaemia are called *counterregulation*, because the hormones involved oppose the action of insulin and therefore are the counterregulatory hormones. The processes of counterregulation were identified in the mid-1970s and early 1980s, using either a bolus injection or continuous infusion of insulin to induce hypoglycaemia (Cryer, 1981; Gerich, 1988). The response to the bolus injection of 0.1 U/kg insulin in a normal subject is shown in Figure 1.4. Blood glucose concentrations decline within minutes of the administration of insulin and reach a nadir after 20–30 minutes, then gradually rise to near normal by two hours after the insulin was administered. The fact that blood glucose starts to rise when plasma insulin concentrations are still ten times the baseline values means that it is not simply the reduction in insulin that reverses hypoglycaemia, but active counterregulation must also occur. Many hormones are released when blood glucose is lowered (see below), but glucagon, the catecholamines, growth hormone and cortisol are regarded as being the most important.

Several studies have determined the relative importance of these hormones by producing isolated deficiencies of each hormone (by blocking its release or action) and assessing the subsequent response to administration of insulin. These studies are exemplified in Figure 1.5 which assesses the relative importance of glucagon, adrenaline (epinephrine) and growth hormone in the counterregulation of short-term hypoglycaemia. Somatostatin infusion blocks glucagon and growth hormone secretion and significantly impairs glucose recovery (Figure 1.5a). If growth hormone is replaced in the same model to produce isolated glucagon deficiency (Figure 1.5b) and glucagon replaced to produce isolated growth hormone deficiency (Figure 1.5c) it is clear that it is glucagon and not growth hormone that is responsible for acute counterregulation. Combined alpha and beta adrenoceptor blockade using phentolamine and propranolol (Figure 1.5d) or adrenalectomy (Figure 1.5e) can be used to evaluate the role of the catecholamines. These and other studies demonstrate that glucagon is the most potent and important counterregulatory hormone while catecholamines provide a backup if

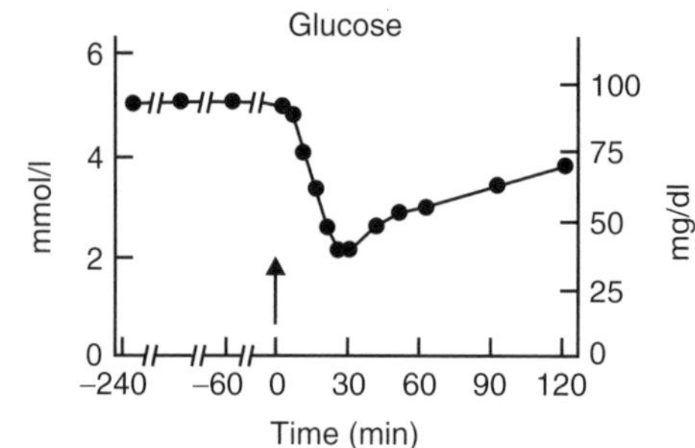

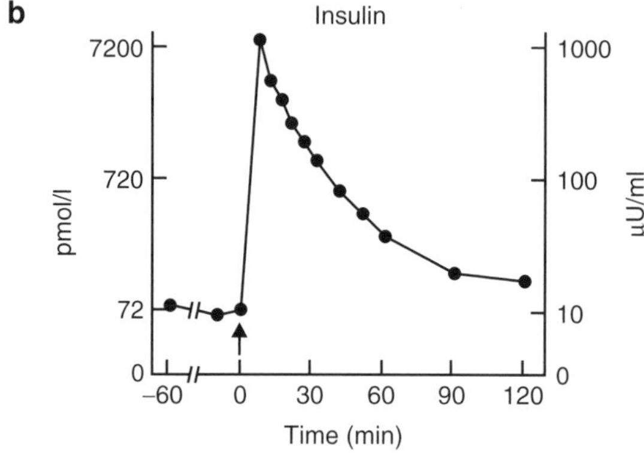

Figure 1.4 (a) Glucose and (b) insulin concentrations after an intravenous injection of insulin 0.1 U/kg at time 0. Reproduced from Garber et al (1976) by permission of *Journal of Clinical Investigation*

glucagon is deficient (for example in type 1 diabetes, Chapters 4 and 5). Cortisol and growth hormone are important only in prolonged hypoglycaemia. Therefore if glucagon and catecholamines are both deficient, as in longstanding type 1 diabetes, counterregulation is seriously compromised, and the individual is literally defenceless against acute hypoglycaemia (Cryer, 1981).

Glucagon and catecholamines increase glycogenolysis and stimulate gluconeogenesis. Catecholamines also reduce glucose utilisation peripherally and inhibit insulin secretion. Cortisol and growth hormone increase gluconeogenesis and reduce glucose utilisation. The role of the other hormones (see below) in counterregulation is unclear, but they are unlikely to make a significant contribution. Finally, there is evidence that in profound hypoglycaemia (blood glucose below 1.7 mmol/l), hepatic

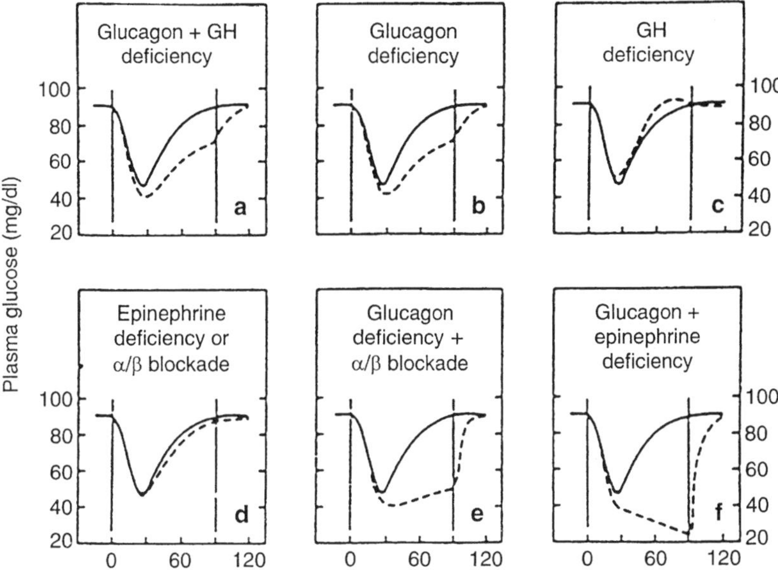

Figure 1.5 Glucose recovery from acute hypoglycaemia. Glucose concentration following an intravenous injection of 0.05 U/kg at time 0; after saline infusion (continuous line) and somatostatin (a), somatostatin and growth hormone (GH) (b), somatostatin and glucagon (c), combined alpha and beta blockade with phentolamine and propranolol infusions or adrenalectomy (d), somatostatin with alpha and beta blockade (e), and somatostatin in adrenalectomised patients (f). Saline infusion (continuous lines); experimental study (broken lines). Reproduced from Cryer (1981) and published by permission of the American Diabetes Association (epinephrine = adrenaline)

glucose output is stimulated directly, although the mechanism is unknown. This is termed *hepatic autoregulation.*

The depth, as well as the duration, of hypoglycaemia is important in determining the magnitude of the counterregulatory hormonal response. Studies using "hyperinsulinaemic clamps" show a hierarchical response of hormone production. In this technique, insulin is infused at a constant rate and a glucose infusion varied to maintain blood glucose concentrations within ±0.2 mmol/l of target concentrations. This permits the controlled evaluation of the counterregulatory hormonal response at varying degrees of hypoglycaemia. It also demonstrates that glucagon, catecholamines and growth hormone start to be secreted at a blood glucose concentration of 3.5–3.7 mmol/l, with cortisol being produced at a lower glucose of 3.0 mmol/l (Mitrakou et al, 1991). The counterregulatory response is initiated before impairment in cerebral function is evident, usually at a blood glucose concentration of approximately 3.0 mmol/l (Heller and Macdonald, 1996).

The magnitude of the hormonal response also depends on the length of the hypoglycaemic episode. The counterregulatory hormonal response commences up to 20 minutes after hypoglycaemia is achieved and continues to rise for 60 minutes (Kerr et al, 1989).

The complex counterregulatory and homeostatic mechanisms described above are thought to be mostly under the control of the central nervous system. Evidence for this comes from studies in dogs, where glucose was infused into the carotid and vertebral arteries to maintain euglycaemia in the brain. Despite peripheral hypoglycaemia, glucagon secretion did not increase and responses of the other counterregulatory hormones were blunted. This, and other studies in rats, led to the hypothesis that the ventromedial nucleus of the hypothalamus (which does not have a blood–brain barrier) acts as a glucose sensor and co-ordinates counterregulation (Borg et al, 1997). However, evidence also exists that other parts of the brain may be involved in mediating counter-regulation. The existence of hepatic autoregulation means that some peripheral control must exist. Studies producing central euglycaemia and hepatic portal venous hypoglycaemia in dogs have provided evidence for hepatic glucose sensors and suggest that these sensors as well as those in the brain are important in the regulation of glucose (Hamilton-Wessler et al, 1994).

HORMONAL CHANGES DURING HYPOGLYCAEMIA

Hypoglycaemia induces a change in various hormones, some of which are responsible for symptom generation (Chapter 2), counterregulation and many of the physiological changes that occur as a consequence of lowering blood glucose. The stimulation of the autonomic nervous system is central to many of these changes.

Activation of the Autonomic Nervous System

The autonomic nervous system comprises sympathetic and parasympathetic components (Figure 1.6). Fibres from the sympathetic division leave the spinal cord with the ventral roots from the first thoracic to the third or fourth lumbar nerves to synapse in the sympathetic chain or visceral ganglia, and the long postganglionic fibres are incorporated in somatic nerves. The parasympathetic pathways originate in the nuclei of cranial nerves III, VII, IX and X, and travel with the vagus nerve. A second component, the sacral outflow, supplies the pelvic viscera via the pelvic branches of the second to fourth spinal nerves. The ganglia in both

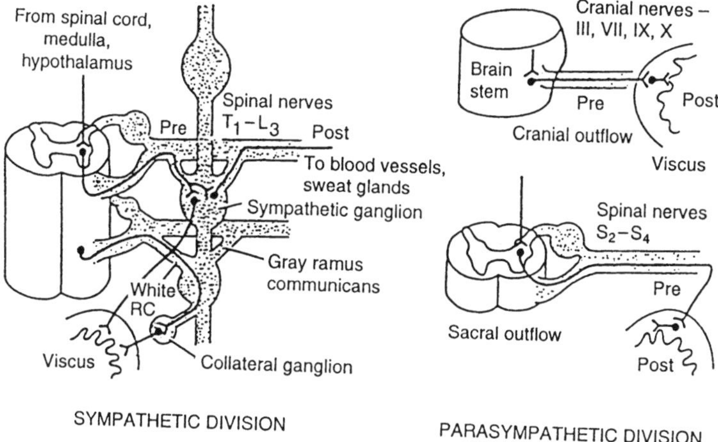

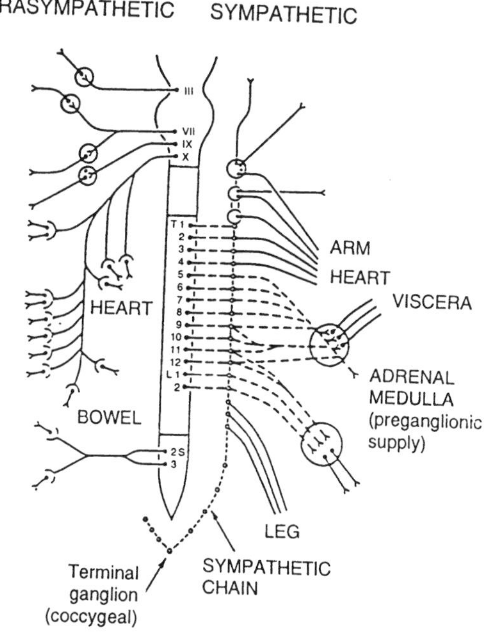

Figure 1.6 Anatomy of the autonomic nervous system. Pre = preganglionic neurones; post = postganglionic neurones; RC = ramus communicans

cases are located near the organs supplied, and the postganglionic neurones are therefore short.

Activation of both divisions of the autonomic system occurs during hypoglycaemia, but is selective. The sympathetic nervous system in particular is responsible for many of the physiological changes observed during hypoglycaemia and the evidence for its activation can be obtained indirectly by observing functional changes such as cardiovascular responses (considered below), measuring plasma catecholamines which gives a general index of sympathetic activation, or by direct recording of sympathetic activity.

Direct recordings are possible from sympathetic nerves supplying skeletal muscle and skin. Sympathetic neural activity in skeletal muscle involves vasoconstrictor fibres which innervate blood vessels and are involved in controlling blood pressure. During hypoglycaemia (induced by insulin), the frequency and amplitude of muscle sympathetic activity are increased as blood glucose falls, with an increase in activity eight minutes after insulin is injected intravenously, peaking at 25–30 minutes coincident with the blood glucose nadir, but persisting for 90 minutes after euglycaemia is restored (Figure 1.7a) (Fagius et al, 1986). During hypoglycaemia, a sudden increase in skin sympathetic activity is seen, which coincides with the onset of sweating. This sweating leads to vasodilatation of skin blood vessels, to which there is also a contribution by a reduction in sympathetic stimulation of the vasoconstrictor compo-

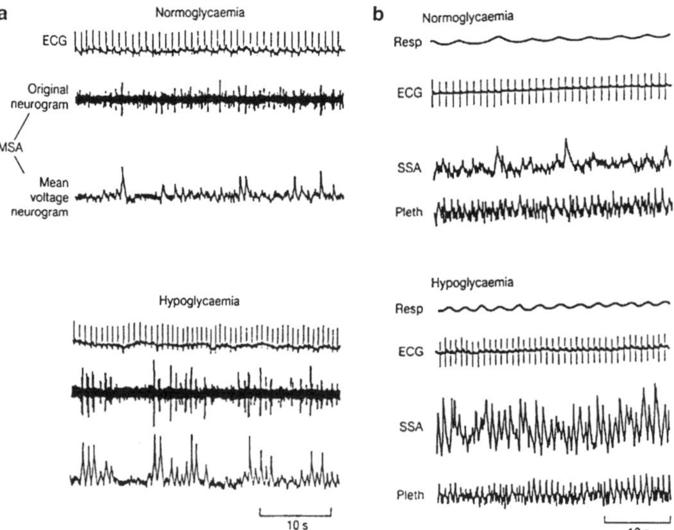

Figure 1.7 (a) Muscle sympathetic activity during normoglycaemia (euglycaemia) and hypoglycaemia. Reproduced from Fagius et al. (1986) and published by permission of the American Diabetes Association. (b) Skin sympathetic activity during normoglycaemia and hypoglycaemia. Reproduced from Berne and Fagius (1986) with permission of *Diabetologia*

nents of skin arterio-venous anastomoses (Figure 1.7b) (Berne and Fagius, 1986). These effects (at least initially) increase total skin blood flow and promote heat loss from the body.

Activation of both muscle and skin sympathetic nerve activity is thought to be centrally mediated. Tissue neuroglycopenia can be produced by 2-deoxy-D-glucose, a glucose analogue, without increasing insulin. Infusion of this analogue causes stimulation of muscle and skin sympathetic activity demonstrating that it is hypoglycaemia and not the insulin used to induce it which is responsible for the sympathetic activation (Fagius and Berne, 1989).

The activation of the parasympathetic nervous system (vagus nerve) during hypoglycaemia cannot be measured directly. The most useful index of parasympathetic function is the measurement of plasma pancreatic polypeptide, the peptide hormone secreted by the PP cells of the pancreas, which is released in response to vagal stimulation.

Neuroendocrine Activation (Box 1.3)

Insulin-induced hypoglycaemia was used to study the function of the pituitary gland as early as the 1940s. The glucose response to insulin was

Box 1.3 Neuroendocrine activation

Hypothalamus	↑ Corticotrophin releasing hormone
	↑ Growth hormone releasing hormone
Anterior Pituitary	↑ Adrenocorticotrophic hormone
	↑ Beta endorphin
	↑ Growth hormone
	↑ Prolactin
	↔ Thyrotrophin
	↔ Gonadotrophins
Posterior Pituitary	↑ Vasopressin
	↑ Oxytocin
Pancreas	↑ Glucagon
	↑ Somatostatin (28)
	↑ Pancreatic polypeptide
	↓ Insulin
Adrenal	↑ Cortisol
	↑ Adrenaline
	↑ Aldosterone
Others	↑ Parathyroid hormone
	↑ Gastrin

used to measure insulin resistance, and thereby evaluate conditions such as Cushing's syndrome and hypopituitarism. The development of assays for adrenocorticotrophic hormone (ACTH) and growth hormone (GH) allowed the direct measurement of pituitary function during hypoglycaemia in the 1960s, and many of the processes governing these changes were unravelled before elucidation of the counterregulatory system. The studies are comparable to those evaluating counterregulation in that potential regulatory factors are blocked to measure the hormonal response to hypoglycaemia with and without the regulating factor.

Hypothalamus and Anterior Pituitary

ACTH, GH and prolactin concentrations increase during hypoglycaemia, but there is no change in thyrotrophin (thyroid stimulating hormone, TSH) or gonadotrophin secretion. The secretion of these pituitary hormones is controlled by releasing factors which are produced in the median eminence of the hypothalamus and secreted into the hypophyseal portal vessels and then pass to the pituitary gland (Figure 1.8). The mechanisms regulating the releasing factors are incompletely under-

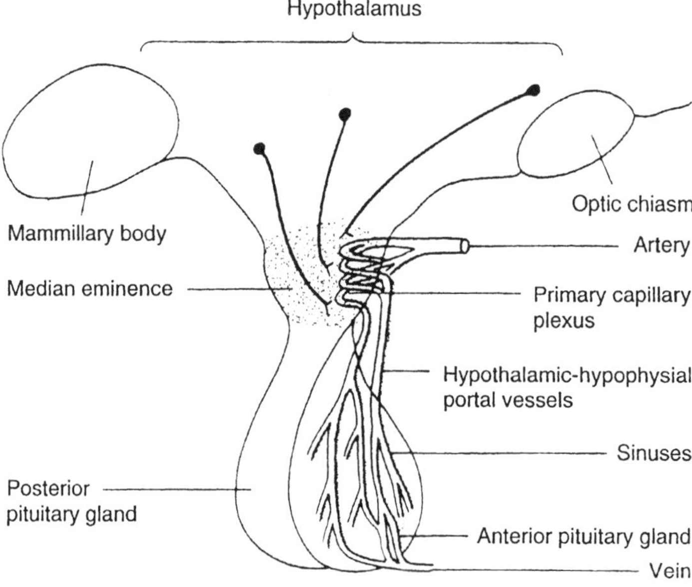

Figure 1.8 Anatomy of the hypothalamus and pituitary gland

stood, but may involve the ventromedial nucleus, one site where brain glucose sensors are situated (Fish et al, 1986).

- *ACTH*: Secretion is governed by release of corticotrophin releasing hormone (CRH) from the hypothalamus; alpha adrenoceptors stimulate CRH release, and beta adrenoceptors have an inhibitory action. A variety of neurotransmitters control the release of CRH into the portal vessels, including serotonin and acetycholine which are stimulatory and GABA which is inhibitory. The increase in ACTH causes cortisol to be secreted from the cortices of the adrenal glands.
- *Beta endorphins* are derived from the same precursors as ACTH and are co-secreted with it. The role of endorphins in counter-regulation is uncertain, but they may influence the secretion of the other pituitary hormones during hypoglycaemia.
- *GH:* Growth hormone secretion is controlled by two hypothalamic hormones: growth hormone releasing hormone (GHRH) which stimulates GH secretion, and somatostatin which is inhibitory. GHRH secretion is stimulated by dopamine, GABA, opiates and through alpha adrenoceptors, while it is inhibited by serotonin and beta adrenoceptors. A study in rats showed that bioassayable GH and GHRH are depleted in the pituitary and hypothalamus respectively after insulin-induced hypoglycaemia (Katz et al, 1967).
- *Prolactin:* The mechanisms are not established. Prolactin secretion is normally under inhibitory control of dopamine, but there is also evidence for releasing factors during hypoglycaemia. Prolactin does not contribute to counterregulation.

Posterior Pituitary

Vasopressin and oxytocin both increase during hypoglycaemia (Fisher et al, 1987). Their secretion is under hormonal and neurotransmitter control in a similar way to the hypothalamic hormones. Vasopressin has glycolytic actions and oxytocin increases hepatic glucose output in dogs, but their contribution to glucose counterregulation in uncertain.

Pancreas

- *Glucagon:* The mechanisms of glucagon secretion during hypoglycaemia are still not fully understood. Although activation of the autonomic nervous system stimulates its release, this pathway has been shown to be less important in humans. A reduction in blood glucose concentration may have a direct effect on the glucagon-secreting pancreatic alpha cells, or the reduced beta cell activity (reduced insulin secretion), which also occurs with low blood glucose, may release the tonic inhibition of glucagon secretion.

- *Somatostatin:* This is thought of as a pancreatic hormone produced from D cells of the islets of Langerhans, but is also secreted in other parts of the gastrointestinal tract. There are a number of structurally different polypeptides derived from prosomatostatin: the somatostatin-14 peptide is secreted from D cells, and somatostatin-28 from the gastrointestinal tract. The plasma concentration of somatostatin-28 increases during hypoglycaemia (Francis and Ensinck, 1987). The normal action of somatostatin is to inhibit the secretion both of insulin and glucagon, but somatostatin-28 inhibits insulin secretion ten times more effectively than glucagon, and thus may have a role in counterregulation by suppressing insulin release.
- *Pancreatic polypeptide:* This peptide has no role in counterregulation, but its release during hypoglycaemia is stimulated by cholinergic fibres through muscarinic receptors and is a useful marker of parasympathetic activity.

Adrenal and Renin–Angiotensin System

The processes governing the increase in cortisol during hypoglycaemia are discussed above. The rise in plasma catecholamines, in particular adrenaline from the adrenal medulla, which occurs when blood glucose is lowered, is controlled by sympathetic fibres in the splanchnic nerve. The increase in renin, and therefore angiotensin and aldosterone, during hypoglycaemia is stimulated primarily by the intra-renal effects of increased catecholamines, mediated through beta adrenoceptors, although the increase in ACTH and hypokalaemia due to hypoglycaemia contributes (Trovati et al, 1988; Jungman et al, 1989). These changes do not have a significant role in counterregulation, although angiotensin II has glycolytic actions in vitro.

PHYSIOLOGICAL RESPONSES

Haemodynamic Changes (Box 1.4)

The haemodynamic changes during hypoglycaemia are mostly due to the activation of the sympathetic nervous system and an increase in circulating adrenaline. An increase in heart rate and cardiac output occurs,

Box 1.4 Haemodynamic changes

↑ Heart rate
↑ Blood pressure (systolic)
↑ Cardiac output
↑ Myocardial contractility
↓ Peripheral resistance

which is mediated through $beta_1$ receptors, but increasing vagal tone counteracts this so the increase is transient (see Chapter 7). Peripheral resistance, estimated from mean arterial pressure divided by cardiac output, is reduced (Hilsted, 1993). A combination of the increase in cardiac output and reduction in peripheral resistance results in an increase in systolic and decrease in diastolic pressure, i.e. widening of pulse pressure without a change in mean arterial pressure.

Changes in Regional Blood Flow (Box 1.5 and Figure 1.9)

- *Cerebral blood flow:* Early work produced conflicting results, but these studies were in subjects receiving insulin shock therapy, and the varying effects of convulsions and altered level of consciousness may have influenced the outcome. Subsequent studies have consistently shown an increase in cerebral blood flow during hypoglycaemia despite the use of different methods of measurement (isotopic, single photon emission computed tomography [SPECT], and Doppler ultrasound). In most of the studies blood glucose concentration was less than 2.0 mmol/l before a change was observed. In animals, hypoglycaemia is associated with loss of cerebral autoregulation (the ability of the brain to maintain cerebral blood flow despite variability in cardiac output) through beta adrenoceptor stimulation, but the exact mechanisms are unknown (Bryan, 1990; Sieber and Traysman, 1992).

Box 1.5 Changes in regional blood flow

↑ Cerebral flow
↑ Total splanchnic flow
↓ Splenic flow
Skin flow variable (early ↑, late ↓)
↑ Muscle flow
↓ Renal flow

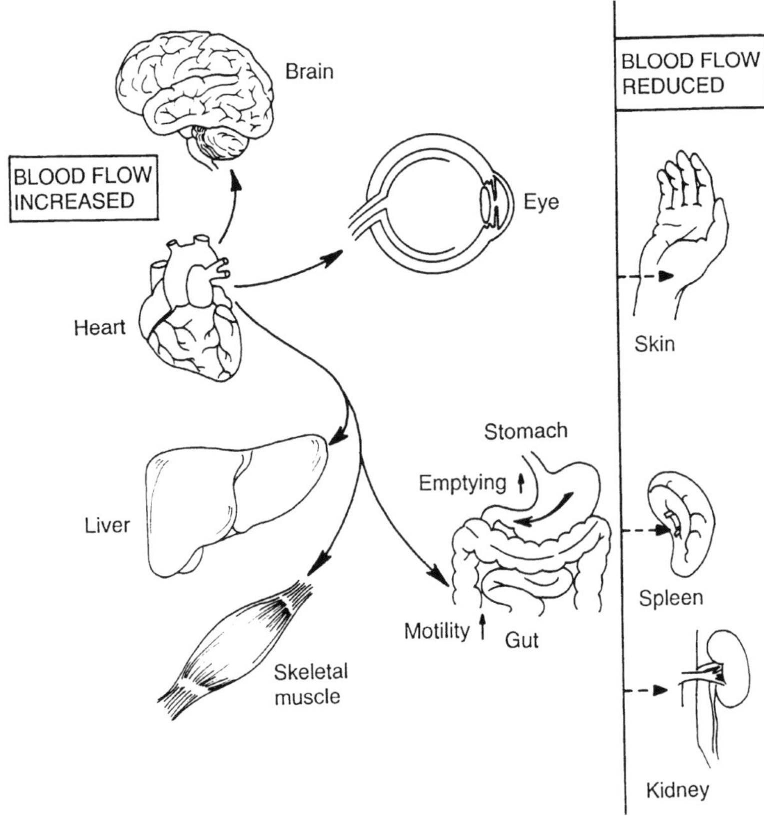

Figure 1.9 Changes in regional blood flow during hypoglycaemia

- *Gastrointestinal system:* Total splanchnic blood flow (that supplying the intestines, liver, spleen and stomach) is increased and splanchnic vascular resistance is reduced as assessed by the bromosulphthalein extraction technique (Bearn et al, 1952). Superior mesenteric blood flow, measured using Doppler ultrasound, increases during hypoglycaemia due to beta adrenoceptor stimulation (Braatvedt et al, 1993). Radioisotope scanning has demonstrated a reduction in splenic activity during hypoglycaemia (Fisher et al, 1990), which is thought to be due to alpha adrenoceptor-mediated reduction in blood flow. All these changes would be expected to increase hepatic blood flow, although this has not been confirmed experimentally.
- *Skin:* The control of blood flow to the skin is complex and different mechanisms predominate in different areas. Studies of the effect of hypoglycaemia on skin blood flow are inconsistent, partly due to

different methods of blood flow measurement and induction of hypoglycaemia, as well as differences in the part of the body studied. Definitive conclusions are therefore not possible. Studies using the dorsum of the foot, cheek and forehead have consistently shown an initial vasodilatation and increase in blood flow followed by later vasoconstriction at a blood glucose of 2.5 mmol/l (Maggs et al, 1994). These findings are consistent with the clinical observation of initial flushing and later pallor, with an early rise in skin blood flow and a later fall.

- *Muscle blood flow:* A variety of techniques have been used to study muscle blood flow and include venous occlusion plethysmography, isotopic clearance techniques and the use of thermal conductivity meters. All studies have consistently shown an increase in muscle blood flow during hypoglycaemia independent of skin blood flow. This change is mediated by $beta_2$ adrenoceptors (Allwood et al, 1959; Abramson et al, 1966).
- *Kidney:* Inulin and sodium hippurate clearance can be used to estimate glomerular filtration rate and renal blood flow respectively. Both decrease during hypoglycaemia (Patrick et al, 1989) and catecholamines and renin are implicated in initiating the changes.

The changes in blood flow in various organs, like the haemodynamic changes, are mostly mediated by the activation of the sympathetic nervous system or circulating adrenaline. The majority either protect vital organs against hypoglycaemia or increase substrate delivery to the brain, liver and skeletal muscles. The increase in cerebral blood flow increases glucose delivery to the brain. Increasing muscle blood flow enhances the release and washout of gluconeogenic precursors. The increase in splanchnic blood flow and concomitant reduction in splenic blood flow serve to increase hepatic blood flow and help to maximise hepatic glucose production. Meanwhile blood is diverted away from organs such as the kidney which are not required in the acute response to this metabolic stress.

Functional Changes (Box 1.6)

- *Sweating:* Sweating is mediated by sympathetic cholinergic nerves, although other neurotransmitters such as vasoactive intestinal peptide and bradykinin may also be involved. The activation of the sympathetic neural activity to the skin as described above results in the sudden onset of sweating. Sweating is one of the first physiological responses to occur during hypoglycaemia and can be demonstrated within 10 minutes of achieving a blood glucose of 2.5

Box 1.6 Functional changes

↑ Sweating (sudden onset)
↑ Tremor
↓ Core temperature
↓ Intraocular pressure
↑ Jejunal activity
↑ Gastric emptying

mmol/l (Maggs et al, 1994). It coincides with the onset of other measures of autonomic activation such as an increase in heart rate and tremor (Figure 1.10).

- *Tremor:* Trembling and shaking are characteristic features of hypoglycaemia and result from an increase in physiological tremor. The rise in cardiac input and the vasodilatation occurring during hypoglycaemia increase the level of physiological tremor and this is exacerbated by the beta adrenoceptor stimulation associated with increased adrenaline concentrations (Kerr et al, 1990). Since adrenalectomy does not entirely abolish tremor, other components such as the activation of muscle sympathetic activity must be involved.
- *Temperature:* Despite a beta adrenoceptor-mediated increase in metabolic rate, core body temperature falls during hypoglycaemia. The mechanisms by which this occurs depend on whether the environment is warm or cold. In a warm environment, heat is lost because of sweating and increased heat conduction from vasodilatation. Hypoglycaemia reduces core temperature by 0.3°C and skin temperature by up to 2°C (depending on which part of the body is measured) after 60 minutes (Maggs et al, 1994). In the cold, shivering is reduced, and this together with vasodilatation and sweating causes a substantial reduction in core temperature (Gale et al, 1983). In rats, mortality was increased in animals whose core temperature was prevented from falling during hypoglycaemia (Buchanan et al, 1991). In humans there is anecdotal evidence from subjects undergoing insulin shock therapy that those who had a rise in body temperature exhibited delayed neurological recovery (Ramos et al, 1968). These findings support the hypothesis that the fall in core temperature reduces metabolic rate, allowing hypoglycaemia to be better tolerated, and thus the changes in body temperature are of survival value. The beneficial effects are likely to be limited, particularly in the cold, where the impairment of cerebral function means subjects may not realise they are cold, causing them to be at risk of severe hypothermia.

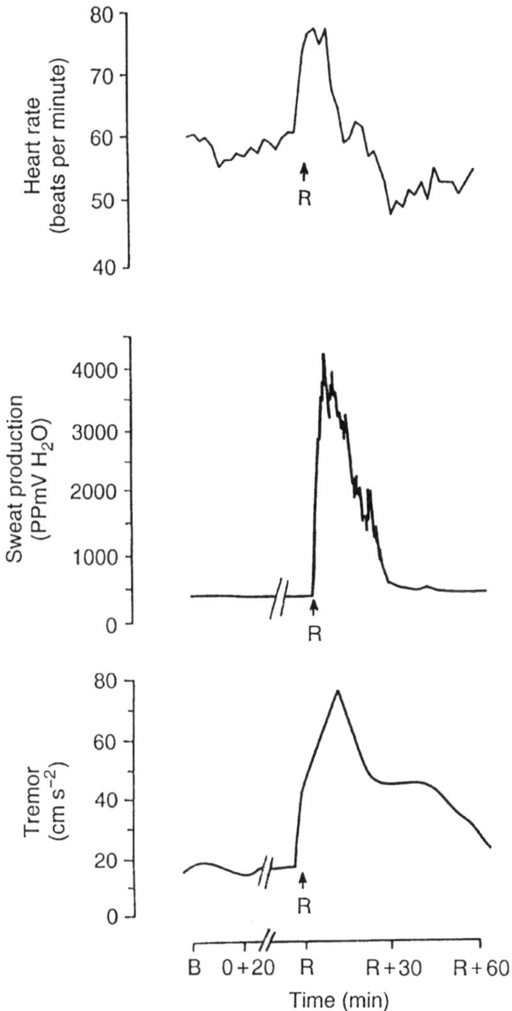

Figure 1.10 Sudden onset of sweating, tremor and increase in heart rate during the induction of hypoglycaemia. Reproduced from *Hypoglycaemia and Diabetes* (eds B.M. Frier and B.M. Fisher) by permission of Edward Arnold (Publishers) Ltd

- Other functional changes include a reduction in intraocular pressure, greater jejunal but not gastric motility and inconsistent abnormalities of liver function tests. An increase in gastric emptying occurs during hypoglycaemia (Schvarcz et al, 1995), which may be protective in that carbohydrate delivery to the intestine is increased, enabling faster glucose absorption and reversal of hypoglycaemia.

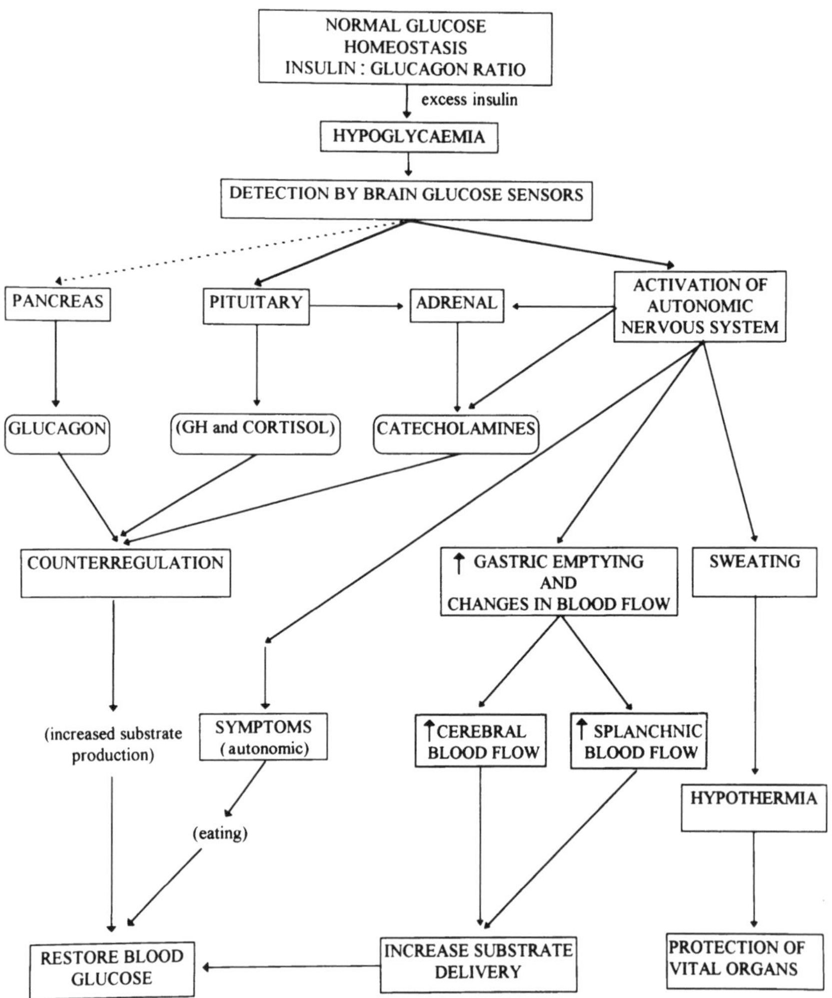

Figure 1.11 Glucose homeostasis and the correction of hypoglycaemia

CONCLUSIONS

- Homeostatic mechanisms exist to maintain glucose concentration within narrow limits despite a wide variety of circumstances.
- The dependence of the central nervous system on glucose has led to a complex series of biochemical, functional and haemo-

continues

continued

dynamic changes aimed at restoring blood glucose concentrations, producing symptoms and protecting the body in general and the central nervous system in particular against the effects of a low blood glucose (Figure 1.11).

- Many symptoms of hypoglycaemia result from the activation of the autonomic nervous system and help to warn the individual that their blood glucose is low. This encourages the ingestion of carbohydrate, so helping to restore blood glucose concentrations in addition to counterregulation.
- Faster gastric emptying and the changes in regional blood flow which also occur as a result of the activation of the autonomic nervous system increase substrate delivery.
- The greater cerebral blood flow increases glucose delivery to the brain (although loss of autoregulation is undesirable), and the increased splanchnic flow results in a greater delivery of gluconeogenic precursors to the liver.
- Activation of the autonomic nervous system also increases sweating, and this, together with the inhibition of shivering predisposes to hypothermia, which may be neuroprotective.

ACKNOWLEDGEMENT

We would like to thank Professor Robert Tattersall for helpful suggestions with the preparation of this chapter.

REFERENCES

Abramson EA, Arky RA and Woeber KA (1966). Effects of propranolol on the hormonal and metabolic responses to insulin-induced hypoglycaemia. *Lancet* **ii**: 1386–8.

Allwood MJ, Hensel H and Papenberg J (1959). Muscle and skin blood flow in the human forearm during insulin hypoglycaemia. *Journal of Physiology* **147**: 269–73.

Auer RN and Siesjö BK (1988). Biological differences between ischemia, hypoglycemia and epilepsy. *Annals of Neurology* **24**: 699–707.

Bearn AG, Billing BH and Sherlock S (1952). The response of the liver to insulin in normal subjects and in diabetes mellitus: hepatic vein catheterisation studies. *Clinical Science* **11**: 151–64.

Bell GI, Karyano T, Buse JB, Burant CF, Takeda T, Lin D, Fukumoto H and Seino S (1990). Molecular biology of mammalian glucose transporters. *Diabetes Care* **13**: 198–208.

Berne C and Fagius J (1986). Skin nerve sympathetic activity during insulin-induced hypoglycaemia. *Diabetologia* **29**: 55–60.

Borg MA, Sherwin RS, Borg WP, Tamborlane WV and Shulman GI (1997). Local ventromedial hypothalamus glucose perfusion blocks counterregulation during systemic hypoglycemia in awake rats. *Journal of Clinical Investigation* **99**: 361–5.

Boyle PJ, Kempers SE, O'Conner AM and Nagy RJ (1995). Brain glucose uptake and unawareness of hypoglycemia in patients with insulin-dependent diabetes mellitus. *New England Journal of Medicine* **333**: 1726–31.

Braatvedt GD, Flynn MD, Stanners A, Halliwell M and Corrall RJM (1993). Splanchnic blood flow in man: evidence for mediation via a beta-adrenergic mechanism. *Clinical Science* **84**: 201–7.

Bryan RM (1990). Cerebral blood flow and energy metabolism during stress. *American Journal of Physiology* **259**: H269–80.

Buchanan TA, Cane P, Eng CC, Sipos GF and Lee C (1991). Hypothermia is critical for survival during prolonged insulin-induced hypoglycemia in rats. *Metabolism* **40**: 330–4.

Cahill GF (1971). Physiology of insulin in man. *Diabetes* **20**: 785–99.

Cryer PE (1981). Glucose counterregulation in man. *Diabetes* **30**: 261–4.

Fagius J and Berne C (1989). Changes of sympathetic nerve activity induced by 2–deoxy-D-glucose infusion in humans. *American Journal of Physiology* **256**: E714–21.

Fagius J, Niklasson F and Berne C (1986). Sympathetic outflow in human muscle nerves increases during hypoglycemia. *Diabetes* **35**: 1124–9.

Fish HR, Chernow B and O'Brian JT (1986). Endocrine and neurophysiologic responses of the pituitary to insulin-induced hypoglycemia: a review. *Metabolism* **35**: 763–80.

Fisher BM, Baylis PH and Frier BM (1987). Plasma oxytocin, arginine vasopressin and atrial natriuretic peptide response to insulin-induced hypoglycaemia in man. *Clinical Endocrinology* **26**: 179–85.

Fisher BM, Gillen G, Hepburn DA, Dargie HJ, Barnett E and Frier BM (1990). Splenic responses to acute insulin-induced hypoglycaemia in humans. *Clinical Science* **78**: 469–74.

Francis BH and Ensinck JW (1987). Differential alterations of the circulating prosomatostatin-derived peptides during insulin-induced hypoglycemia in man. *Journal of Clinical Endocrinology and Metabolism* **65**: 880–4.

Frier BM and Fisher BM, eds (1993). *Hypoglycaemia and Diabetes: Clinical and Physiological Aspects*. Edward Arnold, London.

Gale EAM, Bennet J, Macdonald IA, Holst JJ and Mathews JA (1983). The physiological effects of insulin-induced hypoglycaemia in man: responses at differing levels of blood glucose. *Clinical Science* **65**: 262–71.

Garber AJ, Cryer PE, Santiago JV, Haymond MW, Pagliara AS and Kipnis DM (1976). The role of adrenergic mechanisms in the substrate and hormonal response to insulin-induced hypoglycemia in man. *Journal of Clinical Investigation* **58**: 7–15.

Gerich JE (1988). Glucose counterregulation and its impact on diabetes mellitus. *Diabetes* **37**: 1608–17.

Hamilton-Wessler M, Bergman RN, Halter JB, Watanabe RM and Donovan CM (1994). The role of liver glucosensors in the integrated sympathetic response induced by deep hypoglycemia in dogs. *Diabetes* **43**: 1052–60.

Heller SR and Macdonald IA (1996). The measurement of cognitive function during acute hypoglycaemia: experimental limitations and their effect on the study of hypoglycaemia unawareness. *Diabetic Medicine* **13**: 607–15.

Hilsted J (1993). Cardiovascular changes during hypoglycaemia. *Clinical Physiology* **13**: 1–10.

Jungman E, Konzog C, Holl E, Fassibinder W and Schoffling K (1989). Effect of human atrial natriuretic peptide on blood glucose concentrations and hormone stimulation during insulin-induced hypoglycaemia in healthy man. *European Journal of Clinical Pharmacology* **36**: 593–7.

Katz SH, Dhariwal APS and McCann SM (1967). Effects of hypoglycemia on the content of pituitary growth hormone (GH) and hypothalamic growth hormone releasing factor (GNRH) in the rat. *Endocrinology* **81**: 333–9.

Kerr D, Macdonald IA and Tattersall RB (1989). Influence of duration of hypoglycemia on the hormonal counterregulatory response in normal subjects. *Journal of Clinical Endocrinology and Metabolism* **68**: 118–22.

Kerr D, Macdonald IA, Heller SR and Tattersall RB (1990). A randomised double-blind placebo controlled trial of the effects of Metoprolol CR, Atenolol and Propranolol LA on the physiological responses to hypoglycaemia in the non-diabetic. *British Journal of Clinical Pharmacology* **29**: 685–94.

Maggs DG, Scott AR and Macdonald IA (1994). Thermoregulatory responses to hyperinsulinemic hypoglycemia and euglycemia in humans. *American Journal of Physiology* **267**: R1266–72.

McCall AL (1993). Effects of glucose deprivation on glucose metabolism in the central nervous system. In: *Hypoglycaemia and Diabetes: Clinical and Physiological Aspects*, Frier BM and Fisher BM, eds. Edward Arnold, London: 56–71.

McCall AL, Fixman LB, Fleming N, Tornheim K, Chick W and Ruderman ND (1986). Chronic hypoglycemia increases brain glucose transport. *American Journal of Physiology* **251**: E442–7.

Mitrakou A, Ryan C, Veneman T, Mokan M, Jenssen T, Kiss I, Durrant J, Cryer P and Gerich J (1991). Hierarchy of glycemic thresholds for counterregulatory hormone secretion, symptoms and cerebral dysfunction. *American Journal of Physiology* **266**: E67–74.

Owen OE, Morgan AP, Kemp HG, Sullivan JM, Herrara MG and Cahill GF Jr (1967). Brain metabolism during fasting. *Journal of Clinical Investigation* **46**: 1589–95.

Patrick AW, Hepburn DA, Craig KJ, Thompson I, Swainson CD and Frier BM (1989). The effects of acute insulin-induced hypoglycaemia on renal function in normal human subjects. *Diabetic Medicine* **6**: 703–8.

Ramos E, Zorilla E and Hadley WB (1968). Fever as a manifestation of hypoglycaemia. *Journal of the American Medical Association* **205**: 590–2.

Schvarcz E, Palmér M, Åman J and Berne C (1995). Hypoglycemia increases the gastric emptying rate in healthy subjects. *Diabetes Care* **18**: 674–6.

Sieber FE and Traysman RJ (1992). Special issues: Glucose and the brain. *Critical Care Medicine* **20**: 104–14.

Siegal AM and Kreisberg RA (1975). Metabolic homeostasis: insulin–glucagon interactions. In: *Diabetes Mellitus* (4th edition), Sussman KE and Metz RJS, eds. American Diabetes Association, New York: 29–35.

Sokaloff L (1989). Circulation and energy metabolism of the brain. In: *Basic Neurochemistry*, Siegel G, Agranoff B, Albers RW and Molinoff P, eds. Raven Press, New York: 565–90.

Trovati M, Massucco P, Mularoni E, Cavalot F, Anfossi G, Mattiello L and Emanuelli G (1988). Insulin-induced hypoglycaemia increases plasma concentrations of angiotensin II and does not modify atrial natriuretic polypeptide secretion in man. *Diabetologia* **31**: 816–20.

Wieloch T (1985). Hypoglycemia-induced neuronal damage prevented by an N-Methyl-D-aspartate antagonist. *Science* **230**: 681–3.

2

Symptoms of Hypoglycaemia and Effects on Mental Performance and Emotions

IAN J. DEARY
Department of Psychology, University of Edinburgh

INTRODUCTION

This chapter describes the symptoms which are perceived during acute hypoglycaemia, and the changes in mental functions and emotions that occur during this metabolic state.

Hypoglycaemia is the most feared side-effect of insulin therapy and is the greatest barrier to good glycaemic control. The most obvious benefit to a person of knowing about the symptoms of hypoglycaemia is the ability to recognise the onset of a hypoglycaemic episode as early as possible. This is of key importance in informing and educating people with diabetes. Moreover, if a person with diabetes understands which mental functions are affected by hypoglycaemia they can judge which of their activities may be most threatened in this state.

Hypoglycaemia in Clinical Diabetes. Edited by B. M. Frier and B. M. Fisher.

SYMPTOMS OF HYPOGLYCAEMIA

Identifying the Symptoms

The physiological responses to hypoglycaemia are described in Chapter 1. The response to hypoglycaemia results in physical symptoms, which raises several questions. Can we compile a comprehensive list of symptoms of hypoglycaemia? Which are the more common symptoms of hypoglycaemia? Are there early warning symptoms of hypoglycaemia? Do people differ in how quickly and accurately they detect or recognise hypoglycaemia? Do people differ in the set of symptoms of hypoglycaemia they experience? How can individuals distinguish the symptoms of hypoglycaemia from other bodily changes?

The Total Symptom Complex

The most basic question is: what symptoms do people report when they develop hypoglycaemia?

In humans the symptoms associated with hypoglycaemia were first recorded when insulin became available for the treatment of diabetes (Fletcher and Campbell, 1922). A list of characteristic symptoms was described (Table 2.1). It was noted: that some symptoms appeared before others during hypoglycaemia; that the blood glucose level at which subjects became aware of hypoglycaemia was characteristic for the individual; that there were large individual differences in the levels of blood glucose at which awareness of hypoglycaemia commenced; and that the preceding blood glucose concentration could affect the onset of symptoms.

Lists of common symptoms of hypoglycaemia have been compiled from more recent research. Hepburn (1993) summarised eight population studies of the symptoms of hypoglycaemia experienced by adults and children with insulin-treated diabetes, and Cox et al (1993a) also produced a list of symptoms (Table 2.1). It is evident that the three lists of symptoms do not differ greatly, and that Fletcher and Campbell's early report (1922) had captured many of the symptoms found in subsequent, more structured, investigations. However, their report omitted to mention some symptoms such as tiredness, drowsiness and difficulty concentrating, though it included others—such as pallor (a sign rather than a symptom), incoordination and feelings of temperature change—that are emphasised by others as regularly perceived symptoms. Table 2.1 establishes a useful group of symptoms that are commonly reported in hypoglycaemia.

The way we ask people to describe their symptoms of hypoglycaemia

Table 2.1 Common symptoms associated with hypoglycaemia

Symptoms associated with hypoglycaemia as derived from population studies (after Hepburn, 1993)	Percentage (minimum–maximum) of people reporting the given symptom as associated with hypoglycaemia (after Hepburn, 1993)	Symptoms of hypoglycaemia as noted by Fletcher and Campbell (1922)	Symptoms (and percentage [to nearest 5%]) of people endorsing symptoms as associated with hypoglycaemia; after Cox et al, 1993a, Figure 2)
Sweating	47–84	Sweating	Sweating (80)
Trembling	32–78	Tremulousness	Trembling (65)
Weakness	28–71	Weakness	Fatigue/weak (70)
Visual disturbance	24–60	Diplopia	Blurred vision (20)
Hunger	39–49	Excessive hunger	Hunger (60)
Pounding heart	8–62	Change in pulse rate	Pounding heart (55)
Difficulty with speaking	7–41	Dysarthria, sensory and motor aphasia	Slurred speech (40)
Tingling around the mouth	10–39	–	Numb lips (50)
Dizziness	11–41	Vertigo, faintness, syncope	Light-headed/dizzy (60)
Headache	24–36		Headache (30)
Anxiety	10–44	Nervousness, anxiety, excitement, emotional upset	Nervous/tense (65)
Nausea	5–20	–	–
Difficulty concentrating	31–75	–	Difficulty concentrating (80)
Tiredness	38–46	–	
Drowsiness	16–33	–	Drowsy–sleepy (40)
Confusion	13–53	Confusion, disorientation, "goneness"	
		Pallor	
		Incoordination	Uncoordinated (75)
		Feeling of heat or cold	Cold sweats (40)
		Emotional instability	
			Slowed thinking (70)

can alter what they tell us. The rank order of symptoms alters considerably if patients are asked to indicate the *relevance* of each symptom rather than merely to identify that the symptom is associated with hypoglycaemia (Cox et al, 1993a). With regard to the criterion of relevance, the most useful symptoms in *detecting* hypoglycaemia are:

- sweating
- trembling
- difficulty concentrating
- nervousness, tenseness
- light-headedness, dizziness.

The Initial Symptoms

Another important question is: which hypoglycaemic symptoms appear *early* during an episode? The symptoms of hypoglycaemia that appear first and offer early warning of the onset of hypoglycaemia (Hepburn, 1993) are:

- trembling
- sweating
- tiredness
- difficulty concentrating
- hunger.

This knowledge is obviously useful for the prompt detection and treatment of hypoglycaemia.

The Validity of Symptom Beliefs

The Individuality of Hypoglycaemic Symptom Clusters

A great deal of the interest in symptoms of hypoglycaemia has been stimulated by concerns about patient education. It is helpful to let patients know the range of symptoms found in hypoglycaemia and to inform them of the early warning symptoms reported by other people with diabetes, much like we all tend to know the range of symptoms that are experienced with the common cold. Many surveys and laboratory studies have shown that people differ considerably in the symptoms of hypoglycaemia they experience (Cox et al, 1993a). In addition to learning the generally reported symptoms, individuals with diabetes should be encouraged to learn about their own typical symptoms of hypoglycaemia.

Correctly Interpreting Symptoms as Representing Hypoglycaemia

Symptoms of hypoglycaemia do not appear on top of the bodily equivalent of a blank sheet of paper. Sometimes we experience symptoms when there is nothing wrong with our bodily functions; on the other hand, sometimes we fail to notice any symptoms when the body is malfunctioning. The alert person with diabetes who is on the lookout for hypoglycaemia must make two sorts of decisions. First, symptoms of hypoglycaemia must be detected and correctly identified. It would be dangerous for a patient to ignore symptoms of hypoglycaemia because he/she thought they were related to something else. Secondly, symptoms that have nothing to do with hypoglycaemia must be excluded. Unwanted hyperglycaemia could occur if patients treated themselves for hypoglycaemia when the symptoms had another cause. These two main types of error are a failure to treat hypoglycaemia when blood glucose is low, and inappropriate treatment when blood glucose is acceptable or high (Cox et al, 1985; 1993a) (Figure 2.1).

Blood Glucose Concentration–Symptom Report Correlations

Do patients' reports of symptoms of hypoglycaemia bear any relation to their concurrent blood glucose concentrations? After all, the principal aim of educating people to be aware of symptoms of hypoglycaemia is that they become alert to low and potentially dangerous levels of blood glucose. To answer the above question some researchers have employed a field study approach where people are invited to list any symptoms they are experiencing, and then measure and record their blood glucose concentration several times a day for weeks. As a result of these studies it

		True symptom status	
		Symptom of hypoglycaemia	Non-hypoglycaemic symptom
Perception of symptom by person	Hypo-glycaemic	Appropriate action	Inappropriate anti-hypoglycaemia action
	Non-hypo-glycaemic	Inappropriate inaction (danger of severe hypoglycaemia)	Appropriate non-action (with respect to hypoglycaemia)

Figure 2.1 Consequences of correct and incorrect perception of hypoglycaemic symptoms

is known that each person has some symptoms that are most reliably associated with their actual blood glucose concentrations (Pennebaker et al, 1981). Some of the symptoms that people report during hypoglycaemia are more closely related to their actual blood glucose concentrations than are others, and if we can identify each individual's most informative symptoms, we can instruct people to pay more attention to them.

The following symptoms are most consistently associated with actual blood glucose concentrations (Pennebaker et al, 1981):

- hunger (in 53% of people)
- trembling (in 33%)
- weakness (in 27%)
- light-headedness (in 20%)
- pounding heart and fast heart rate (both 17%).

The same symptoms are not informative for everyone. There were 27% of people for whom weakness was significantly associated with hypoglycaemia, but there were 7% in whom it was a good symptom of hyperglycaemia! Most people reported more than three symptoms that were strongly associated with the measured blood glucose concentration.

It is evident that an individual's symptoms are idiosyncratic. If we can help a patient to identify the symptoms of hypoglycaemia peculiar to themselves which relate to actual blood glucose concentrations, then, by attending to these symptoms, the person should be especially accurate in recognising hypoglycaemia. People who have one or more reliable symptom(s) of hypoglycaemia correctly recognise half of their episodes of hypoglycaemia (defined as a blood glucose less than 3.9 mmol/l [Cox et al, 1993a]). Those who have four or more reliable symptoms recognise a blood glucose below 3.9 mmol/l three-quarters of the time. The field study method has suggested that attention to the following symptoms was particularly useful in detecting actual low blood glucose concentrations:

- nervousness/tenseness
- slowed thinking
- trembling
- light-headedness/dizziness
- difficulty concentrating
- pounding heart
- lack of coordination.

Classifying Symptoms of Hypoglycaemia

Until now the symptoms of hypoglycaemia have been treated as a homogeneous whole. Can these symptoms be divided into different groups?

Hypoglycaemia has effects on more than one part of the body, and the symptoms of hypoglycaemia reflect this. First, the direct effects of a low blood glucose concentration on the brain—especially the cerebral cortex—cause *neuroglycopenic* symptoms. Secondly, *autonomic* symptoms result from activation of parts of the autonomic nervous system. Finally, there may be some *non-specific* symptoms that are not directly generated by either of these two mechanisms. It is only recently that scientific investigations have taken place to confirm the idea that these separable groups of hypoglycaemic symptoms exist.

As suggested above, during the body's reaction to hypoglycaemia there are at least two distinct groups of symptoms (Hepburn et al, 1991):

- *Autonomic*, with symptoms such as trembling, anxiety, sweating and warmness
- *Neuroglycopenic*, with symptoms such as drowsiness, confusion, tiredness, inability to concentrate and difficulty speaking.

This information can assist with patient education by supplying evidence for separable groups of symptoms, and by indicating which symptoms belong to each group. Some neuroglycopenic symptoms, such as inability to concentrate, weakness and drowsiness, are among the earliest detectable symptoms, but patients tend to rely more on autonomic symptoms when detecting the onset of hypoglycaemia. Paying more attention to the potentially useful, early neuroglycopenic symptoms could help with the early detection of hypoglycaemia.

Similar groups of symptoms of hypoglycaemia have been discovered by asking people to recall the symptoms they typically noticed during hypoglycaemia. However, in addition to the two groups described above, a general feeling of malaise is added (Deary et al, 1993):

- *Autonomic*: e.g. sweating, palpitations, shaking and hunger
- *Neuroglycopenic*: e.g. confusion, drowsiness, odd behaviour, speech difficulty and incoordination
- *General malaise*: e.g. headache and nausea.

These 11 symptoms are so reliably reported by people and so clearly separable into these three groups, that they are used as the "Edinburgh Hypoglycaemia Scale" (Deary et al, 1993). Table 2.2 shows how different researchers have found similar groups of autonomic and hypoglycaemic symptoms.

In addition to the above studies that used patients' self-reported symptoms, physiological studies have also confirmed that the symptoms of hypoglycaemia can be divided into autonomic and neuroglycopenic groups. Symptoms such as sweating, hunger, pounding heart, tingling,

Table 2.2 Different authors' lists of autonomic and neuroglycopenic symptoms of hypoglycaemia

Autonomic			Neuroglycopenic	
Deary et al (1993)	Towler et al (1993)	Weinger et al (1995)	Deary et al (1993)	Towler et al (1993)
Sweating	Sweaty	Sweating	Confusion	Difficulty thinking/ confused
Palpitation	Heart pounding	Pounding heart, fast pulse	Drowsiness	Tired/drowsy
Shaking	Shaky/ tremulous	Trembling	Odd behaviour	
Hunger	Hungry		Speech difficulty	Difficulty speaking
	Tingling		Incoordination	
	Nervous/ anxious	Tense		Weak
		Breathing hard		Warm

nervousness and feeling shaky/tremulous (autonomic symptoms) can be reduced or even prevented by drugs which block neurotransmission within the autonomic nervous system (Towler et al, 1993), confirming that these symptoms are caused by the autonomic response to hypoglycaemia. Symptoms such as warmth, weakness, difficulty thinking/confusion, feeling tired/drowsy, feeling faint, difficulty speaking, dizziness and blurred vision (neuroglycopenic symptoms) are not prevented by drugs which block the autonomic nervous system. Therefore, neuroglycopenic symptoms are not mediated via the autonomic nervous system and are thought to be caused by the direct effect of glucose deprivation on the brain. This type of research has also observed that people tend to rely on autonomic symptoms to detect hypoglycaemia, even when neuroglycopenic symptoms are just as prominent (Towler et al, 1993). Once more, this suggests that more emphasis should be placed on education of the potential importance of neuroglycopenic symptoms for the early warning of hypoglycaemia.

Symptoms in Children

Children often have difficulty in recognising symptoms of hypoglycaemia, and they show marked variability in symptoms between episodes of hypoglycaemia (Macfarlane and Smith, 1988). Trembling and sweating are often the first symptoms recognised by children. From interviews with the parents of children (aged up to 16 years) with type 1 diabetes, and with some of their children, more is known about the frequency of symptoms of hypoglycaemia in children (McCrimmon et al, 1995; Ross et al, 1998) (Table 2.3). The most frequently reported sign that parents observed was pallor (noted by 88%). The parents frequently reported symptoms of behavioural disturbance such as irritability, argumentativeness and aggression. This latter group of symptoms is not prominent in adults, although the Edinburgh Hypoglycaemia Scale includes "odd behaviour" as an adult neuroglycopenic symptom. Others had previously noted the prominence of symptoms such as irritability, aggression and disobedience in the parents' reports of their children's

Table 2.3 Symptoms of hypoglycaemia in children (derived from Ross et al, 1998)

Symptom	Frequency of rating (%)		Correlation between parents' and children's intensity ratings[a]
	Parents' reports	Children's reports	
Tearful	73	47	0.40[d]
Headache	73	65	0.33[d]
Irritable	85	65	0.16
Unco-ordinated	62	56	0.18
Naughty	47	31	0.23[b]
Weak	79	83	0.21[b]
Aggressive	75	62	0.26[c]
Trembling	79	88	0.25[b]
Sleepiness	63	69	0.27[c]
Nightmares	33	19	0.33[d]
Sweating	76	73	0.28[c]
Slurred speech	53	45	0.28[c]
Blurred vision	52	55	0.30[c]
Tummy pain	67	41	0.36[d]
Feeling sick	63	53	0.32[c]
Hungry	74	84	0.19
Yawning	48	45	0.20[b]
Odd behaviour	65	50	0.22[b]
Warmness	57	68	0.13
Restless	61	57	0.21[b]
Daydreaming	70	48	0.14
Argumentative	64	50	0.21[b]
Pounding heart	21	44	0.02
Confused	75	70	0.41[d]
Tingling lips	20	24	−0.01
Dizziness	66	87	0.28[c]
Tired	83	76	0.26[c]
Feeling awful	92	79	0.20

[a]Correlations: p of z (corrected for ties) 1.0 represents perfect agreement; 0 represents no agreement.
[b] $p < 0.05$, [c] $p < 0.01$, [d] $p < 0.001$.

symptoms of hypoglycaemia (Macfarlane and Smith, 1988; Macfarlane et al, 1989). Parents tend to under-report the subjective symptoms of hypoglycaemia, such as weakness and dizziness, but generally there is good agreement between parents and their children about the most prominent symptoms of childhood hypoglycaemia (McCrimmon et al, 1995; Ross et al, 1998).

Separate groups of autonomic and neuroglycopenic symptoms were not found in children (McCrimmon et al, 1995; Ross et al, 1998). These symptoms are reported together by children and are not distinguished as separate groups, whereas the group of symptoms related to behavioural disturbance is clearly reported as a distinct group. In a refinement of the earlier study by McCrimmon et al (1995), Ross et al (1998) found that parents could distinguish between autonomic and neuroglycopenic symptoms.

By contrast, elderly patients with type 2 diabetes treated with insulin commonly report *neurological* symptoms of hypoglycaemia which may be misinterpreted as features of cerebrovascular disease, such as transient ischaemic attacks (Jaap et al, 1998). The age-specific differences in the groups of hypoglycaemic symptoms, classified using statistical techniques (Principal Component Analysis) are shown in Table 2.4. Health professionals and carers who are involved in the treatment and education of diabetic patients should be aware of which symptoms are common at either end of the age spectrum.

From Symptom Perception to Action

People with diabetes are better at estimating their blood glucose in natural, everyday, as opposed to clinical laboratory, settings (Cox et al, 1985). In some ways this is surprising as natural hypoglycaemia often occurs at a time when it is unexpected. In this situation, attention toward symptoms will not be as actively directed toward detection as in the laboratory setting where it is usually anticipated. Furthermore, hypoglycaemia in everyday life occurs on the background of other bodily feelings

Table 2.4 Classification of symptoms of hypoglycaemia using Principal Components Analysis in patients with insulin-treated diabetes depending on age group

Children (pre pubertal)	Adults	Elderley
Autonomic/ neuroglycopenic	Autonomic	Autonomic
	Neuroglycopenic	Neuroglycopenic
Behavioural	Non-specific malaise	Neurological

and must be separated from other causes of the same symptoms. For example, exercise and various acute illnesses can provoke sweating in people with diabetes, independently of their association with hypoglycaemia.

In a real-life situation a person must *detect* symptoms of hypoglycaemia and then *interpret* them. Failure to detect symptoms can lead to a failure to treat hypoglycaemia, but detection without the correct interpretation of the cause of the symptoms is equally dangerous. Furthermore, it is obvious that someone who does interpret symptoms correctly as being caused by hypoglycaemia, but who does not take action to treat the low blood glucose, will be at the same risk. These and other steps toward the avoidance of severe hypoglycaemia demonstrate the key role of education about symptoms in people with diabetes (Gonder-Frederick et al, 1997).

Symptom Generation

Figure 2.2 outlines the stages that intervene between low blood glucose occurring in an individual and the implementation of effective treatment (Gonder-Frederick et al, 1997). It is interesting to note how important behavioural factors are in generating states of low blood glucose. Episodes of low blood glucose are most likely to come about because of changes in routine aspects of diabetes management, such as taking extra insulin, eating less food or taking more exercise (Clarke et al, 1997). These factors predict more than 85% of episodes of hypoglycaemia in people with diabetes.

In the presence of an intact physiological response to a low blood glucose, autonomic and neuroglycopenic symptoms, and symptoms of general malaise are generated (Figure 2.2). The degree of hypoglycaemia, the person's quality of glycaemic control and any recent episodes of hypoglycaemia may all affect the magnitude of the body's physiological response. Recent, preceding hypoglycaemia can reduce the symptomatic and counterregulatory hormonal responses to subsequent hypoglycaemia, resulting in a diminished awareness of symptoms. This effect of "antecedent" hypoglycaemia is described in Chapter 5.

At the second stage in Figure 2.2 comes the actual generation of physical symptoms. Among the variables which can influence this stage is the prior ingestion of caffeine, which has been shown to enhance the intensity of the autonomic and neuroglycopenic symptoms of experimentally induced hypoglycaemia (Debrah et al, 1996). Caffeine may act by increasing the intensity of symptoms of hypoglycaemia to perceptible levels, much as a magnifying glass enables one to read otherwise too-small print.

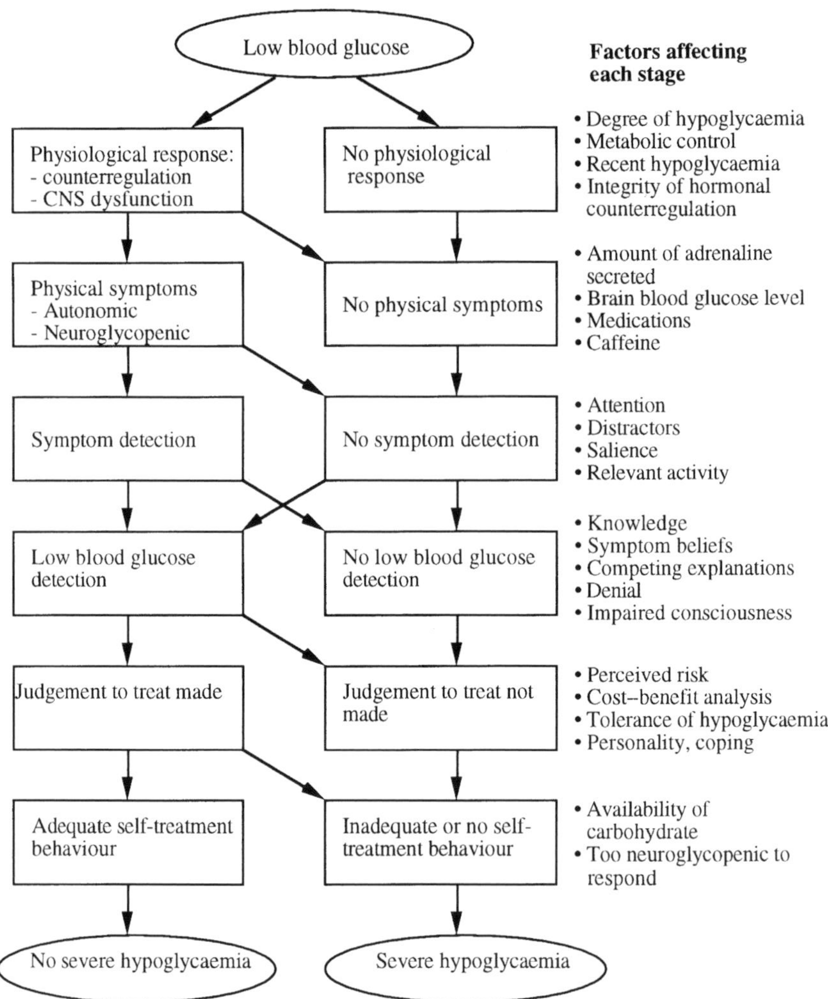

Figure 2.2 A model for the occurrence and avoidance of severe hypoglycaemia (after Gonder-Frederick et al, 1997). Note on the right-hand side of each stage the factors that affect its occurrence

Symptom Detection

The occurrence of physiological changes in the body does not guarantee that a person will detect symptoms (Gonder-Frederick et al, 1997). If attention is directed to physical changes, people are more likely to detect symptoms than if their attention is held elsewhere. Everyone has had the experience of feeling less discomfort, and being less likely to detect a physical symptom, when being distracted by something diverting. The personal relevance of the symptom may affect detection; for example, a person with heart disease may be very likely to detect palpitations (Cox et al, 1993a). The activity of the person at the time of the physiological change is obviously important. Hypoglycaemic symptoms will be more obvious to the person engaged in active mental effort, such as sitting an examination, than to the person relaxing and watching television. A doctor engaged in microsurgery may be very sensitive to the onset of tremor.

The autonomic symptoms of hypoglycaemia are often emphasised in the detection of hypoglycaemia. However, a strong case can be made for an equal emphasis on neuroglycopenic symptoms (Gonder-Frederick et al, 1997) because:

- performance on mental tasks deteriorates during hypoglycaemia, and subjective awareness of this decrement begins at very mild levels of hypoglycaemia
- the difference in glycaemic thresholds for the onset of autonomic and neuroglycopenic symptoms is so small that it is unlikely to be detected when blood glucose declines rapidly
- neuroglycopenic symptoms are as strongly related to actual blood glucose concentrations as are autonomic symptoms (Cox et al, 1993a)
- people with insulin-treated diabetes cite autonomic and neuroglycopenic symptoms with equal frequency as the primary warning symptoms of hypoglycaemia (Hepburn et al, 1991).

Low Blood Glucose Detection—Symptom Interpretation

The correct detection of a symptom of hypoglycaemia does not always lead to correct interpretation (Figure 2.2). After correctly detecting relevant symptoms people fail to detect about 26% of episodes of low blood glucose (Gonder-Frederick et al, 1997). There are several factors that could break a perfect relationship between detection and recognition, and some are discussed below. However, it should be appreciated that symptom detection (internal cues) is not mandatory for the detection of a low blood glucose. Self-testing of blood glucose, or the information of family members (external cues) can lead to the successful recognition of hypoglycaemia without the patient having detected the episode by symptomatic perception (see Box 2.1).

Correct knowledge about symptoms of hypoglycaemia is necessary for the detection of a low blood glucose. The lack of such knowledge among elderly people with diabetes in particular gives cause for concern (Mutch

Box 2.1 Identification of hypoglycaemia

- Internal cues–autonomic, neuroglycopenic and non-specific symptoms
- External cues–relationship of insulin injection to meals, exercise and experience of self-management
- Blood glucose monitoring
- Information from observers (e.g. relatives, friends, colleagues)

and Dingwall-Fordyce, 1985). Of 161 diabetic people between ages 60 and 87, all of whom were injecting insulin or taking a sulphonylurea, only 22% had ever been told the symptoms of hypoglycaemia and 9% knew no symptoms at all! The percentages of the insulin-treated diabetic patients who knew that the following symptoms were associated with hypoglycaemia were:

- sweating (82%)
- palpitations (62%)
- confusion (53%)
- hunger (51%)
- inability to concentrate (50%)
- speech problems (41%)
- sleepiness (33%).

In the midst of this ignorance, much hypoglycaemia may not be treated because of a lack of knowledge of the symptoms of hypoglycaemia which would aid their recognition.

Most, if not all, of the symptoms of hypoglycaemia could be explained by other physical conditions. Therefore, correct symptom detection could be usurped by incorrect attribution of the cause. For example, having completed some strenuous activity, an athlete may attribute the symptoms of sweating and palpitations to physical exertion. An obvious problem in detecting a low blood glucose is the fact that the organ responsible for the detection and interpretation of symptoms—the brain, especially the cerebral cortex—is impaired. Thus, impaired concentration and lowered consciousness levels can beget even more severe hypoglycaemia.

Symptom Scoring Systems

The controversy about the effect of human insulin on symptom awareness (Chapter 5) stimulated the development of scoring systems for hypoglycaemia to allow comparative studies between insulin species.

This produced scoring systems such as the Edinburgh Hypoglycaemia Scale (Deary et al, 1993), and any such system must be validated for research application. It is important to note that the *nature* and *intensity* of individual symptoms are as important, if not more important, as the *number* of symptoms generated by hypoglycaemia. The concepts involved are discussed in detail by Hepburn (1993).

ACUTE HYPOGLYCAEMIA AND COGNITIVE FUNCTIONING

Symptoms are subjective reports of bodily sensations. With respect to hypoglycaemia some of these reports—especially neuroglycopenic symptoms—pertain to altered cognitive (mental ability) functioning. Do reports of 'confusion' and 'difficulty thinking' (Table 2.2) concur with objective mental test performance in hypoglycaemia? Before experimental hypoglycaemia became an accepted investigative tool in diabetes, expert clinical observers noted impairments of cognitive functions despite clear consciousness during hypoglycaemia (Fletcher and Campbell, 1922; Wilder, 1943). Cognitive functions include the following sorts of mental activity: orientation and attention, perception, memory (verbal and non-verbal), language, construction, reasoning, executive function, and motor performance. Early studies (Russell and Rix-Trot, 1975) established that the following abilities become disrupted below blood glucose levels of about 3.0 mmol/l:

- fine motor co-ordination
- mental speed
- concentration
- some memory functions.

The hyperinsulinaemic glucose clamp technique allows more controlled experiments of acute hypo- and hyperglycaemia. However, although this technique is used in most studies of cognitive function in hypoglycaemia, it does not mimic the physiological or temporal characteristics of "natural" or intercurrent episodes of hypoglycaemia experienced by people with type 1 diabetes. From laboratory experiments using the glucose clamp technique it was found that blood glucose concentrations between 3.1 and 3.3 mmol/l (Holmes, 1987; Deary, 1993):

- slowed reaction times (this experiment involves making a fast response when a light appears on a computer screen. Hypoglycaemia had more effect on reaction times when the reaction involved making a decision)

- slowed mental arithmetic
- impaired verbal fluency (in this test one has to think of words beginning with a given letter, and probably involves the frontal lobes of the brain)
- impaired performance in parts of the Stroop test (in this test one has to read aloud a series of ink colours when words are printed in a different colour from that of the name, e.g. the word RED printed in green ink).

Some mental functions were spared during hypoglycaemia, e.g.

- simple motor (like the speed of tapping) and sensory skills
- the speed of reading words aloud.

By 1993 over 16 studies had investigated cognitive functions during acute, mild–moderate hypoglycaemia (Deary, 1993). The levels of blood glucose ranged from 2.0 to 3.7 mmol/l. The way that hypoglycaemia was induced varied among studies, as did methods of blood sampling (e.g. arterialised or venous blood). Moreover, the ability levels of the people in different studies varied, and there was much heterogeneity in the test batteries used to assess mental performance. An authoritative statement as to the mental functions disrupted during hypoglycaemia is still not possible. However, in at least one or more of the studies a number of tests were significantly impaired during hypoglycaemia (Box 2.2).

Box 2.2 Cognitive function tests impaired during acute hypoglycaemia

- trail making (involving visual scanning and mental flexibility)
- digit symbol (speed of replacing a list of numbers with abstract codes)
- reaction time (especially involving a decision)
- mental arithmetic
- verbal fluency
- Stroop test
- grooved pegboard (a test of fine manual dexterity)
- pursuit rotor (a test of eye–hand co-ordination)
- letter cancellation (striking out occurrences of a given letter in a page of letters)
- delayed verbal memory
- backward digit span (repeating back a list of numbers backwards)
- story recall

Few areas of mental function are preserved at normal levels during acute hypoglycaemia. There is a general dampening of many abilities that involve conscious mental effort. In the face of so many deleterious effects, what mental functions remain intact during acute hypoglycaemia? At blood glucose concentrations similar to those indicated above, the following mental tests are not significantly impaired:

- finger tapping
- forward digit span (repeating back a list of numbers in the same order)
- simple reaction time
- elementary sensory processing.

Thus tests which involve speeded responses and which are more cognitively complex and attention-demanding tend to show impairment during hypoglycaemia (Deary, 1993). Heller and Macdonald (1996) have concluded that:

- even quite severe degrees of hypoglycaemia do not impair simple motor functions
- choice reaction time (where a mental decision of some kind is needed before reacting to a stimulus) is affected at higher blood glucose concentrations than simple reaction time
- speed of responding is sometimes slowed in a task in which accuracy is preserved
- many aspects of mental performance become impaired when blood glucose falls below about 3.0 mmol/l
- there are important individual differences; some people's mental performance is already impaired above a blood glucose of 3.0 mmol/l, whereas others continue to function well at lower levels
- the speed of response of the brain in making decisions slows down during hypoglycaemia (Tallroth et al, 1990; Jones et al, 1990)
- it can take as long as 40 to 90 minutes after blood glucose returns to normal for the brain to recover fully (Blackman et al, 1992; Lindgren et al, 1996).

Memory is an important domain of mental function which has received very little formal study during hypoglycaemia, but the limited evidence that is available suggests that many memory functions are relatively preserved.

Determining whether mental performance is impaired at all during mild to moderate hypoglycaemia, while a person is still fully conscious, is only the beginning of this line of investigation. The next question to ask is whether some particular functions are more susceptible and some less so? Figure 2.3 encapsulates this and illustrates three other questions about the cognitive effects of acute hypoglycaemia that are of importance:

1. What factors affect the degree of cognitive impairment during hypoglycaemia, other than the level of blood glucose?
2. Do impairments in laboratory cognitive tasks have a bearing on mental performance in real life?
3. Which basic brain functions are disturbed during acute hypoglycaemia?

Influences on the Degree of/Threshold for Cognitive Dysfunction During Acute Hypoglycaemia

Although people experience impairment of mental performance during hypoglycaemia, some do not change or may even improve (Pramming et al, 1986; Hoffman et al, 1989). It is not yet certain whether such individual differences in responses are stable (Gonder-Frederick et al, 1994; Driesen

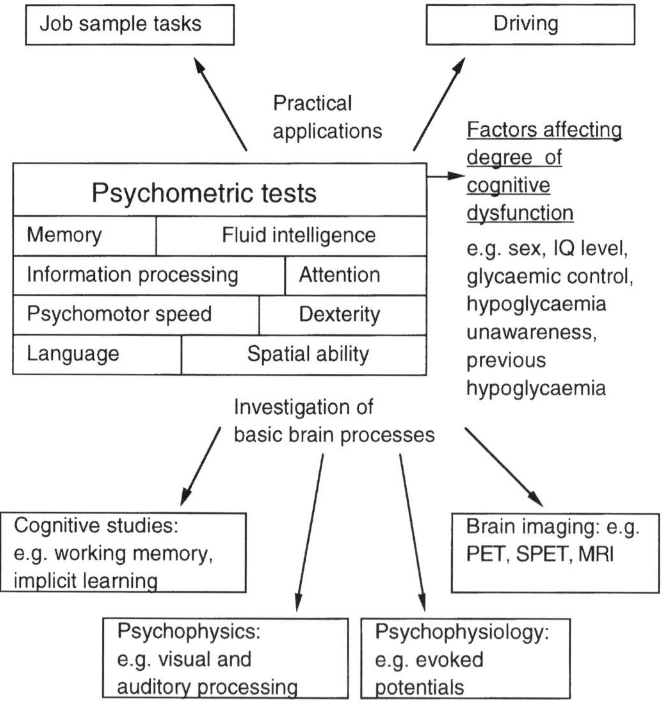

Figure 2.3 Cognitive effects of hypoglycaemia (after Deary, 1998)

et al, 1995). The following factors might increase a person's degree of cognitive impairment during acute hypoglycaemia:

- male sex (Draelos et al, 1995)
- impaired hypoglycaemia awareness (Gold et al, 1995b)
- type 1 diabetes (Wirsen et al, 1992)
- high IQ (Gold et al, 1995a).

Does glycaemic control affect the cognitive impact of hypoglycaemia? People with type 1 diabetes on intensified insulin therapy attain glycaemic control that is nearer to normal than most people treated with conventional insulin treatment. As a result, the frequency of severe hypoglycaemia is increased and is associated with a greater risk of impaired hypoglycaemia awareness. Neuroendocrine responses to hypoglycaemia are reduced in magnitude and begin at lower absolute blood glucose concentrations than in people with less strict glycaemic control. However, the hypoglycaemic threshold for cognitive dysfunction may not change in a similar fashion. Diabetic patients on intensive insulin therapy reported autonomic and neuroglycopenic symptoms at blood glucose concentrations of about 2.4 and 2.3 mmol/l respectively, whereas in those with less strict glycaemic control and in non-diabetic individuals, these symptoms commenced at between 2.8 and 3.0 mmol/l. However, in all three groups, the accuracy and speed in a reaction time test deteriorated significantly at blood glucose concentrations between 2.8 and 3.0 mmol/l (Amiel et al, 1991; Maran et al, 1995). Therefore, people with insulin-treated diabetes who have strict glycaemic control, have the misfortune that the deterioration in their mental performance begins before the onset of warning symptoms of hypoglycaemia. By contrast, neurophysiological responses (P300 event-related potentials), which have been linked to various measures of cognitive function, occur at lower blood glucose concentrations, suggesting that cerebral adaptation has occurred (Ziegler et al, 1992). The effects of quality of glycaemic control, antecedent hypoglycaemia and impaired hypoglycaemia awareness on the mental performance responses to hypoglycaemia, and the relation of these responses to the perceptions of the symptoms of hypoglycaemia, are important topics still under study (see Chapters 5 and 6). The interrelation of these factors makes the field complex, and progress is further hampered by the lack of consensus agreement on a validated battery of cognitive tests for use in hypoglycaemia.

Are the Cognitive Changes During Acute Hypoglycaemia Important and Valid?

Do the impairments of mental test performance actually have implications for real-life functions? In addition, are the mental changes during hypoglycaemia a result of impairments in basic brain functions?

One common, important and potentially dangerous area of real-life functioning is driving (see Chapter 11), which involves many cognitive abilities including psychomotor control and divided attention. Cox and colleagues (1993b) employed a sophisticated driving simulator and had people "drive" on this during controlled hypoglycaemia using a glucose clamp technique. At moderate hypoglycaemia (blood glucose 2.6 mmol/l) the diabetic patients committed significant driving errors including:

- more swerving and spinning
- poor steering
- poor road positioning and more time off the road.

During hypoglycaemia the patients often drove very slowly, possibly using a compensatory mechanism to avoid errors. Despite this, more global errors of driving were committed and about half of the participants, despite demonstrating seriously impaired ability to drive, said they felt competent to drive irrespective of their low blood glucose! It cannot be stated with certainty that the findings obtained in a driving simulator will apply to real-life driving. However, studies that examine the *practical* cognitive effects of hypoglycaemia are invaluable and more are required.

Just as more studies that examine the practical cognitive aspects of hypoglycaemia would be useful, so would more studies of the brain's processing efficiency. Cognitive tests typically involve a mélange of inseparable mental processes, yet, very specific aspects of the human brain's activities can be measured in the clinical laboratory (Massaro, 1993). Basic, specific aspects of visual and auditory processing have been examined during acute hypoglycaemia in non-diabetic humans. Standard tests of visual acuity—those that are measured by an optometrist—are not affected by hypoglycaemia, but other aspects of vision are affected (McCrimmon et al, 1996). These include:

- contrast sensitivity (the ability to discriminate faint patterns)
- inspection time (the ability to see what is in a pattern when it is shown for a very brief period of time)
- visual change detection (the ability to spot a small, quick change in a pattern)
- visual movement detection (the ability to spot brief movement in a pattern).

This means that the ability to see the environment changes in important ways during hypoglycaemia. Visual acuity is preserved, as tested by the ability to read black letters on a white background. However, most visual activity is not like that; many of the things we see happen quickly and in relatively poor light. When the level of contrast falls, or discriminations must be made under pressure of time, visual processing is impaired during hypoglycaemia. However, at about the same degree of hypoglycaemia, the ability to distinguish one colour from another does not appear to be impaired (Hardy et al, 1995). Speed of auditory processing also appears to be impaired by hypoglycaemia, and the ability to discriminate the loudness of two tones is disrupted (McCrimmon et al, 1997). This suggests that the ability to understand language may be compromised during hypoglycaemia.

ACUTE HYPOGLYCAEMIA AND EMOTIONS

Mood change is part of the experience of hypoglycaemia. Moods are emotion-like experiences that are quite general rather than applied to specific situations. Psychologists recognise three basic moods:

- energetic arousal (a tendency to feel lively and active rather than tired and sluggish)
- tense arousal (a tendency to feel anxious and nervous versus relaxed and calm)
- hedonic tone (a tendency to feel happy versus sad).

When people are asked to rate their mood states during hypoglycaemia induced in the laboratory, changes occur in all of these basic mood states. People feel less energetic, more tense, and less happy (Gold et al, 1995c; McCrimmon et al, 1999a). In addition, some people become more irritable and have angry feelings during hypoglycaemia (Merbis et al, 1996; McCrimmon et al, 1999b). The feeling of low energy takes over half an hour to be restored to normal levels, whereas the feelings of tenseness and unhappiness disappear when blood glucose returns to normal. The prolonged feeling of low energy after hypoglycaemia may affect work performance, so that when hypoglycaemia has been treated, an immediate return to the normal state should not be expected.

In addition to some people experiencing a low, tense, washed-out, angry mood state, hypoglycaemia alters the way some people look at their life problems. When junior doctors were asked to assess their career prospects during controlled hypoglycaemia, they were more pessimistic (McCrimmon et al, 1995) and if a general state of pessimism is common during hypoglycaemia, it would be a poor state from which to make personal decisions. It is possible that the change in mood states during hypoglycaemia is one of the causes of adults admitting to more "odd behaviour" (Deary et al, 1993). Altered mood may also account in part for symptoms of behavioural disturbance that are so prominent in the responses to hypoglycaemia of children with diabetes (McCrimmon et al, 1995).

In addition to emotional responses as a result of hypoglycaemia, some people have emotional responses in anticipation of hypoglycaemia. In Edinburgh one young man with insulin-treated diabetes developed a phobic anxiety state; his phobia was of becoming comatose as a result of hypoglycaemia (Gold et al, 1997a). Such a case is exceptional, but many people with diabetes are frightened of hypoglycaemia (see Chapter 11). The Hypoglycaemia Fear Survey (HFS) measures this tendency (Cox et al, 1987). The HFS comes in two parts. The first asks people several questions concerning how much they worry about hypoglycaemia (e.g. "Do you worry if you have no one around you during a [hypoglycaemic] reaction?"). The second part asks several questions about what people do to avoid hypoglycaemia (e.g. "Do you eat large snacks at bedtime?"). People with greater fear of hypoglycaemia (Polonsky et al, 1992; Hepburn et al, 1994):

- have more anxious personalities in general
- are more likely to confuse symptoms of anxiety for those of hypoglycaemia
- report having had more episodes of hypoglycaemia.

It is not yet known whether people who experience more hypoglycaemia become worriers about it, or whether people who are worriers in general just worry more about hypoglycaemia as well. Perhaps both are true. However, it does seem likely that the experience of more severe hypoglycaemia in the past and the development of impaired awareness of hypoglycaemia lead to increased worry about subsequent hypoglycaemia (Gold et al, 1997b).

CONCLUSIONS

- Because people with diabetes are closely involved in their own treatment it is important that they and their educators know about the main side-effects and sequelae of the disorder and its treatments.
- Accurate knowledge of the symptoms of hypoglycaemia may be used to avoid the dangers of hypoglycaemia.
- The progressively more serious impairment in cognitive function that occurs as blood glucose declines, provides knowledge about the brain's compromised state during hypoglycaemia:

continues

continued

basic functions like visual processing deteriorate and driving becomes dangerously error-prone. Performance on a host of mental tests becomes worse during hypoglycaemia.

- Some of the neuroglycopenic symptoms of hypoglycaemia are thought to be subjective impressions of impaired cognitive function: these impressions are fully supported by the results of objective cognitive testing.
- Moderate hypoglycaemia may induce a state of anxious tension, unhappiness and low energy, and even irritability and anger. Thus hypoglycaemia importantly touches the emotions as well as inducing bodily symptoms and affecting mental performance.

REFERENCES

Amiel SA, Pottinger RC, Archibald HR, Chusney G, Cunnah DTF, Prior PF, Gale EAM (1991). Effect of antecedent glucose control on cerebral function during hypoglycemia. *Diabetes Care* **14**: 109–18.

Blackman JD, Towle VL, Sturis J, Lewis GF, Spire J-P, Polonsky KS (1992). Hypoglycemic thresholds for cognitive dysfunction in IDDM. *Diabetes* **41**: 392–9.

Clarke WL, Cox DJ, Gonder-Frederick LA, Julian D, Schlundt D, Polonsky W (1997). The relationship between nonroutine use of insulin, food, and exercise and the occurrence of hypoglycemia in adults with IDDM and varying degrees of hypoglycemia awareness and metabolic control. *Diabetes Education* **23**: 55–8.

Cox DJ, Clarke WL, Gonder-Frederick L, Pohl S, Hoover C, Snyder A, Zimbelman L, Carter WL, Bobbitt S, Pennebaker J (1985). Accuracy of perceiving blood glucose in IDDM. *Diabetes Care* **8**: 529–36.

Cox DJ, Irvine A, Gonder-Frederick L, Nowacek G, Butterfield J (1987). Fear of hypoglycemia: quantification, validation and utilization. *Diabetes Care* **10**: 617–21.

Cox DJ, Gonder-Frederick L, Antoun B, Cryer PE, Clarke WL (1993a). Perceived symptoms in the recognition of hypoglycemia. *Diabetes Care* **16**: 519–27.

Cox D, Gonder-Frederick L, Clarke W (1993b). Driving decrements in type 1 diabetes during moderate hypoglycemia. *Diabetes* **42**: 239–43.

Deary IJ (1993). Effects of hypoglycaemia on cognitive function. In: Frier BM and Fisher BM (eds), *Hypoglycaemia and Diabetes: Clinical and Physiological Aspects*. London: Edward Arnold pp. 80–92.

Deary IJ (1998). The effects of diabetes on cognitive function. In Marshall SM, Home PD, Rizza RA (eds), *Diabetes Annual* **11**: 97–118.

Deary IJ, Hepburn DA, MacLeod KM, Frier BM (1993). Partitioning the symptoms of hypoglycaemia using multi-sample confirmatory factor analysis. *Diabetologia* **36**: 771–7.

Debrah T, Sherwin RS, Murphy J, Kerr D (1996). Effect of caffeine on recognition of and physiological responses to hypoglycaemia in insulin-dependent diabetes. *Lancet* **347**: 19–24.

Draelos MT, Jacobson AM, Weinger K, Widom B, Ryan CM, Finkelstein DM, Simonson DC (1995). Cognitive function in patients with insulin-dependent diabetes mellitus during hyperglycemia and hypoglycemia. *The American Journal of Medicine* **98**: 135–44.

Driesen NR, Cox DJ, Gonder-Frederick L, Clarke W (1995). Reaction time impairment in insulin-dependent diabetes: task complexity, blood glucose levels, and individual differences. *Neuropsychology* **9**: 246–54.

Fletcher AA, Campbell WR (1922). The blood sugar following insulin administration and the symptom complex-hypoglycemia. *Journal of Metabolic Research* **2**: 637–49.

Gold AE, Deary IJ, MacLeod KM, Frier BM (1995a). The effect of IQ level on the degree of cognitive deterioration experienced during acute hypoglycemia in normal humans. *Intelligence* **20**: 267–90.

Gold AE, MacLeod KM, Deary IJ, Frier BM (1995b). Hypoglycemia-induced cognitive dysfunction in diabetes mellitus: effect of hypoglycemia unawareness. *Physiology and Behavior* **58**: 501–11.

Gold AE, MacLeod KM, Frier BM, Deary IJ (1995c). Changes in mood during acute hypoglycemia in healthy subjects. *Journal of Personality and Social Psychology* **68**: 498–504.

Gold AE, Deary IJ, Frier BM (1997a). Hypoglycaemia and non-cognitive aspects of psychological function in insulin-dependent (type 1) diabetes mellitus (IDDM). *Diabetic Medicine* **14**: 111–18.

Gold AE, Frier BM, MacLeod KM, Deary IJ (1997b) A structural equation model for predictors of severe hypoglycaemia in patients with insulin-dependent diabetes mellitus. *Diabetic Medicine* **14**: 309–15.

Gonder-Frederick L, Cox D, Driesen NR, Ryan CM, Clarke W (1994). Individual differences in neurobehavioral disruption during mild and moderate hypoglycemia in adults with IDDM. *Diabetes* **43**: 1407–12.

Gonder-Frederick L, Cox D, Kovatchev B, Schlundt D, Clarke W (1997). A biopsychobehavioral model of risk of severe hypoglycemia. *Diabetes Care* **20**: 161–9.

Hardy KJ, Scase MO, Foster DH, Scarpello JH (1995). Effect of short term changes in blood glucose on visual pathway function in insulin dependent diabetes. *British Journal of Ophthalmology* **79**: 38–41.

Heller SR and Macdonald IA (1996). The measurement of cognitive function during acute hypoglycaemia: experimental limitations and their effects on the study of hypoglycaemia unawareness. *Diabetic Medicine* **13**: 607–15.

Hepburn DA (1993). Symptoms of hypoglycaemia. In: Frier BM and Fisher BM (eds), *Hypoglycaemia and Diabetes: Clinical and Physiological Aspects*. London: Edward Arnold 93–103.

Hepburn DA, Deary IJ, Frier BM, Patrick AW, Quinn JD, Fisher BM (1991). Symptoms of acute insulin-induced hypoglycemia in humans with and without IDDM. Factor-analysis approach. *Diabetes Care* **14**: 949–57.

Hepburn DA, Deary IJ, MacLeod KM, Frier BM (1994). Structural equation modeling of symptoms, awareness and fear of hypoglycemia, and personality in patients with insulin-treated diabetes. *Diabetes Care* **17**: 1273–80.

Hoffman RG, Speelman DJ, Hinnen DA, Conley KL, Guthrie RA, Knapp RK (1989). Changes in cortical functioning with acute hypoglycemia and hyperglycemia in type 1 diabetes. *Diabetes Care* **12**: 193–7.

Holmes CS (1987). Metabolic control and auditory information processing at altered glucose levels in insulin dependent diabetes. *Brain and Cognition* **6**: 161–74.

Jaap AJ, Jones GC, McCrimmon RJ, Deary IJ, Frier BM (1998).Perceived symptoms of hypoglycaemia in elderly type 2 diabetic patients treated with insulin. *Diabetic Medicine* **15**: 398–401.

Jones TW, McCarthy G, Tamborlane WV, Caprio S, Roessler E, Kraemer D, Starick-Zych K, Allison T, Boulware SD, Sherwin RS (1990). Mild hypoglycemia and impairment of brainstem and cortical evoked potentials in healthy subjects. *Diabetes* **39**: 1550–5.

Lindgren M, Eckert B, Stenberg G, Agardh C-D (1996). Restitution of neurophysiological functions, performance, and subjective symptoms after moderate insulin-induced hypoglycaemia in non-diabetic men. *Diabetic Medicine* **13**: 218–25.

Maran A, Lomas J, Macdonald IA, Amiel SA (1995). Lack of preservation of higher brain function during hypoglycaemia in patients with intensively-treated IDDM. *Diabetologia* **38**: 1412–18.

Massaro DW (1993). Information processing models: microscopes of the mind. *Annual Review of Psychology* **44**: 383–425.

Macfarlane PI, Smith CS (1988). Perceptions of hypoglycaemia in childhood diabetes mellitus: a questionnaire study. *Practical Diabetes* **5:** 56–58.

Macfarlane PI, Walters M, Stutchfield P, Smith CS (1989). A prospective study of symptomatic hypoglycaemia in childhood diabetes. *Diabetic Medicine* **6**: 627–30.

McCrimmon RJ, Gold AE, Deary IJ, Kelnar CJH, Frier BM (1995). Symptoms of hypoglycemia in children with IDDM. *Diabetes Care* **18**: 858–61.

McCrimmon RJ, Deary IJ, Huntly BJP, MacLeod KJ, Frier BM (1996). Visual information processing during controlled hypoglycaemia in humans. *Brain* **119**: 1277–87.

McCrimmon RJ, Deary IJ, Frier BM (1997). Auditory information processing during acute insulin-induced hypoglycaemia in non-diabetic human subjects. *Neuropsychologia* **35:** 1547–53.

McCrimmon RJ, Deary IJ, Frier BM (1999a). Appraisal of mood and personality during hypoglycaemia. *Physiology and Behavior* **67**: 27–33.

McCrimmon RJ, Ewing FME, Frier BM, Deary IJ (1999b). Anger-state during acute insulin-induced hypoglycaemia. *Physiology and Behavior* **67**: 35–39.

Merbis MAE, Snoek FJ, Kanc K, Heine RJ (1996). Hypoglycaemia induces emotional disruption. *Patient Education and Counseling* **29**: 117–22.

Mutch WJ, Dingwall-Fordyce I (1985). Is it a hypo? Knowledge of symptoms of hypoglycaemia in elderly diabetic patients. *Diabetic Medicine* **2**: 54–6.

Pennebaker JW, Cox DJ, Gonder-Frederick L, Wunsch MG, Evans WS, Pohl S (1981). Physical symptoms related to blood glucose in insulin-dependent diabetics. *Psychosomatic Medicine* **43**: 489–500.

Polonsky WH, Davis CL, Jacobson AM, Anderson BJ (1992).Correlates of hypoglycemic fear in type 1 and type 2 diabetes mellitus. *Health Psychology* **11**: 199–202.

Pramming S, Thorsteinsson B, Theilgaard A, Pinner EM, Binder C (1986). Cognitive function during hypoglycaemia in type 1 diabetes mellitus. *British Medical Journal* **292**: 647–50.

Ross LA, McCrimmon RJ, Frier BM, Kelnar CJH, Deary IJ (1998). Hypoglycaemic symptoms reported by children with type 1 diabetes mellitus and by their parents. *Diabetic Medicine* **15**: 836–43.

Russell PN, Rix-Trot HM (1975). An exploratory study of some behavioural consequences of insulin-induced hypoglycaemia. *New Zealand Medical Journal* **81**: 337–40.

Tallroth G, Lindgren M, Stenberg G, Rosen I, Agardh C-D (1990). Neurophysiological changes during insulin-induced hypoglycaemia and in the recovery period following glucose infusion in type 1 (insulin-dependent) diabetes mellitus and in normal man. *Diabetologia* **33:** 319–23.

Towler DA, Havlin CE, Craft S, Cryer P (1993). Mechanism of awareness of hypoglycemia: perception of neurogenic (predominantly cholinergic) rather than neuroglycopenic symptoms. *Diabetes* **42**: 1791–8.

Weinger K, Jacobson AM, Draelos MT, Finkelstein DM, Simonson DC (1995). Blood glucose estimation and symptoms during hyperglycemia and hypoglycemia in patients with insulin-dependent diabetes mellitus. *American Journal of Medicine* **98**: 22–31.

Wilder J (1943). Psychological problems in hypoglycemia. *American Journal of Digestive Diseases* **10**: 428–35.

Wirsen A, Tallroth G, Lindgren M, Agardh C-D (1992). Neuropsychological performance differs between type 1 diabetic and normal men during insulin-induced hypoglycaemia. *Diabetic Medicine* **9**: 156–65.

Ziegler D, Hubinger A, Muhlen H, Gries FA (1992). Effects of previous glycaemic control on the onset and magnitude of cognitive dysfunction during hypoglycaemia in type 1 (insulin-dependent) diabetic patients. *Diabetologia* **35**: 828–34.

3

Frequency, Causes and Treatment of Hypoglycaemia

ROBERT B. TATTERSALL
Queen's Medical Centre, Nottingham

INTRODUCTION

Whenever a doctor or layman talks about their life on insulin, the No. 1 topic is always hypoglycaemia and its life-disrupting effects. For example, the late Charles Fletcher, a well known chest physician and television doctor who was on insulin for over 50 years, wrote:

> "My main problem has always been hypoglycaemia. At first I was nearly always aware of it by day and woke by night, because of the adrenaline response. But, particularly in the past 20 years, it gradually became more difficult ... Sometimes diplopia, dysphasia, weariness, or inability to think may lead me to do a blood sugar. But I often become too muddled to know what is wrong, and I have had to thank my wife, my children, and many generations of housemen, registrars, and secretaries for spotting these low levels ... I can no longer safely sleep away from home by myself, although these nocturnal attacks have been much less frequent since I have regularly measured my blood sugar before going to bed ... One difficulty I've had has been the ignorance of most of my contemporary medical colleagues about hypoglycaemia." (Fletcher, 1980)

The freelance journalist and one-time cricket correspondent of *The Financial Times*, Teresa McLean, writes:

Hypoglycaemia in Clinical Diabetes. Edited by B. M. Frier and B. M. Fisher.

> "Hypos are easily cured. It is hard to believe that such a dangerous and often spectacular disorder can be put right by swallowing a lump of sugar ... Always at the back of my mind I am waiting for hypoglycaemia. And I wait for it with dread ... Some hypos are mainly physical, some are mainly mental and some are both. They share a common core of ghastliness, but the ones I hate most are the mental ones ... I am not violent or aggressive when hypo. Instead, I am without personality; a corpse performing a malignant parody of myself." (McLean, 1985)

Both these people in different walks of life have had scores or even hundreds of hypos during their combined 80 years on insulin. In fact, since 1922 hypoglycaemia has always been the commonest side-effect of insulin treatment, although, until the 1970s, it is surprisingly difficult to find indications of its frequency or even evidence that it was of as much interest to diabetologists as to their patients. For example, in a review in 1933 Wauchope wrote:

> "Severe reactions are comparatively rare especially when one considers the variability of diet and activity, the swift fall in blood sugar that may follow a dose of insulin, the changing susceptibility of the body, and lastly the vast possibilities for human error." (Wauchope, 1933)

The demand for figures was articulated by Franz Ingelfinger, the editor of the *New England Medical Journal*, who in a 1977 editorial asked:

> "What is the frequency of fatalities, serious sequelae and hospital admissions attributable to the tight control treatment of diabetes?" (Ingelfinger, 1977)

The past two decades have seen an unprecedented interest in the clinical and physiological aspects of hypoglycaemia because of:

- the ability to measure counterregulatory hormones, which has led to a greater understanding of the physiological defence mechanisms
- concern that innovations such as insulin pen devices and pumps might increase the frequency of hypoglycaemia
- a renewed belief, finally proved by the Diabetes Control and Complications Trial (DCCT) that "tight control" prevents diabetic complications but at the price of an increase in hypoglycaemia (The Diabetes Control and Complications Trial Research Group, 1993).

DEFINITIONS

Blood glucose is tightly regulated in health, and spontaneous hypoglycaemia in the non-diabetic individual is very rare. By contrast, insulin-induced hypoglycaemia in the diabetic patient is common and can be classified as:

- biochemical (blood glucose below a defined but arbitrary concentration)
- mild symptomatic (self-treatment by the patient)
- severe symptomatic (help needed from another person)
- profound (causing coma or convulsions).

This classification seems straightforward but is hard to apply in practice. Asymptomatic (biochemical) hypoglycaemia is common, especially at night (*vide infra*), but usually goes unnoticed because it can only be identified by measuring blood glucose which, if done by the patient, may be unreliable and, unless very frequent, may miss most nadirs. Inpatient profiles overcome these problems but are labour-intensive and unrepresentative of normal life. Mild episodes are difficult to assess because the symptoms are non-specific and their relationship to blood glucose levels are variable and unreliable (Pramming et al, 1990). One would think that patients would always remember a severe episode but these may not be recalled because of retrograde amnesia or emotional denial. Patients and their partners or relatives may disagree about the frequency of attacks and particularly about whether the patient is usually aware of low blood glucose (Heller et al, 1995). Semantic misunderstandings between doctor and patient are also common; a surprising number of patients, when asked whether they have had any hypos, will reply "no" because they assume that a hypo means a coma. "Unconscious" may be misunderstood to mean unaware of the surroundings rather than in the medical sense of coma, and "had a fit" may mean twitching movements, a vacant expression or aggressive behaviour rather than a true convulsion. It may seem pedantic, but when talking to patients it is important to make clear exactly what you are asking. Thus, you could say, "How often have you felt the symptoms of low blood glucose during the past week?" or "How often have you been low during the past week?" You could then continue, "Since I last saw you, how many times have you had a low blood glucose reaction where someone else has had to help you?"

Definitions in published papers are often not explicit. In general, severe hypoglycaemia (SH) is defined as an episode in which self-treatment is not possible and external help is required, but sometimes the adjective "severe" is restricted to episodes which result in coma or a convulsion.

Biochemical Hypoglycaemia

It is a truism that insulin replacement is unphysiological because it does not mimic the minute-to-minute modulation of insulin secretion that normally occurs in relation to meals, exercise and fasting. Continuous blood glucose monitoring invariably shows that diabetic patients treated with injections of subcutaneous insulin, have wide excursions (or, put another way, a much larger standard deviation of blood glucose) compared to non-diabetic people, even if they have a mean blood glucose concentration or haemoglobin A1c within the non-diabetic range. Thus, during a representative day they will have some abnormally high and some abnormally low levels. This variability will exist even if the patient is very careful with diet and exercise and however many times they measure their blood glucose. What is surprising is how many of these nadirs are asymptomatic and unrecognised by the patient.

Thorsteinsson et al (1986) measured seven point blood glucose profiles during the day (on samples sent by post in capillary tubes) in 79 patients on twice-daily insulin and 20 patients on continuous subcutaneous insulin infusion (CSII). Values below 3.0 mmol/l increased non-linearly with decreasing median blood glucose concentration. For a median blood glucose of 5.0 mmol/l (i.e. normoglycaemia), values below 3.0 mmol/l would be expected 10% of the time. With twice-daily insulin there was a 40% chance that the low value would occur at 1100 hours, whereas on CSII low blood glucose concentrations were distributed evenly throughout the day. As expected, hypoglycaemia was more common before, rather than after, meals in both groups. This study allowed an estimate of the frequency of hypoglycaemia for a given median blood glucose (Figure 3.1). As a consequence, if it is considered that only 2% of all diurnal blood glucose concentrations below 3.0 mmol/l are acceptable, a median value of 11.0 mmol/l has to be the treatment goal.

Thorsteinsson et al (1986) studied patients during their ordinary lives but could not measure duration of hypoglycaemia, since only seven measurements were made in the day during waking hours. Arias et al (1985) used a portable continuous blood glucose monitor so that patients could walk about the hospital during the study, and found that nine of 10 patients on CSII and five of nine patients taking four injections had at least one blood glucose below 2.8 mmol/l during the 24 hours. In four patients on CSII, hypoglycaemia was present for three to seven hours of the 24, whereas in only one patient on four times daily insulin did the total duration of hypoglycaemia exceed three hours. Despite the prolonged hypoglycaemia in the CSII group, only six of the 23 episodes were symptomatic.

If daytime insulin replacement does not mimic normal physiology, the

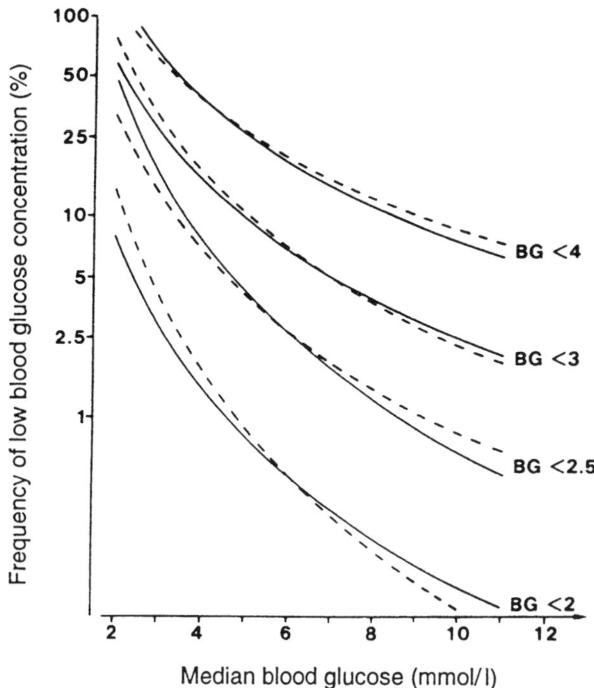

Figure 3.1 Correlation between the median blood glucose concentration and the frequencies of blood glucose concentrations below 4, 3, 2.5 and 2 mmol/l in patients with type 1 diabetes. Conventional insulin therapy: continuous lines; continuous subcutaneous insulin infusion: broken lines. Reproduced from Thorsteinsson et al (1986) by permission of *Diabetic Medicine*

night is an even greater problem (Box 3.1). Absorption of all long-acting, modified (cloudy) insulins produces a parabolic curve with a peak in the middle of the night rather than the constant basal level of the non-diabetic state. This is compounded by the variability of absorption of modified insulins which, in the same subject, may lead to a difference in plasma free insulin concentrations of 50% on two different nights. Thus it is not surprising to find a high frequency of biochemical hypoglycaemia at night (Table 3.1). In one of the first systematic overnight studies Gale and Tattersall (1979) found at least one blood glucose value below 2.0 mmol/l in half of 39 diabetic patients treated with insulin, and in three-quarters of these episodes the hypoglycaemia lasted for three or more hours. Bendtson et al (1988) did a similar study in 23 patients on multiple injections of insulin and 25 on CSII. Thirty per cent on multiple injections and 44% on CSII had at least one blood glucose value below 3.0 mmol/l during the night, with a mean duration of hypoglycaemia of

Box 3.1 Nocturnal hypoglycaemia

Nocturnal hypoglycaemia:

- occurs in 10–56% of overnight profiles
- is asymptomatic in 25–70% of episodes
- may last up to six hours

The time of the nadir depends on the insulin regimen and time of the main evening meal.

two hours (range 1–6) on multiple injections and four hours (range 1–7) on CSII. In patients on twice-daily insulin regimens, a third had a blood glucose <3.0 mmol/l during the night and one in ten a value below 2.0 mmol/l (Pramming et al, 1985). A striking finding in all these studies was that less than a quarter of the hypoglycaemic patients had symptoms; those who did wake were as likely to have a normal or a high blood glucose. While the sleeping patient may be unaware of the low blood glucose, an observer can often identify the hypoglycaemia by physical signs such as sweating, increased muscle tone or restlessness during sleep (see Chapter 11).

The time of the nocturnal glucose nadir depends on the time of the evening meal (often at 1800 hours in the UK but rarely before 2000 hours in Southern Europe) and the time of injection of the intermediate or long-acting insulin (before the main evening meal in conventional, twice-daily insulin regimens and at bedtime in basal-bolus regimens). In the study of Gale and Tattersall (1979) in which patients were taking twice-daily insulin, the commonest time for hypoglycaemia was at 0300 hours, and at 0400 hours in the study by Pramming et al (1985). By contrast, in patients on a basal-bolus regimen, there appear to be two times of risk with "early night" hypoglycaemia between 2300 and 0100 hours and "early morning" hypoglycaemia between 0400 and 0730 hours. For example, in the study of Vervoort et al (1996), five out of 31 patients became hypoglycaemic in the early night, and seven out of 31 in the early morning, but none between 0100 and 0400 hours.

It would be useful for patients, their partners or the parents of a diabetic child to be able to predict whether hypoglycaemia was likely to occur in general or on a particular night. When patients are taking twice-daily insulin, advice based on the studies of Gale and Tattersall (1979) and Dornan et al (1981) is that measurement of a blood glucose at 0300 hours is the most profitable. However, on multiple injection regimens Bendtson et al (1988) found that a value at 0300 hours would have detected only 13% of episodes, so detection of nocturnal hypoglycaemia

Table 3.1 Frequency of biochemical nocturnal hypoglycaemia in patients with insulin-treated diabetes

Reference	Adults (A) or children (C)	Number of patients	Treatment[a]	Percentage with glucose (mmol/l) below			Percentage asymptomatic	Mean glycated haemoglobin (%)
				3.0	2.5	2.0		
Gale and Tattersall (1979)	A	39	BD insulin			56	64	N/A
Dornan et al (1981)	A	82	Conventional	–	–	27	27	9.5 (A1)
Pramming et al (1985)	A	58	BD insulin	29	22	9	9	9.1 (A1c)
Whincup and Milner (1987)	C	71	BD insulin	34	–	11	N/A	
		31	OD insulin	10	–	–	N/A	
Bendtson et al (1988)	A	23	Multiple injections	30	9	9	57	8.3 (A1)
		25	CSII	44	36	12	66	7.0 (A1c)
Shalwitz et al (1990)	C	135	"Conventional"	14	7	2	?100	10.3 (A1)
Vervoort et al (1996)	A	31	Basal-bolus	29			67	8.6 (A1c)

[a]OD = once daily, BD = twice daily, CSII = Continuous subcutaneous insulin infusion. Conventional therapy is a combination of soluble and isophane insulins, twice daily

with basal-bolus insulin regimens requires different times of measurement of blood glucose during the night.

Rather than waking the patient during the night, it would be more convenient if it were possible to predict nocturnal hypoglycaemia on the basis of a blood glucose last thing at night or first thing in the morning. Unfortunately, the findings for adults and children are conflicting. Pramming et al (1985) reported that if blood glucose was below 6.0 mmol/l at 2300 hours, the risk of nocturnal biochemical hypoglycaemia was 80%, while if it was above 6.0 mmol/l, the risk was 12%. In children with diabetes, Whincup and Milner (1987) showed a positive predictive value of 83% for a blood glucose below 7.0 mmol/l at 2200 hours. Bendtson et al (1988) found that a value below 6.0 mmol/l at 2300 hours was associated with 100% chance of nocturnal hypoglycaemia in patients on multiple insulin injections but had no predictive value in those on CSII. In the study of Vervoort et al (1996) a bedtime blood glucose predicted "early night" but not "early morning" hypoglycaemia, whereas a fasting glucose below 5.5 mmol/l was indicative of preceding "early morning" hypoglycaemia.

FREQUENCY OF SEVERE HYPOGLYCAEMIA (SH)

Adults (Table 3.2)

A simplified summary of the prevalence of hypoglycaemic coma in adults on conventional therapy is the so-called "rule of thirds" (Gale, 1986: Box 3.2). However, severe hypoglycaemia causing neuroglycopenia can occur without coma, and in adults severe hypoglycaemia is defined by the need to have external help to effect recovery.

Two studies were done in the late 1970s when most patients were on one or two daily injections, relatives were rarely provided with glucagon, and home blood glucose monitoring was in its infancy. In a one-year prospective study by Potter et al (1982) in the accident and emergency department of a British hospital, there were 200 attendances for SH in patients on insulin: 96 presented once, while 34 others were seen on a total of 104 occasions. It was calculated that 9% of patients on insulin had at least one episode of SH per year. This was a minimum because severe episodes treated at home or elsewhere were excluded. In a retrospective study of 172 consecutive patients in Paris, Goldgewicht et al (1983) found that mild hypoglycaemia had occurred at least once a month in 58% and a quarter had experienced at least one episode requiring assistance during the previous year. These results were greeted with alarm and some scepticism. However, a study performed in Denmark in 1984 (but

Table 3.2 Frequency of severe hypoglycaemia in adults

Reference	Year	Country	No. of Patients	Percentage with SH in previous year	Incidence (episodes/100 patient years)	Percentage on three or more injections
Potter et al (1979)	1979	England	1229	9	–	None
Goldgewicht et al (1983)	1979	France	172	26	–	17
Pramming et al (1991)	1984	Denmark	411		140	Very few
Muhlhauser et al (1985b)	1980–3	Germany and Austria	384	10	–	Very few
			50 (CSII)	9	–	–
The DCCT Research Group (1987)	1984–6	USA	132 (conventional)	9.8	17	None
			146 (strict)	26	54	100
MacLeod et al (1993)	1991–2	Scotland	600	29.2	160	10.8
Gold et al (1994)	1993	Scotland	29 (unaware)	66	280	< 30
			31 (aware)	26	50	

Box 3.2 Hypoglycaemic coma: "The Rule of Thirds" (Gale, 1986)

1. One in three patients will have a hypoglycaemic coma at some point in their diabetic life
2. One in three of these (i.e. 10% of the total) will have had a coma in the previous year
3. One in three of these (i.e. 2–3% of the total) have a very real disruption of their lives from recurrent hypoglycaemic coma

not published until 1991) found that mild hypoglycaemia occurred at a rate of 1.8 episodes per patient per week with 1.4 severe episodes per patient per year (Pramming et al, 1991). During their life on insulin, 36% of Danish patients had been unconscious from hypoglycaemia and 3.5% had been comatose on more than 10 occasions. A striking finding was that only 6% of severe episodes were treated in a hospital emergency department, confirming that hospital records of SH are an unreliable index of its frequency. This is even more true now that most relatives have glucagon or a glucose gel at home (see below).

The prevalence of SH with conventional treatment appears to be similar from country to country. Apparent differences can usually be explained by different definitions, different methods of data collection (hospital records, retrospective questionnaires, or interviews with relatives), the inclusion of patients with insulin-treated type 2 diabetes, and whether the denominator (the number with diabetes in the background population) is known or assumed.

Children and Adolescents (Table 3.3)

As with adults, the reported frequency of SH in children is rather variable (Table 3.3). The earliest study came from a clinic which, unusually for the 1970s, aimed for strict glycaemic control, and was reassuring in that during 18 months only 4% of children had suffered SH (Goldstein et al, 1981). Severe reactions were confined to children who had a glycated haemoglobin within the non-diabetic range. Prevalence rates of SH in one year were reported in large North American series, one from Montreal and one from the Joslin Clinic in Boston, at 6.8 and 12% respectively (Bergada et al, 1989; Bhatia and Wolfsdorf, 1991). Even more alarming figures have been reported from another study in Canada and one from Sweden. In Toronto, of 311 children with a mean age of 11.6 years and diabetes duration of 4.6 years, 31% had experienced at least one coma or

Table 3.3 Incidence of severe hypoglycaemia in children and adolescents with type 1 diabetes

Reference	Country	Episodes per patient per year
Goldstein et al, 1981	USA	0.03
Bergada et al, 1989	Canada	0.07
Egger et al, 1991	Switzerland	0.07
Bhatia and Wolfsdorf, 1991	USA	0.12
Davis et al, 1997	Australia	0.15
Daneman et al, 1989	Canada	0.16
Macfarlane et al, 1989	UK	0.2
Dorchy et al, 1997	Belgium	0.02
Barkai et al, 1998	Hungary	0.4
Aman et al, 1989	Sweden	0.4
Adolescents in the DCCT		
The DCCT Research Group, 1997	USA	0.28 (Conventional)
	USA	0.86 (Intensive)

convulsion since diagnosis and in 16% this had occurred in the year of study (Daneman et al, 1989). In a group of 92 children in Sweden, 17% had been unconscious with convulsions in the previous year and 44% had reported an episode which needed assistance (Aman et al, 1989). In a more recent Swedish study, Nordfeldt and Ludvigsson (1997) reported that the annual incidence of coma did not increase despite an improvement in HbA1c from 8.1% in 1992 to 6.9% in 1994, but there was a slight increase in SH from 1.01 to 1.26 events per patient per year. The authors conclude that using multiple injections (90% of these children were taking four injections per day), near normal HbA1c can be achieved without a pronounced increase in SH. They suggest that the much better results in Sweden than in the DCCT can be explained by the fact that this regimen has been used in Sweden for many years, whereas it was a culture shock for both the patients and investigators in the DCCT.

The American paediatrician, Travis (1989), has questioned whether an annual rate of SH of 4% or 16% is the norm, commenting that the lower figure is disturbing and the higher frightening. As with adults there is good evidence that absence of endogenous secretion of C-peptide and near normal glycated haemoglobin are important risk factors. Thus, severe hypoglycaemia is rare in the 12 months after diagnosis (Davis et al, 1997). More worrying is that in many series the rate of SH is highest in very young children. This may partly relate to the difficulty of defining SH in young children who are dependent on parents or adult carers for treatment and may be unable to identify symptoms of hypoglycaemia. In the series of Davis et al (1997) the rate of SH for children less than six years of age was 0.49 episodes per year compared to 0.16 for children over six. The same was true in other studies of children with diabetes (Daneman et al, 1989; Barkai et al, 1998). The concern is that the brains of infants and young children are particularly vulnerable to hypoglycaemia which may cause permanent cognitive impairment.

DOES INTENSIVE TREATMENT INCREASE THE RISK OF SH?

The answer is almost certainly "Yes, by two or three times". The evidence comes from three studies; the Diabetes Control and Complications Trial (DCCT), the Stockholm Study, and the Bucharest–Dusseldorf Study.

The Diabetes Control and Complications Trial (Table 3.4 and Box 3.3)

This was a prospective randomised trial in the USA and Canada to finally settle the question, asked repeatedly since the first use of insulin in 1922, whether near normoglycaemia will prevent the development or progression of microvascular complications. Patients were randomly allocated to conventional or intensive treatment. "Conventional" treatment was the typical way in which patients with type 1 diabetes were managed in the USA in 1980 when the study was devised. Patients were taking one or two injections of insulin per day, did not do home blood glucose

Table 3.4 Hypoglycaemia in the Diabetes Control and Complications Trial (DCCT)

Adults	Conventional (n = 730)		Intensive (n = 711)		Relative risk
	Cumulative at 9 years (%)	Rate/100 patient years	Cumulative at 9 years (%)	Rate/100 patient years	
Hypoglycaemia requiring assistance	41.4	18.7	72.8	61.2	3.28
Coma and/or seizure	25.5	5.4	47.4	16.3	3.02
Adolescents	Conventional (n = 103)		Intensive (n = 92)		
Hypoglycaemia requiring assistance	45	27.8	82	85.7	2.97
Coma and/or seizure	25	9.7	63	26.7	2.93

Box 3.3 The DCCT

In the DCCT severe hypoglycaemia on intensive treatment was:

- three times more frequent than in those on conventional treatment
- more common in adult men than women
- more common in adolescents than adults
- in any year an intensively treated patient had a 1 in 3 chance of hypoglycaemia requiring assistance and a 1 in 10 chance of a coma
- less common in those with residual C-peptide secretion

monitoring and had a three-monthly review at which investigators and patients were masked to the HbA1c result unless it was over 13%. The upper limit of the non-diabetic range for the HbA1c assay used was 6% and the average level in the conventionally treated group was 9%. "Intensive" therapy was either CSII or four injections of insulin daily with frequent home blood glucose monitoring, monthly clinic visits and an attempt to reach near normoglycaemia.

Two important points need to be made about this protocol:

1. Patients were self-selected (often from newspaper advertisements) and were presumably highly motivated. Patients in the intensive group were seen every month for 6–9 years by a doctor, diabetes nurse, dietitian and psychologist. This degree of supervision and advice was, and still is, atypical in the USA and UK.
2. Because the intensively treated group had an average HbA1c of 7%, compared to 9% in the conventional group, one cannot conclude that only intensive treatment produces good glycaemic control. Given the same tools and supervision, many patients on one or two injections of insulin daily might have achieved as good control as those on four injections.

In March 1984, 278 subjects were recruited for the feasibility phase and after one year those on intensive therapy had a threefold higher rate of SH (26% vs 10%; The DCCT Research Group, 1987). The rate was particularly high in those who had a history of hypoglycaemic coma before the study and the protocol was amended to exclude any patient who had a history of two or more episodes of hypoglycaemic coma or convulsions in the previous two years. Had this not been done, the eventual frequency of SH would probably have been much higher.

For the main study 1441 patients with type 1 diabetes aged 13–39 years, and without significant complications, were recruited from 29 centres between 1983 and 1989. In the first report in 1991, 55% of the intensive group had recorded at least one episode of SH in three years compared to 31% of the conventional group. Three-quarters of the hypoglycaemic comas or convulsions had occurred in the intensive group (The DCCT Research Group, 1991). In the final analysis the rate of SH in intensively treated patients was 61.2 per 100 patient years and 18.7 per 100 patient years in the conventionally treated group (The DCCT Research Group, 1997 and Table 3.4). After 6.5 years of follow-up, two-thirds of intensively treated patients had experienced at least one episode of SH, compared to a third of the conventionally treated patients. Men on intensive treatment were nearly twice as likely to have SH as women. Furthermore, adolescents had more SH than adults in either treatment arm, with no gender difference. Patients with residual C-peptide secretion had a significantly lower risk of SH on either treatment. The increased risk of SH was seen in all but two of the 29 clinics, and in 19 clinics the relative risk for intensive vs conventional treatment was greater than two. Not surprisingly the risk of SH was greater the lower the HbA1c, although this did not account for all the differences between groups. For example, a patient who entered the DCCT with a HbA1c of 9.5% which was reduced to 7.5% with intensive therapy had a risk of SH of 56.7 per 100 patient years. Against this, a conventionally treated patient with a HbA1c of 7.5% who entered the trial at the same level had a risk of only 31.5 per 100 patient years. At every level of HbA1c, the subjects receiving intensive therapy had a higher risk of SH.

The Stockholm Study

This trial, which began in 1986, had the same aim as the DCCT but was much smaller with only 96 subjects, 44 of whom were randomised to intensified and 52 to standard treatment. Mean HbA1c was 7.2% in the intensified and 8.7% in the standard group (non-diabetic range for their assay was 3.9–5.7%). During the first five years of the study, the intensified group had a mean of 1.1 episodes of SH per patient per year compared to 0.4 in the standard group (Reichard et al, 1991).

The Bucharest–Dusseldorf Study

Both the DCCT and the Stockholm study showed a two- to three-fold increase in the frequency of SH on intensive treatment and this must be regarded as a conservative estimate because these were highly motivated patients in research studies. It is likely that attempts to force down the

HbA1c in unselected patients in ordinary clinical practice would lead to still higher rates of SH. In addition, in the DCCT the most hypoglycaemia-prone patients, those with a history of two or more previous hypoglycaemic comas, were excluded. Nevertheless, Muhlhauser and colleagues in Dusseldorf have always claimed that improved glycaemic control need not necessarily be associated with more hypoglycaemia, because:

> "Intensification of insulin therapy usually aims at a more physiologic substitution of insulin, i.e. separate application of basal and prandial insulin requirements. Thus, it should be associated by a smoothing of glucose swings and hence not necessarily by an increased risk of hypoglycaemia." (Muhlhauser, 1988)

This appeared to be supported by the Bucharest–Dusseldorf study (Muhlhauser et al, 1987) in which the rates of SH in the first year were 6% and 12% respectively in the intensively and conventionally treated groups but fell to 3–4% in the second year. In this study, 300 patients were randomised into groups receiving three different treatment regimens; the first was the traditional way of managing diabetes in Romania in which patients were admitted to hospital for seven days to begin or "re-stabilise" insulin therapy. Most patients were taking twice-daily insulin, were not taught to adjust their insulin dosage and did neither blood nor urine tests. The 100 patients in this "traditional" group (11 newly diagnosed) had a mean HbA1 of 12.5% at entry and during the first year four died (one of hypoglycaemia and three of infections complicated by ketoacidosis). Thirteen patients had 16 episodes of ketoacidosis during the year and 173 hospital admissions totalling 1447 days. Six patients had one or more episodes of severe hypoglycaemia. By contrast, the 100 patients randomised to the intensive treatment and teaching programme had 67 hospital admissions in the first year totalling 630 days and only two had ketoacidosis. However, 12 had at least one episode of severe hypoglycaemia. In the second year (in which the conventionally treated patients were converted to intensive therapy) the rate of SH fell to 3–4% in both groups and ketoacidosis to 0–2%. These are impressive results in a large group of 14–40 year-old people with type 1 diabetes living in difficult conditions in communist Romania. However, the median duration of diabetes was only 5–6 years and the eventual mean HbA1 was 9% (normal range 5.4–7.6%). Why the results in Romania should be better than those in the DCCT has been the subject of spirited discussion. Muhlhauser suggests it is because the Bucharest patients were treated by one specialist team and admitted for five days of intensive education and hypoglycaemia training whereas, in the DCCT, they were looked after in 29 different centres (possibly by doctors who were more skilled at clinical research than at clinical medicine). Santiago (1988), on behalf of the DCCT, suggested that the most obvious explanation was that patients in the Bucharest–Dusseldorf study were less well controlled than those in the DCCT.

RISK FACTORS FOR HYPOGLYCAEMIA (BOX 3.4)

From the evidence presented so far it will be clear that certain types of patient are at increased risk of hypoglycaemia.

The vulnerability of children in general and those below the age of six years in particular is not surprising. It is difficult to regiment children, and to expect them or their parents to manage diabetes as conscientiously and competently as a volunteer in the DCCT is unreasonable. It was, however, achieved by Nordfeldt and Ludvigsson (1997) who emphasise that their population was unselected and included children from broken homes and those with serious psychosocial problems. They emphasise that they treated the family and the psyche in addition to the blood glucose. Another factor is that in childhood the subjective distinction between autonomic and neuroglycopaenic symptoms has not yet developed and that a common indication of hypoglycaemia is usually behavioural change, with reliance on adult carers to provide treatment (McCrimmon et al, 1995).

Adolescents are another difficult and hypoglycaemia-prone group. In the DCCT the frequency of SH was 85.7 per 100 patient years in

Box 3.4 Risk factors for severe hypoglycaemia

- Intensive insulin therapy
- Near normoglycaemia (low glycated haemoglobin)
- Previous history of severe hypoglycaemia
- Sleep
- Long duration of diabetes
- Impaired hypoglycaemia awareness
- Irregular life style
- Alcoholism or binge drinking
- Increasing age
- Social class
- Special groups – extremes of age
  – adolescents
  – pregnancy (insulin-treated patients)

intensively treated and 27.8 per 100 patient years in conventionally treated subjects (The DCCT Research Group, 1997). This is presumably associated with their higher insulin dose together with greater irregularities in diet, exercise and life style, and experimentation with alcohol. A study in Germany has shown that the lower the social class and the greater the patient's determination to achieve strict glycaemic control, the higher the risk of SH (Muhlhauser et al, 1998).

Patients who abuse alcohol are probably at risk of SH and certainly at greater risk of developing brain damage. Contrary to what is stated in many medical textbooks, ethanol does not cause hypoglycaemia directly; the doses needed to induce hypoglycaemia are large and require depletion of hepatic glycogen stores. No effect of moderate alcohol intake on blood glucose could be shown in patients with insulin-treated diabetes who ate their usual meals (Moriarty et al, 1993). What ethanol does do is blunt the warning symptoms of hypoglycaemia (Kerr et al, 1990). The combination of excessive alcohol consumption and hypoglycaemia can lead to irreversible coma (Arky et al, 1968).

It is axiomatic that the best way of preventing SH is to be able to recognise the early warning symptoms. Patients who cannot do this—up to 50% with diabetes for over 30 years (Pramming et al, 1991) and up to 25% of the generality of patients with insulin-treated diabetes—will be at particular risk, especially on intensive therapy. The problem of hypoglycaemia unawareness is discussed in detail in Chapter 5. Important though the perception of the onset of hypoglycaemia is in preventing severe episodes, it does not explain everything. In the study of Clarke et al (1995) 16% of unaware patients had no SH in one year while 26% of aware patients experienced SH.

There is no definitive psychological profile of the patient who is most likely to have hypoglycaemic, as opposed to ketoacidotic, "brittle diabetes". My own experience is that they come from both ends of the personality spectrum—the extremely casual and slapdash and the obsessional perfectionist (Tattersall, 1997).

CAUSES OF HYPOGLYCAEMIA (TABLE 3.5)

When patients are questioned retrospectively in an attempt to explain a particular episode of hypoglycaemia, there is a danger of spurious attribution. The determination of some investigators to find a cause or judge the patient, and the willingness of others to accept what the patient says, probably explains the differences between studies.

Table 3.5 Attributed causes of severe hypoglycaemia

Reference	Unknown (%)	Patient error (%)	Too much insulin (%)
Potter et al (1982)	38	26	13
Rump et al (1987)	31	44	15
Feher et al (1989)	19	70	17

No Cause Found

Most of these attacks are probably explained by altered awareness or a mismatch between the absorption of food and insulin or most commonly a combination of the two. During the past 30 years much research has been done on the pharmacokinetics of insulin and the facts are clear, but curiously neglected in patient education and clinical practice. A good review has been written by Galloway and Chance (1994). What is needed to mimic physiological insulin secretion are sharp short-lived peaks of insulin with meals and a low but constant level of basal insulin when fasting, especially during the night. The purification of insulin and developments in genetic engineering have produced short-acting insulins which more nearly approach the ideal, but purification has had the opposite effect on modified or long-acting insulins which are not only shorter-acting, but have a high intra- and inter-individual coefficient of variation of absorption. When one reads that:

> "In some patients there is a large, seemingly unavoidable variation in serum insulin and glucose response to insulin injected at the same dose and site." (Galloway and Chance, 1994)

it is hardly surprising that some patients have inexplicable hypoglycaemia.

Patient Errors

The well-controlled patient with an HbA1c within the non-diabetic range is in a delicate equilibrium which will be upset and lead to hypoglycaemia if meals are missed or exercise taken without reducing the insulin dose or increasing the intake of food. Bhatia and Wolfsdorf (1991) attributed two-thirds of episodes to "lapses in the application of the basic principles of diabetes self-care", an unduly harsh verdict which, I think, understates the difficulties of the daily balancing act of the person with type 1 diabetes. Tchobroutsky (1981) was more sympathetic and attributed the frequency of SH to "the difficulty of playing the game in spite of good knowledge, tools and rational behaviour". Simulation experiments show how difficult the "diabetic game" actually is. In a one-week experiment to mimic the life style of the person with insulin-treated diabetes, a group of 12 doctors, nurses, dietitians and occupational therapists missed their prescribed snacks on an astonishing 32 occasions (causing "minor hypoglycaemia") and meals were omitted three times (causing "major hypoglycaemia"). Bearing in mind the training and qualifications of the group, their performance as pseudo-diabetic patients could only be rated as "fair" (Welborn and Duncan, 1980). If health care professionals cannot do better in an experiment lasting only a week, what hope is there that the person who has type 1 diabetes for life will achieve better compliance, as tedium quickly becomes a major problem?

Exercise

Exercise increases insulin sensitivity, lowers insulin dosage, controls weight, improves general health and strength and is encouraged as part of the treatment regimen. The effect of exercise on blood glucose can be simply stated as follows: if levels of insulin in the blood are low, there is an increase in hepatic glucose production which leads to a progressive rise in blood glucose. By contrast, if the patient is "well insulinised", hepatic glucose production is inhibited and peripheral glucose utilisation is stimulated so that unless more food is taken, hypoglycaemia will result. The principles are easy to state but putting them into practice is much more difficult, because what happens to blood glucose depends on: the intensity of exercise, its duration, whether it is spontaneous or planned, the time of day, previous food intake, plasma insulin concentration, insulin regimen and the injection site.

The absorption of short-acting insulin is accelerated if exercise starts immediately after the injection, but not if it is delayed for 35 minutes. This does not depend on whether the injection is given into an exercised limb, and shifting the site from the thigh to the abdominal wall before exercise involving the legs may actually increase the risk of hypoglycaemia (Kemmer and Berger, 1984). The effect of exercise on depot insulins has received less attention; in dogs, protamine zinc insulin is absorbed much faster by exercise eight hours after injection and, in humans, exercise three hours after an injection of isophane insulin more than doubles plasma insulin concentrations while the exercise continues (Thow et al, 1989). Frid et al (1990) showed that when "accidental" intramuscular injection of insulin into the thigh was followed by exercise on a bicycle, there was a pronounced increase in insulin absorption compared to injection in a subcutaneous site.

There are so many variables involved that rigid rules cannot be laid down on how the patient with insulin-treated diabetes should cope with exercise. Some manipulation will inevitably be necessary and each patient must find out how he or she reacts by trial and error. In one study 22 patients with type 1 diabetes cycled 250 km down the Rhine Valley; all reached their destination without incident but individuals used very different strategies to keep their diabetes under control. Reduction of basal insulin dosage ranged from 50% to 90% and carbohydrate consumption was doubled or trebled (Thurm and Harper, 1992). Hardy and Gill (1991) surveyed the problem in their adolescent diabetic clinic. Three-quarters of the 55 patients (27 male; 28 female) took regular exercise for an average of 4.2 hours per week. Virtually all took precautions against hypoglycaemia; 71% altered their diet, 7% changed their insulin dose and 22% adjusted both. Only 9% of those taking regular exercise said that recurrent hypoglycaemia had been a problem. The practical guidelines suggested by Hardy and Gill are shown in Box 3.5.

Another problem which has not received much attention is late post-exercise hypoglycaemia which is typically nocturnal and occurs between 6 and 15 hours after the end of strenuous exercise. It is not limited to patients with good metabolic control and can occur after a single bout of exertion in patients who are unused to exercise or in those making the transition from the untrained to the trained state.

Renal Failure

In diabetic patients with advancing renal failure, insulin requirements usually fall and this may be accompanied by frequent and severe hypoglycaemia. Muhlhauser et al (1991) found that, at comparable levels of HbA1c, patients with type 1 diabetes and a raised serum creatinine had a fivefold higher incidence of SH than matched patients with normal serum creatinine. Apart from failure to reduce insulin dosage to compensate for the reduced clearance of insulin, other factors which might predispose diabetic patients with renal failure to SH include anorexia, low body weight, gastroparesis, visual impairment and possibly the use of antihypertensive agents such as beta adrenoceptor blockers or angiotensin converting enzyme inhibitors.

Coincidental Endocrine Disease

Any condition which reduces the concentration of anti-insulin hormones will increase insulin sensitivity and theoretically predispose to severe hypoglycaemia.

Addison's disease is more common in patients with type 1 diabetes than in the general population and usually presents with declining insulin requirements and hypoglycaemia. Hypopituitarism presents in

Box 3.5 Guidelines for insulin-treated diabetic patients participating in sport or physical exercise

1. Consult your GP or clinic doctor before starting on an exercise programme. It is a good idea to wear something which says you have diabetes.
2. If unaccustomed to exercise, build it up slowly, preferably under qualified supervision.
3. Measure your blood glucose before, during and after exercise until you are familiar with the effects of a given level and duration of exercise.
4. If your blood glucose is over 17 mmol/l or you have ketones in your urine, you should avoid exercise as, under these circumstances, exercise could cause ketoacidosis.
5. If your blood glucose is less than 6.5 mmol/l and your exercise is to be moderate or heavy (tennis, jogging, cycling, hillwalking, football, swimming, etc) you should take 25–50 g of carbohydrate (three to six digestive biscuits, a sandwich with milk or a Mars Bar) at the start and then 10–15 g every half to one hour and monitor your blood glucose carefully. If the exercise is vigorous, you should eat more afterwards as well.
6. If you enjoy regular vigorous exercise, you may find it useful to reduce the dose of short-acting insulin before the exercise (depending on the exercise, the dose may need to be reduced to half normal or further and a small reduction of your intermediate-acting insulin may also be necessary).
7. These guidelines are necessarily vague as everybody is different and there are many different degrees of exertion which can be performed for vastly different times. The best way to learn is to experiment for yourself—at first, this requires very frequent blood glucose monitoring but most people quickly learn what suits them.

Adapted from Hardy & Gill, 1991

the same way and SH was a major problem in patients in whom pituitary ablation had been performed for the treatment of proliferative retinopathy in the 1960s and 1970s. In the series of Nabarro et al (1979), three of the six deaths were caused by hypoglycaemia in men who lived alone. One cause of hypopituitarism which is unique to women is ante-partum pituitary infarction (Sheehan's syndrome). This usually occurs during the third trimester and is characterised by severe deep midline headache lasting between one and three days which, in diabetic women, is associated with a sudden decrease in insulin requirement (Scalch and Burday, 1971). In survivors, the diagnosis may be delayed for several years (range 1–18 years) after pregnancy.

Malabsorption and Gastroparesis

Coeliac disease (gluten-sensitive enteropathy) is more common in patients with type 1 diabetes and is often diagnosed late, either because symptoms are absent, mild or non-specific or because increased frequency of bowel action may be ascribed to "diabetic diarrhoea" associated with autonomic neuropathy. Features which may suggest coeliac disease are abdominal pain and distension, loose stools, glossitis, aphthous ulceration, peripheral oedema and anaemia. In retrospect, the most prominent symptom is often loss of weight and, unless the insulin dose is reduced, the condition may result quite dramatically in episodes of SH (Walsh et al, 1978). A gluten-free diet usually resolves the problem.

Delay in gastric emptying with dilatation of the stomach ("gastroparesis diabeticorum") is usually considered to be associated with severe autonomic neuropathy. Gross gastroparesis is rare but invariably leads to erratic glycaemic control with periods of hypo- and hyperglycaemia. More subtle abnormalities of gastric emptying are probably relatively common, may contribute to hypoglycaemia and are often unrecognised (Kong et al, 1996).

Factitious Hypoglycaemia

Factitious hypoglycaemia in insulin-treated diabetes is probably rare but, when it does occur, may be unsuspected and undetected for a long time. Hypoglycaemia, or the threat of it, can provide a manipulative adolescent with a weapon second to none. Situations which in the non-diabetic child or young adult would be manipulated by the complaint of abdominal pain or a half-hearted drug overdose, may be dealt with through the medium of hypoglycaemia, a threat ignored by those on the receiving end only at the risk of coma or convulsions. Usually the manipulative use of hypoglycaemia is overt in children but O'Brien et al (1985) and Orr et al (1986) have reported small series of patients in which considerable detective work and clinical acumen were needed to uncover the factitious nature of recurrent hypoglycaemia in diabetic adults and adolescents.

Psychological Factors

It is clear that psychological factors must play a part in the frequency of hypoglycaemia. For example, one of my patients said that the sensation of mild to moderate hypoglycaemia was better than an orgasm, which led her to court it. Conversely, other patients are so terrified that they may get into a situation where they cannot distinguish between symptoms of hypoglycaemia and anxiety.

Gonder-Frederick et al (1997) have devised what they call a biopsychobehavioural model which aims to understand, predict and reduce the risk of SH. I am not convinced that this very complex scheme is helpful, but Gonder-Frederick and her colleagues do make some important points. For example, they note that some patients, particularly those who indulge in high-risk behaviours in other areas of life, may, even if they recognise a low blood glucose, decide to take a risk and not treat themselves. Conversely, others with a high fear of hypoglycaemia may overestimate the risk and treat themselves prematurely and unnecessarily. Clinicians will doubtless recognise such personality types. The same group have also devised a blood glucose awareness training programme, a behavioural approach which is said to improve patients' ability to recognise symptoms (particularly in patients who have impaired awareness of hypoglycaemia) and take appropriate action to avoid hypoglycaemia (Cox et al, 1994).

HYPOGLYCAEMIA AND TYPE 2 DIABETES

A detailed description of hypoglycaemia and type 2 diabetes is beyond the scope of this chapter. Sulphonylurea-induced hypoglycaemia is well recognised (Campbell, 1993), and although it is less common than insulin-induced hypoglycaemia, it may cause significant morbidity and mortality. Risk factors for hypoglycaemia from sulphonylureas are described in Box 3.6, and measures to reduce hypoglycaemia in patients on sulphonylureas are described in Box 3.7.

Hypoglycaemia occurs more frequently in patients with type 2 diabetes who are receiving insulin treatment than during treatment with sulphony-

Box 3.6 Risk factors for hypoglycaemia from gliclazide and glibenclamide

- Age (not dose)
- Previous history of cardiovascular disease or stroke
- Impairment of renal function
- Reduced food intake
- Alcohol ingestion
- Interaction with other drugs (see Chapter 4)

Box 3.7 Avoidance of sulphonylurea-induced hypoglycaemia

- Use short-acting drugs (tolbutamide, gliclazide, glipizide)
- Check renal, hepatic and cardiac function
- Consider stopping drugs if HbA1c is within the non-diabetic range
- Reduce dose or discontinue if food intake is substantially reduced

lureas (Heller, 1993). Elderly patients treated with insulin may be experiencing hypoglycaemia which is misdiagnosed as cerebrovascular disease because neurological abnormalities may be associated with hypoglycaemia in this age group. Advanced age does not appear to diminish or delay the counterregulatory responses to hypoglycaemia (see Chapter 4).

TREATMENT

It goes without saying that prevention is better than cure and all newly diagnosed patients with type 1 diabetes need to be thoroughly educated about the potential risks of hypoglycaemia. It has been suggested that "since the early subjective symptoms are subtly but uniquely different for each individual ... a controlled episode of hypoglycaemia should be deliberately induced and then treated" (MacCuish, 1993). I disagree for two reasons; one is that, using ordinary subcutaneous injections as opposed to an insulin clamp, it is not easy to induce hypoglycaemia in a newly diagnosed patient. In my experience, it often takes several hours while the patient and nurse wait anxiously for hypoglycaemia to occur. The second reason is that most patients get good autonomic warning symptoms in the first year or so after diagnosis and SH in patients started on insulin as an outpatient is remarkably rare (Wilson et al, 1986). The problem of impaired awareness of hypoglycaemia does not usually commence until diabetes has been present for five or more years, by which time much of the initial education will probably have been forgotten. Hence I suggest re-education between five and ten years after diagnosis.

I agree with MacCuish (1993) that, in practical terms, the treatment of hypoglycaemia is best regarded as a spectrum of increasing therapeutic complexity with at one end the simple self-selection of oral carbohydrate and at the other, acute medical therapy in an intensive care unit (Table 3.6). The simplest treatment when the patient recognises early warning symptoms is to eat carbohydrate which must be palatable, concentrated

Table 3.6 The therapeutic spectrum of hypoglycaemia; complexity of treatment depends primarily on duration

Duration of hypoglycaemia				
Minutes				Hours
By patient	By family	By paramedics	In Hospital A&E Department	In Intensive Care
Oral carbohydrate (> 20 g)	Oral carbohydrate (liquid/solid) Hypostop Glucagon 1 mg im	Glucagon 1 mg im or iv 25 g glucose iv	25 g glucose iv Glucagon 1 mg iv	Mannitol (20%, 20 ml) Dexamethasone (16–24 mg/day) Dextrose/insulin infusion Oxygen Anticonvulsants Sedation

Adapted from MacCuish, 1993
im = intramuscular; iv = intravenous.

and portable. Glucose tablets (Dextrosol) are usually recommended in the UK, barley sugar in the USA and, in France, lumps of sugar (sucrose) which are found on the table in every bar or cafe. Chocolate or fizzy drinks with a high glucose content are also suitable, although I have known patients who got into trouble because in the heat of the moment they consumed a can of "diet" or low-calorie beverage rather than an ordinary sugar-containing drink!

The second level is when the patient is clearly hypoglycaemic but cannot or will not take fast-acting carbohydrate. As noted by Charles Fletcher (see Introduction), people on insulin will often not admit to being hypoglycaemic and may react to attempts to give them carbohydrate as though they were being asked to swallow poison. Liquid glucose solutions are often unsatisfactory because the patient can spit them out and what results is a sticky mess. It is better to use a glucose gel such as Hypostop (Diabetic Bio-diagnostics) which can be squeezed like toothpaste into the buccal cavity. Some doubts have been expressed about the effectiveness of Hypostop but in many patients it seems to work and many relatives prefer to try it before resorting to glucagon. It should not be used in comatose patients. Jam or honey may be just as effective.

Glucagon promotes hepatic glycogenolysis and the glycaemic response to 1 mg is essentially the same whether it is injected subcutaneously, intramuscularly or intravenously (Muhlhauser et al, 1985a). The great advantage of glucagon is that it can be given by relatives or friends after minimal training. Paramedics can also use it at the patient's home or in an ambulance. The disadvantages are that it takes longer (approximately 10 min) than intravenous glucose to restore consciousness and does not work in patients with deficient or absent hepatic glycogen stores (alcoholics or people with cachexia). Unfortunately, even where glucagon is available, relatives or friends may not use it. In the study of Muhlhauser et al (1985b), 53 of 123 episodes of SH were treated by relatives or friends with glucagon, 30 by assisting physicians and 44 required hospital admission. When it was available but not used, it was because those who knew how to use it were absent (20 cases) or too anxious (24 cases). In children with diabetes, Daneman et al (1989) found that glucagon was used in only a third of households in which it was available—presumably because relatives were too frightened or poorly educated—reading the instruction leaflet while the child is convulsing is too late! Another problem is its limited shelf life; Ward et al (1990) found that nearly three-quarters of patients knew about glucagon but only 20% had a supply which was in date. Its effect is less certain if coma has been prolonged. In a study of 100 patients brought to a hospital outpatient department, glucagon was immediately effective in only 41% of patients whose mean estimated duration of coma was 50 minutes (MacCuish et al, 1970).

Anyone who has observed the effect of intravenous dextrose in waking an unconscious patient "on the end of the needle" would have no doubt that it is the most spectacular and effective treatment. Within five minutes the traditional dose of 50 ml of 50% solution raises blood glucose from below 1.0 to 12.5 mmol/l (Collier et al, 1987) (Figure 3.2). The main problem is the difficulty of giving an intravenous injection to a patient who is thrashing about. Extravasation outside the vein causes painful phlebitis and, because of its hypertonicity, even an intravascular injection can cause phlebitis or thrombosis. This may be a particular issue in the young diabetic woman with brittle diabetes who "needs her veins".

"IRREVERSIBLE" HYPOGLYCAEMIC COMA

This is a subject in which opinion and anecdote are more prominent than facts or controlled observations. The frequency of the condition is unknown. When insulin coma therapy was used as a treatment for mental illness, Kay (1961) estimated "one prolonged coma to 2000 normal ones". You may be surprised to read a description of a "normal" coma. Kay writes:

> A man aged 38 failed to go into coma with doses of insulin up to 800 units given intramuscularly in spite of adequate hypoglycaemia and all its

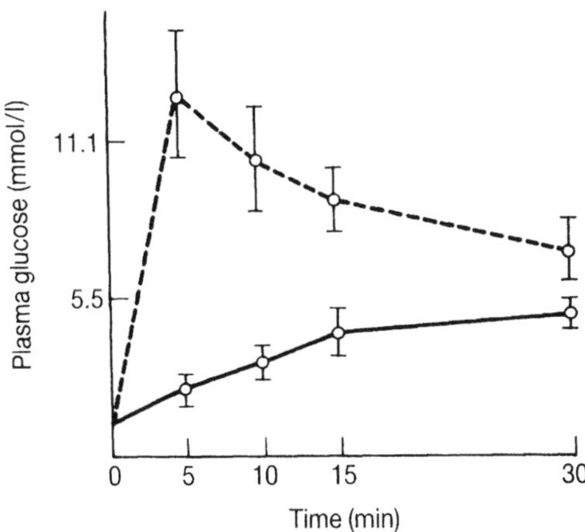

Figure 3.2 Glycaemic profiles in hypoglycaemic diabetic patients after intravenous injection of 1 mg glucagon (continuous line) or 25 g dextrose (broken line). Each treatment group contains 24 patients and the results are expressed as means with 95% confidence limits. Reproduced from Collier et al (1987), and published by permission of the American Diabetes Association

> attendant discomforts. Finally, he was given 800 units of insulin intravenously. The prodromata to coma were shortened and his resistance broken through. He went rapidly into a profound coma from which he was aroused by intravenous infusion of glucose solution. When assured that he had "had a coma", he asked if that was "all that it was" and confessed his previous fear. Thereafter he went regularly into coma on an intramuscular dose of 350–450 units of insulin.

The usual scenario is that a known patient with type 1 diabetes is admitted to hospital deeply unconscious, having been found at home. Blood glucose is 1.0–2.0 mmol/l but, in spite of 50% glucose intravenously, the patient fails to recover consciousness. Other causes of coma such as poisoning with alcohol or opiates, subarachnoid haemorrhage or other intracranial catastrophes must be excluded. A CT brain scan must be obtained urgently but while waiting one should start treatment for presumed cerebral oedema with sedation and 200 ml of 20% mannitol intravenously over 20 min. Dexamethasone 6 mg should be injected every six hours and blood glucose maintained in the range 10–15 mmol/l.

The most difficult decision is to know how long to continue treatment. I have been told of patients who have made a full recovery after being unconscious for several days but have also been involved in keeping alive patients who subsequently turned out to have severe brain damage.

CONCLUSIONS

- Hypoglycaemia is a frequent problem for people with diabetes.
- Hypoglycaemia can be classified into degrees of severity depending on the physical effects and the need for help from another person to restore a normal blood glucose.
- Severe hypoglycaemia (requiring help from another person) is common in children, adolescents and adults with type 1 diabetes; the risk is increased with intensive insulin regimens.
- Multiple risk factors for hypoglycaemia have been identified, but in many episodes of hypoglycaemia no cause can be identified.
- Treatment can be regarded as a spectrum of increasing therapeutic complexity depending on the clinical status of the patient.
- "Irreversible" hypoglycaemic coma remains a difficult clinical problem, and cerebral oedema should be sought.

REFERENCES

Aman J, Karlsson I and Wranne L (1989). Symptomatic hypoglycaemia in childhood diabetes: a population-based questionnaire study. *Diabetic Medicine* **6**: 257–61.

Arias P, Kerner W, Zier H, Navascues I and Pfeiffer EF (1985). Incidence of hypoglycemic episodes in diabetic patients under continuous subcutaneous insulin infusion and intensified conventional insulin treatment: Assessment by means of semiambulatory 24-hour continuous blood glucose monitoring. *Diabetes Care* **8**: 134–40.

Arky RA, Veverbrants E and Abramson EA (1968). Irreversible hypoglycemia. A complication of alcohol and insulin. *Journal of the American Medical Association* **206**: 575–8.

Barkai L, Vamosi I and Lukacs K (1998). Prospective assessment of severe hypoglycaemia in diabetic children and adolescents with impaired and normal awareness of hypoglycaemia. *Diabetologia* **41**: 898–903.

Bendtson I, Kverneland A, Pramming S and Binder C (1988). Incidence of nocturnal hypoglycaemia in insulin-dependent diabetic patients on intensive therapy. *Acta Medica Scandinavica* **223**: 543–8.

Bergada I, Suissa S, Dufresne J and Schiffrin A (1989). Severe hypoglycemia in IDDM children. *Diabetes Care* **12**: 239–44.

Bhatia V and Wolfsdorf JI (1991). Severe hypoglycemia in youth with insulin-dependent diabetes mellitus: frequency and causative factors. *Pediatrics* **88**: 1187–93.

Campbell IW (1993). Hypoglycaemia and type 2 diabetes: sulphonylureas. In: *Hypoglycaemia and Diabetes: Clinical and Physiological Aspects*, Frier BM, Fisher BM, eds. Edward Arnold, London: 387–92.

Clarke WJ, Cox DJ, Gonder-Frederick LA, Julian D, Schlundt D and Polonsky W (1995). Reduced awareness of hypoglycemia in adults with IDDM. A prospective study of hypoglycemic frequency and associated symptoms. *Diabetes Care* **18**: 517–22.

Collier A, Steedman DJ, Patrick AW, Nimmo GR, Matthews DM, MacIntyre CA, Little K and Clarke BF (1987). Comparison of intravenous glucagon and dextrose in treatment of severe hypoglycemia in an Accident and Emergency Department. *Diabetes Care* **10**: 712–15.

Cox DJ, Gonder-Frederick L, Julian DM and Clarke W (1994). Long-term follow-up of blood glucose awareness training. *Diabetes Care* **17**: 1–5.

Daneman D, Frank M, Perlman K, Tamm J and Ehrlich R (1989). Severe hypoglycemia in children with insulin-dependent diabetes mellitus: frequency and predisposing factors. *Journal of Pediatrics* **115**: 681–5.

Davis EA, Keating B, Byrne GC, Russell M and Jones TW (1997). Hypoglycemia: Incidence and clinical predictors in a large population-based sample of children and adolescents with IDDM. *Diabetes Care* **20**: 22–5.

Dorchy H, Roggemans M-P and Willems D (1997). Glycated hemoglobin and related factors in diabetic children and adolescents under 18 years of age: a Belgian experience. *Diabetes Care* **20**: 2–6.

Dornan TL, Peckar CO, Mayon-White VA, Knight AH, Moore RA, Hockaday TDR, Bron AJ and Turner RC (1981). Unsuspected hypoglycaemia, haemoglobin A1 and diabetic control. *Quarterly Journal of Medicine* **197**: 31–8.

Egger M, Gschwend S, Davey Smith G and Zuppinger K (1991). Increasing incidence of hypoglycemic coma in children with IDDM. *Diabetes Care* **14**: 1001–5.

Feher MD, Grout P, Kennedy A, Elkeles RS and Touquet R (1989). Hypoglycaemia in an inner city accident and emergency department: a 12 month survey. *Archives of Emergency Medicine* **6**: 183–8.

Fletcher C (1980). One way of coping with diabetes. *British Medical Journal* **i**: 115–16.

Frid A, Ostman J and Linde B (1990). Hypoglycemia risk during exercise after intramuscular injection of insulin in thigh in IDDM. *Diabetes Care* **13**: 473–7.

Gale EAM (1986). The frequency of hypoglycaemia in insulin treated diabetic patients. In *Diabetes 1985*, Serrano Rios M, Lefebvre PJ, eds. Elsevier, Amsterdam: 934–7.

Gale EAM and Tattersall RB (1979). Unrecognised nocturnal hypoglycaemia in insulin-treated diabetics. *Lancet* **i**: 1049–52.

Galloway JA and Chance RE (1994). Improving insulin therapy: Achievements and challenges. *Hormone and Metabolic Research* **26**: 591–8.

Gold AE, MacLeod KM and Frier BM (1994). Frequency of severe hypoglycemia in patients with type I diabetes with impaired awareness of hypoglycemia. *Diabetes Care* **17**: 697–703.

Goldgewicht TC, Slama G, Papoz L and Tchobroutsky G (1983). Hypoglycaemic reactions in 172 type 1 (insulin-dependent) diabetic patients. *Diabetologia* **24**: 95–9.

Goldstein DE, England JD, Hess R, Rawlings SS and Walker B (1981). A prospective study of symptomatic hypoglycemia in young diabetic patients. *Diabetes Care* **4**: 601–5.

Gonder-Frederick L, Cox D, Kovatchev B, Schlundt D and Clarke W (1997). A biopsychobehavioral model of risk of severe hypoglycemia. *Diabetes Care* **20**: 661–9.

Hardy KJ, Kenyon R and Gill GV (1991). Sport for all? *Practical Diabetes* **8**: 235–7.

Heller SR (1993). Hypoglycaemia and type 2 diabetes: insulin therapy. In: *Hypoglycaemia and Diabetes: Clinical and Physiological Aspects*, Frier BM, Fisher BM, eds. Edward Arnold, London: 393–400.

Heller SR, Chapman J, McCloud J and Ward J (1995). Unreliability of reports of hypoglycaemia by diabetic patients. *British Medical Journal* **310**: 440.

Ingelfinger FJ (1977). Debates on diabetes. *New England Journal of Medicine* **296**: 1228–9.

Kay WW (1961). The treatment of prolonged insulin coma. *J.Ment.Sci.* **107**: 194–238.

Kemmer FW and Berger M (1984). Exercise in diabetes: part of treatment, part of life. In: *Recent Advances in Diabetes*, Nattrass M, Santiago JV, eds. Churchill Livingstone, Edinburgh: 137–43.

Kerr D, Macdonald IA, Heller SR and Tattersall RB (1990). Alcohol causes hypoglycaemic unawareness in healthy volunteers and patients with type 1 (insulin-dependent) diabetes. *Diabetologia* **33**: 216–21.

Kong M-F S-C, Macdonald IA and Tattersall RB (1996). Gastric emptying in diabetes. *Diabetic Medicine* **13**: 112–19.

MacCuish AC (1993). Treatment of hypoglycaemia. In: *Hypoglycaemia and Diabetes: Clinical and Physiological Aspects*, Frier BM, Fisher BM, eds. Edward Arnold, London: 212–21.

MacCuish AC, Munro JF and Duncan LJP (1970). Treatment of hypoglycaemic coma with glucagon, intravenous dextrose, and mannitol infusion in a hundred diabetics. *Lancet* **ii**: 946–9.

Macfarlane PI, Walters M, Stutchfield P and Smith CS (1989). A prospective study of symptomatic hypoglycaemia in childhood diabetes. *Diabetic Medicine* **6**: 627–30.

MacLeod KM, Hepburn DA and Frier BM (1993). Frequency and morbidity of severe hypoglycaemia in insulin-treated diabetic patients. *Diabetic Medicine* **10**: 238–45.

McCrimmon RJ, Gold AE, Deary IJ, Kelnar CJH and Frier BM (1995). Symptoms of hypoglycemia in children with IDDM. *Diabetes Care* **18**: 858–61.

McLean T (1985). *Metal Jam: The Story of a Diabetic*. Hodder & Stoughton, London.

Moriarty KT, Maggs DG, Macdonald IA and Tattersall RB (1993). Does ethanol cause hypoglycaemia in overnight fasted patients with type 1 diabetes? *Diabetic Medicine* **10**: 61–5.

Muhlhauser I (1988). The frequency of severe hypoglycaemia during intensive insulin therapy: Dusseldorf experience. *Diab.Nutr.Metab.* **1**: 77–82.

Muhlhauser I, Koch J and Berger M (1985a). Pharmacokinetics and bioavailability of injected glucagon: Differences between intramuscular, subcutaneous, and intravenous administration. *Diabetes Care* **8**: 39–42.

Muhlhauser I, Berger M, Sonnenberg G, Koch J, Jorgens V, Schernthaner G, Scholz V and Padagogin D (1985b). Incidence and management of severe hypoglycemia in 434 adults with insulin-dependent diabetes mellitus. *Diabetes Care* **8**: 268–73.

Muhlhauser I, Bruckner I, Berger M, Cheta D, Jorgens V, Ionescu-Tirgoviste C, Scholz V and Mincu I (1987). Evaluation of an intensified insulin treatment and teaching programme as routine management of type 1 (insulin-dependent) diabetes. The Bucharest–Dusseldorf Study. *Diabetologia* **30**: 681–90.

Muhlhauser I, Toth G, Sawicki PT and Berger M (1991). Severe hypoglycemia in type 1 diabetic patients with impaired kidney function. *Diabetes Care* **14**: 344–6.

Muhlhauser I, Overmann H, Bender R, Bott U and Berger M (1998). Risk factors of severe hypoglycaemia in adult patients with type I diabetes—a prospective population based study. *Diabetologia* **41**: 1274–82.

Nabarro JDN, Mustaffa BE, Morris DV, Walport MJ and Kurtz AB (1979). Insulin deficient diabetes. Contrasts with other endocrine deficiencies. *Diabetologia* **16**: 5–12.

Nordfeldt S and Ludvigsson J (1997). Severe hypoglycemia in children with IDDM. A prospective population study, 1992–1994. *Diabetes Care* **20**: 497–503.

O'Brien IAD, Lewin IG, Frier BM, Rodman H, Genuth S and Corrall RJM (1985). Factitious diabetic instability. *Diabetic Medicine* **2**: 392–4.

Orr DP, Eccles T and Lawlor R (1986). Surrepitious insulin administration in adolescents with insulin-dependent diabetes mellitus. *Journal of the American Medical Association* **256**: 3227–30.

Potter J, Clarke P, Gale EAM, Dave SH and Tattersall RB (1982). Insulin-induced hypoglycaemia in an accident and emergency department: the tip of an iceberg? *British Medical Journal* **285**: 1180–2.

Pramming S, Thorsteinsson B, Bendtson I, Ronn B and Binder C (1985). Nocturnal hypoglycaemia in patients receiving conventional treatment with insulin. *British Medical Journal* **291**: 376–9.

Pramming S, Thorsteinsson B, Bendtson I and Binder C (1990). The relationship between symptomatic and biochemical hypoglycaemia in insulin-dependent diabetic patients. *Journal of Internal Medicine* **228**: 641–6.

Pramming S, Thorsteinsson B, Bendtson I and Binder C (1991). Symptomatic hypoglycaemia in 411 type 1 diabetic patients. *Diabetic Medicine* **8**: 217–22.

Reichard P, Britz A and Rosenqvist U (1991). Intensified conventional insulin treatment and neuropsychological impairment. *British Medical Journal* **303**: 1439–42.

Rump A, Stahl M, Caduff F and Berger W (1987). 173 cases of insulin-induced hypoglycemia admitted to hospital. *Deutsche Medizinische Wöchenschrift* **112**: 1110–16.

Santiago JV (1988). The frequency of severe hypoglycaemia during intensive insulin therapy: The North American Viewpoint. *Diabetes, Nutrition and Metabolism* **1**: 82–6.

Scalch DS and Burday SZ (1971). Antepartum pituitary insufficiency in diabetes mellitus. *Annals of Internal Medicine* **74**: 357–60.

Shalwitz RA, Farkas-Hirsch R, White NH and Santiago JV (1990). Prevalence and consequences of nocturnal hypoglycemia among conventionally treated children with diabetes mellitus. *Journal of Pediatrics* **116**: 685–9.

Tattersall RB (1997). Brittle diabetes revisited. *Diabetic Medicine* **14**: 99–110.

Tchobroutsky G (1981). Metabolic control and diabetic complications. In: *Handbook of Diabetes Mellitus*, Volume 5, Brownlee M, ed. John Wiley and Sons, Chichester: 3–39.

The Diabetes Control and Complications Trial Research Group (1987). Diabetes Control and Complications Trial (DCCT): results of a feasibility study. *Diabetes Care* **10**: 1–19.

The Diabetes Control and Complications Trial Research Group (1991). Epidemiology of severe hypoglycemia in the Diabetes Control and Complications Trial. *American Journal of Medicine* **90**: 450–9.

The Diabetes Control and Complications Trial Research Group (1993). The effect of intensive treatment of diabetes on the development and progression of long-term complications in insulin-dependent diabetes mellitus. *New England Journal of Medicine* **329**: 977–86.

The Diabetes Control and Complications Trial Research Group (1997). Hypoglycemia in the Diabetes Control and Complications Trial. *Diabetes* **46**: 271–86.

Thorsteinsson B, Pramming S, Lauritzen T and Binder C (1986). Frequency of daytime biochemical hypoglycaemia in insulin-treated diabetic patients: relation to daily median blood glucose concentrations. *Diabetic Medicine* **3**: 147–51.

Thow JC, Johnson AB, Antsiferov M and Home PD (1989). Exercise augments the absorption of isophane (NPH) insulin. *Diabetic Medicine* **6**: 342–5.

Thurm U and Harper PN (1992). I'm running on insulin. Summary of the history of the International Diabetic Athletes Association. *Diabetes Care* **15**(Suppl 4): 1811–13.

Travis LB (1989). Hypoglycemia in insulin-dependent diabetes mellitus. *Journal of Pediatrics* **115**: 740–1.

Vervoort G, Goldschmidt HMG and van Doorn LG (1996). Nocturnal blood glucose profiles in patients with type 1 diabetes mellitus on multiple (> 4) daily insulin injection regimens. *Diabetic Medicine* **13**: 794–9.

Walsh CH, Cooper BT, Wright AD, Malins JM and Cooke WT (1978). Diabetes mellitus and coeliac disease: A clinical study. *Quarterly Journal of Medicine* **47**: 89–100.

Ward CM, Stewart AW and Cutfield RG (1990). Hypoglycaemia in insulin dependent diabetic patients attending an outpatients' clinic. *New Zealand Medical Journal* **103**: 339–41.

Wauchope GM (1933). Hypoglycaemia: A critical review. *Quarterly Journal of Medicine* **26**: 117–56.

Welborn TA and Duncan N (1980). Diabetic staff simulation of insulin-dependent diabetic life. *Diabetes Care* **3**: 679–81.

Whincup G and Milner RDG (1987). Prediction and management of nocturnal hypoglycaemia in diabetes. *Archives of Disease in Childhood* **62**: 333–7.

Wilson RM, Clarke P, Barkes H, Heller SR and Tattersall RB (1986). Starting insulin treatment as an outpatient: Report of 100 consecutive patients followed for a year. *Journal of the American Medical Association* **256**: 877–80.

4

Counterregulatory Deficiencies in Diabetes

DAVID KERR
The Royal Bournemouth Hospital, Bournemouth

INTRODUCTION

People who have diabetes face a daunting task. They are exhorted to strive for normoglycaemia to try to avoid the long-term complications of diabetes and premature mortality while, in the short term, they wish to avoid acute hypoglycaemia associated with insulin therapy (Table 4.1). Doctors and nurses often underestimate the frequency of hypoglycaemia, the anxiety it causes to patients and their relatives and the disruption to everyday life (Table 4.2). From the patient's perspective, the psychological consequences of recurrent hypoglycaemia can range from mild inconvenience to a phobic avoidance of a low blood glucose. While a resigned acceptance that some hypoglycaemic episodes are an inevitable consequence of insulin therapy may be realistic, fear of a low blood glucose can lead a patient to eschew attempts at improving their glycaemic

Table 4.1 Therapeutic goals in diabetes (Dreyer, personal communication)

Ranking by professionals		Ranking by patients
3	Quality of life	1
2	Perspective in life (secondary prevention)	2 (in some years)
1	Expectation of life	3 (later life)

Hypoglycaemia in Clinical Diabetes. Edited by B. M. Frier and B. M. Fisher.

Table 4.2 Doctors' and patients' perceptions of the difficulties associated with living with diabetes in order of magnitude

Doctors' perception		Patients' perception
1	Injections/blood testing	4
2	Diet/change in lifestyle	3
3	Fear of complications	2
4	Hypoglycaemia	1

control, to the frustration of all members of the specialist diabetes team (Cox et al, 1987).

Over a lifetime of diabetes, it has been estimated that a typical insulin-treated patient will have suffered on average 70 severe (i.e. requiring help from someone else), and more than 3500 mild episodes of hypoglycaemia. Despite hypoglycaemia being so common, death or serious permanent sequelae are surprisingly rare (see Chapter 7).

To protect against severe and prolonged hypoglycaemia, complex physiological systems have evolved which are activated as blood glucose levels fall below the normal range (Chapter 1). The functional aim of these systems is to restore blood glucose to normal (glucose counterregulation) even in the face of sustained hyperinsulinaemia, which commonly occurs in patients with type 1 diabetes.

NORMAL GLUCOSE COUNTERREGULATION

This is described in detail in Chapter 1. Under normal circumstances, the brain uses glucose as its predominant fuel and is almost completely dependent upon a continuous supply of glucose from the peripheral circulation (Figure 4.1). Consequently, to protect the delivery of glucose to the brain, a characteristic hierarchy of responses are activated as peripheral blood glucose falls below normal (Mitrakou et al, 1991). In general, glucose counterregulation consists of three elements:

- suppression of endogenous insulin production
- release of hormones that counteract the effects of insulin on glucose production by the liver and glucose uptake by muscle
- activation of the autonomic nervous system with the development of characteristic warning symptoms (Chapter 2).

During profound hypoglycaemia (blood glucose <2.0 mmol/l) glucose delivery to the brain is enhanced as a consequence of increasing cerebral blood flow. Normal glucose counterregulation also includes hepatic autoregulation, whereby the liver is able to respond to hypoglycaemia by

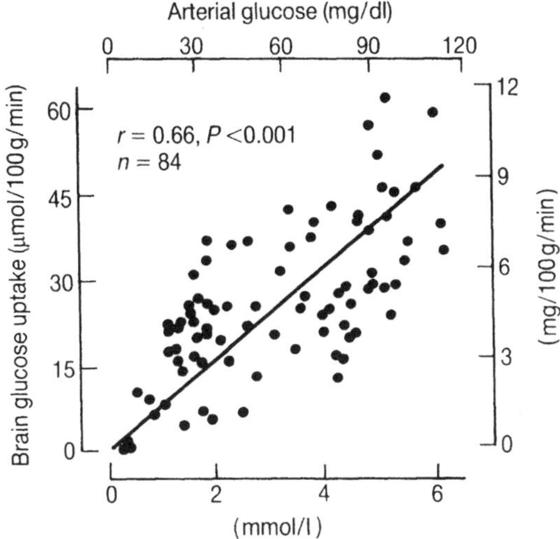

Figure 4.1 Relationship between brain glucose uptake and arterial plasma glucose concentrations in humans: $r = 0.66$; $P < 0.001$; $n = 84$. Reproduced from Cryer and Gerich (1985) by permission of the *New England Journal of Medicine*

increasing glucose production in the absence of detectable hormonal stimulation. Hepatic autoregulation only appears to have an influential role in glucose counterregulation during more profound hypoglycaemia.

As described in Chapter 1, hormonal counterregulation is mediated principally by glucagon and adrenaline, with both hormones directly increasing the production of glucose by the liver as a consequence of breakdown of hepatic glycogen stores (glycogenolysis) and the manufacture of glucose by gluconeogenesis. Adrenaline also promotes muscle glycogenolysis, proteolysis and lipolysis to provide substrates (lactate, alanine and glycerol) for further gluconeogenesis (Figure 4.2).

The key organ in co-ordinating the hormonal responses to hypoglycaemia is the brain (Figure 4.3). Although numerous neural areas have been proposed as the control centres for counterregulation, it is likely that neurones located within the ventro-medial nuclei of the hypothalamus are essential for integrating the hormonal responses to a fall in peripheral blood glucose (Borg et al, 1994). However, there is debate as to whether specific "glucoreceptors", involved in initiating the counterregulatory response, exist outside the brain, and possibly within the liver.

As blood glucose falls below normal, the hormonal responses are not "all or nothing". Individual hormones have specific blood glucose thresholds at which levels begin to rise above their baseline values (Figure 4.4). For example, the glycaemic threshold for the release of glucagon and

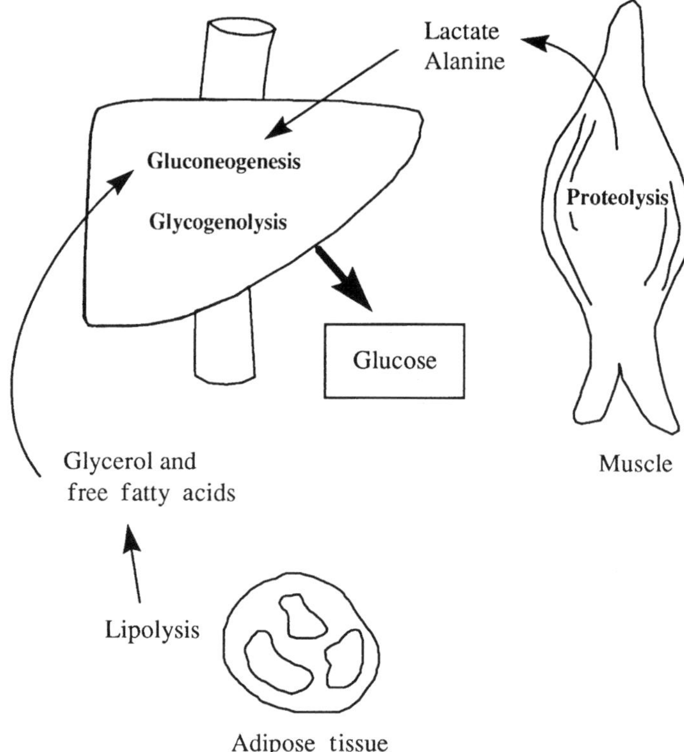

Figure 4.2 Principal metabolic effects of counterregulation in response to hypoglycaemia

adrenaline is around 3.8 mmol/l and for cortisol is 3.3 mmol/l, both levels being well above the threshold for the development of warning symptoms (3.0 mmol/l) and impairment of higher brain (cognitive) function (2.8 mmol/l) (Mitrakou et al, 1991). At or below 2.0 mmol/l, cerebral blood flow begins to increase to enhance glucose delivery to the central nervous system (Kerr et al, 1993a). These thresholds are not fixed but can be altered upwards or downwards according to the prevailing quality of glycaemic control. They are not, however, influenced by the rate of fall of blood glucose within the hyper- or euglycaemic range.

COUNTERREGULATORY FAILURE IN DIABETES

The best defence against hypoglycaemia is its early recognition allowing appropriate action to be taken, i.e. eat some carbohydrate. In many

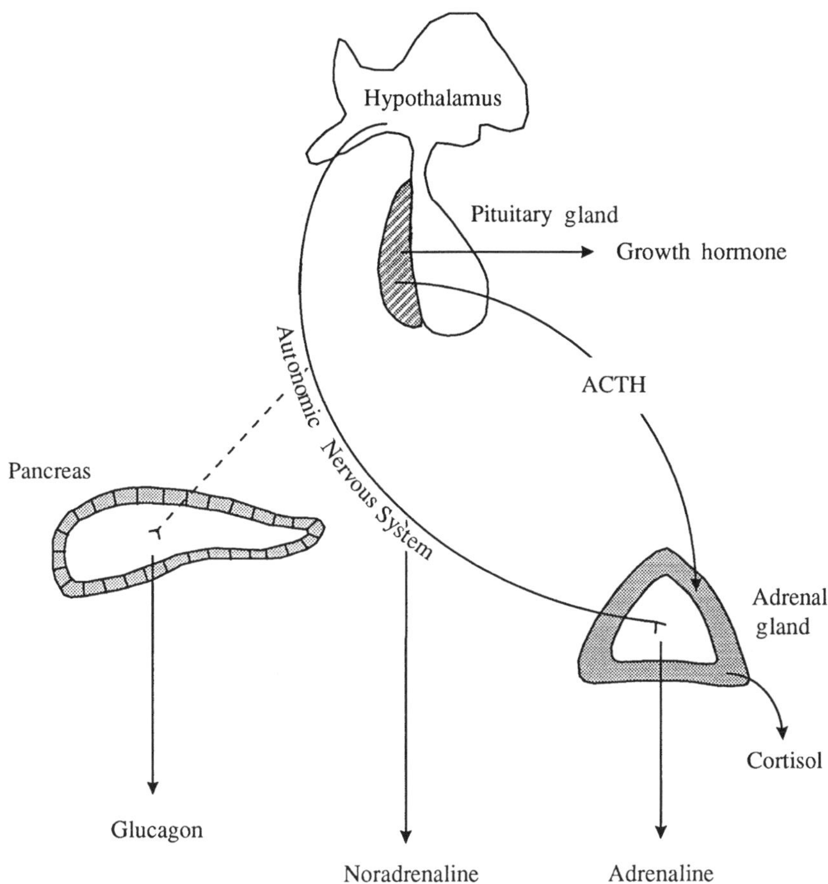

Figure 4.3 The brain is the key regulatory organ involved in glucose counterregulation

patients (up to 25%) with type 1 diabetes, their ability to detect the onset of hypoglycaemia becomes diminished or lost completely, i.e. they develop the syndrome of impaired hypoglycaemia awareness (Chapter 5). Individuals who develop loss of the usual warning symptoms are more or less completely dependent upon efficient glucose counterregulation to protect them from exposure to recurrent, severe hypoglycaemia. Unfortunately, when this problem is associated with hypoglycaemia, it may be compounded by defects in glucose counterregulation (Gerich and Bolli, 1993).

Theoretically, defects in hormonal counterregulation can result as a consequence of:

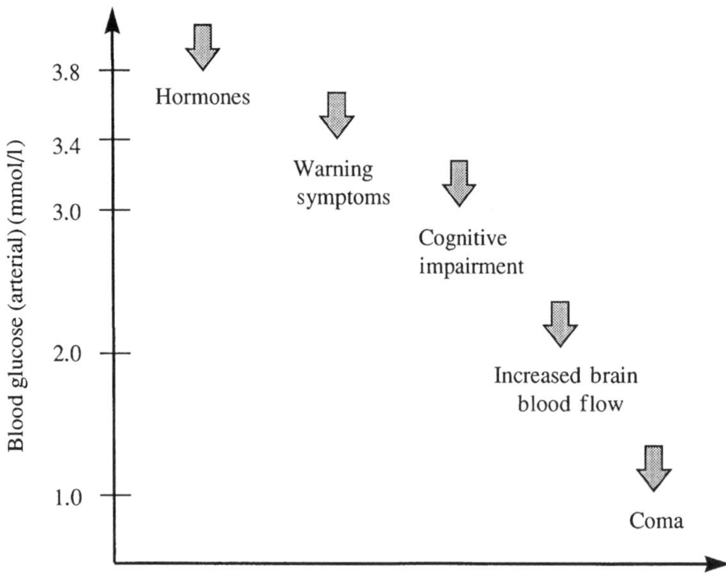

Figure 4.4 Blood glucose thresholds for release of counterregulatory hormones, onset of warning symptoms and cognitive impairment as blood glucose falls below normal

- release of inadequate amounts of hormone
- alteration (elevation) of the blood glucose threshold at which the hormones are released, i.e. a more profound hypoglycaemic stimulus is required before hormonal secretion increases above baseline
- diminished tissue sensitivity to a given plasma concentration of hormone.

DEFECTIVE HORMONAL GLUCOSE COUNTERREGULATION

Glucagon

In non-diabetic humans, glucagon is the key counterregulatory hormone within the first 30 minutes after blood glucose falls below normal. Glucagon is released from pancreatic alpha cells, directly as a consequence of local tissue glucopenia and indirectly, by autonomic nervous system stimulation via three different sympatho-adrenal inputs to the pancreas:

- via pancreatic parasympathetic nerves
- via the effects of circulating adrenaline
- via pancreatic sympathetic nerves.

It is unclear whether local (pancreatic) tissue glucopenia or autonomic activation is the key process involved in stimulating the release of glucagon during hypoglycaemia. Both mechanisms may be involved but it is noteworthy that pharmacological blockade of the autonomic nervous system can reduce glucagon responses by up to 75% (Havel and Ahren, 1997).

In people with type 1 diabetes, the glucagon secretory response to hypoglycaemia is diminished and subsequently lost within a few years of the onset of diabetes (Gerich et al, 1973), although it can be released in response to other stimuli, e.g. exercise or infusion of arginine (Gerich and Bolli, 1993). This indicates that the failure of the glucagon response is hypoglycaemia-specific. When glucagon secretion is deficient, the liver becomes exquisitely sensitive to insulin, with greater suppression of hepatic glucose production for a given plasma insulin level, even if there is compensatory hyper-secretion of other counterregulatory hormones. In diabetic patients with coexistent autonomic neuropathy, glucagon release is even more severely compromised (Hilsted, 1993) (Figure 4.5).

In people with type 1 diabetes, the failure of glucagon to be released in response to hypoglycaemia develops quickly, possibly within the first year after the clinical onset of the disorder. Various pathological mechanisms have been proposed to explain the defect in glucagon counterregulation (Box 4.1). Glucagon can be released in response to exercise or other stimuli, suggesting that the defect is not caused simply by a reduction in pancreatic islet cell mass. Similarly, the absence of an appropriate glucagon response to hypoglycaemia from within a few months to five years of the onset of diabetes, makes autonomic neuropathy an unlikely aetiological factor. Insulin is a potent inhibitor of glucagon release and supraphysiological levels of insulin have been shown to impair glucagon release in response to moderate hypoglycaemia (Kerr et al, 1991). Thus, hyperinsulinaemia, which inevitably is associated with the exogenous administration of insulin to treat type 1 diabetes, may also be implicated in the pathogenesis of glucagon counterregulatory failure.

Alternatively, it is possible that chronic hyperglycaemia may directly impair pancreatic alpha cell function through glucose toxicity similar to the effect which this has on beta cell function. Nevertheless, improvements in glycaemic control, following introduction of intensive insulin therapy, invariably fail to restore the glucagon responses to hypoglycaemia (Amiel, 1991). The early appearance of an impaired response of

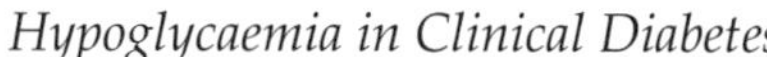

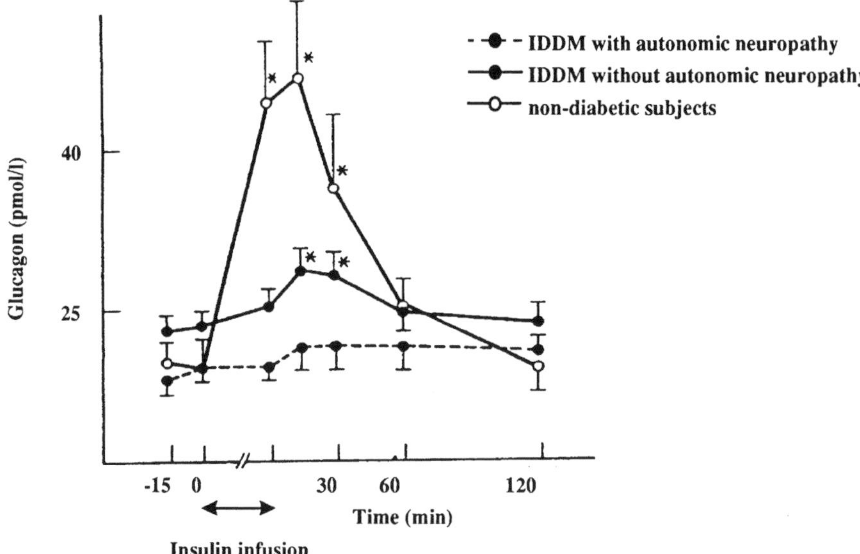

Figure 4.5 Influence of coexisting autonomic neuropathy on glucagon response to hypoglycaemia in patients with type 1 diabetes (IDDM = insulin dependent diabetes mellitus). Reproduced from Hilsted et al, 1982; Reproduced with permission of The Endocrine Society

Box 4.1 Possible mechanisms involved in the pathogenesis of defective glucagon response to hypoglycaemia in type 1 diabetes

- Reduction in pancreatic alpha cell mass
- Autonomic neuropathy
- Local effect of insulin on alpha cell function
- Generalised hyperinsulinaemia
- Chronic hyperglycaemia
- Increased pancreatic production of somatostatin
- Accumulation of amylin
- Local effect of insulin-like growth factor-1

glucagon, together with a temporal dissociation from deficiencies in other counterregulatory hormones, argues against this abnormality being mediated from within the central nervous system. The near-normal glucagon responses to hypoglycaemia found in patients with type 1 diabetes who have undergone pancreatic transplantation also suggests that the defect is related specifically to the diabetic pancreas (Kendall et al, 1997).

Blunting of the normal glucagon response to hypoglycaemia can be achieved by infusion of insulin-like growth factor-1 (IGF-1), the putative mediator of the somatotrophic action of growth hormone, in non-diabetic humans (Kerr et al, 1993b) (Figure 4.6). Whether IGF-1 is involved in the pathogenesis of glucagon counterregulatory failure is unclear.

Impairment of the glucagon response to hypoglycaemia results in greater suppression of hepatic glucose production by insulin. Since the ability of insulin to increase glucose utilisation is unaltered, glucose uptake by muscle and other tissues will exceed hepatic glucose production for much longer, resulting in more profound and prolonged hypoglycaemia. Whether or not the lack of a glucagon response is by itself sufficient to increase the frequency of severe hypoglycaemia is unclear; most patients with recurrent severe hypoglycaemia have impairment both of glucagon and adrenaline responses.

Catecholamines

It is unknown how common catecholamine counterregulatory failure is in type 1 diabetes, but like glucagon deficiency, it is related to the

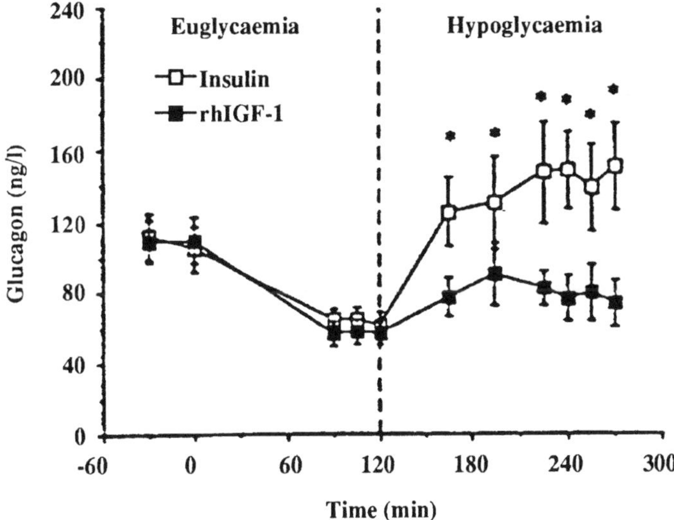

Figure 4.6 Infusion of insulin-like growth factor 1 abolishes the expected rise in glucagon when blood glucose was lowered to and maintained at 2.8 mmol/l in healthy volunteers. (Kerr et al [1993b]). Reproduced by permission of The American Society for Clinical Investigation

duration of diabetes and the prevailing quality of glycaemic control. Estimates suggest a defect in the catecholamine response to hypoglycaemia exists in up to 45% of people with type 1 diabetes of long duration (Gerich and Bolli, 1993).

The mechanism responsible for catecholamine counterregulatory failure is unknown but is likely to differ from that underlying the glucagon deficiency. In some diabetic patients, autonomic neuropathy may coexist with the deficient adrenaline response to hypoglycaemia. In other individuals, adrenaline response may become sub-optimal as a result of:

- elevation of the glycaemic threshold for sympathoadrenal activation (i.e. more profound hypoglycaemia is required)
- recurrent exposure to hypoglycaemia *per se*
- a defect in the neural centre responsible for the recognition and initiation of glucose counterregulation
- peripheral autonomic neuropathy affecting the neural innervation of the adrenal gland.

The adrenaline response to hypoglycaemia can be subnormal in patients with type 1 diabetes who have no clinical evidence of autonomic neuropathy and also in individuals with secondary (pancreatic) diabetes. Like glucagon, adrenaline secretory deficiency is stimulus-specific to hypoglycaemia, remaining intact in response to exercise. The isolated failure of plasma adrenaline concentrations to rise in response to hypoglycaemia does not appreciably impair glucose counterregulation but when combined with glucagon deficiency (as occurs in patients with long-standing type 1 diabetes), the risk of severe and prolonged hypoglycaemia is significantly increased (Figure 4.7).

Cortisol and Growth Hormone

Growth hormone (GH) and cortisol are thought to become important glucose-raising hormones only after hypoglycaemia has been prolonged for more than one hour. Defects in cortisol and GH release can cause profound and prolonged hypoglycaemia because of a reduction in hepatic glucose production and, to a lesser extent, by exaggeration of insulin-stimulated glucose uptake by muscle.

Abnormalities in growth hormone and cortisol secretion in response to hypoglycaemia are characteristic of long-standing type 1 diabetes, affecting up to a quarter of patients who have had diabetes for more than 10 years (Table 4.3). In rare cases, coexistent endocrine failure such as Addison's disease or hypopituitarism predisposes patients to severe hypoglycaemia. Pituitary failure, although uncommonly associated with type 1 diabetes, occasionally develops in young women as a consequence

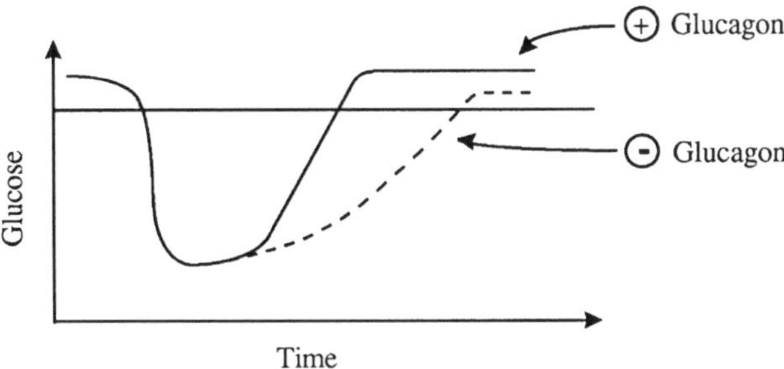

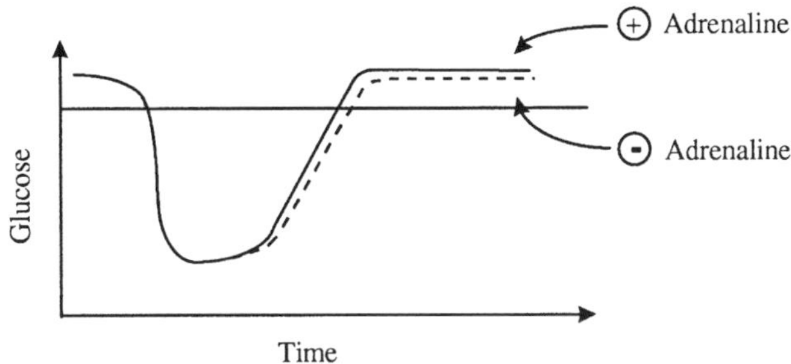

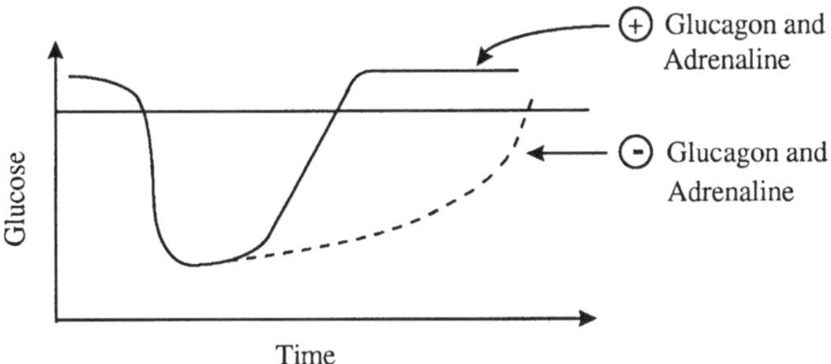

Figure 4.7 Schematic representation of the consequences of defective glucagon, adrenaline or a combined defect of glucagon and adrenaline release during recovery from hypoglycaemia

of ante-partum pituitary infarction (Flynn et al, 1988) (see Chapter 3). As an intact hypothalamic–pituitary–adrenal axis is important for adequate counterregulation, this axis should be formally assessed in any individual with "brittle diabetes" presenting with unexplained, recurrent hypoglycaemia (Hardy et al, 1994).

Table 4.3 Frequency of abnormal counterregulatory responses to hypoglycaemia in patients with type 1 diabetes (reproduced from Gerich and Bolli, 1993, by permission)

Duration of diabetes	Glucagon (%)	Adrenaline (%)	Cortisol (%)	Growth hormone (%)
<1 year	27	9	0	0
1–5 years	75	25	0	0
5–10 years	100	44	11	11
>10 years	92	66	25	25

DURATION OF DIABETES AND COUNTERREGULATORY FAILURE

Numerically, defects in hormonal counterregulation mentioned earlier, as a consequence of long duration of diabetes, have the greatest clinical significance. At diagnosis of type 1 diabetes, hormonal counterregulation is usually normal but within five years glucagon responses to hypoglycaemia become markedly impaired or even absent (Figure 4.8), although a glucagon response can occur if the hypoglycaemic stimulus is sufficiently profound (Frier et al, 1988; Hvidberg et al, 1998). After 10 years of diabetes, patients usually have a sub-optimal adrenaline response to compound the absent glucagon response to a fall in blood glucose (White et al, 1985). Thus, patients with type 1 diabetes of long duration are at risk of severe and prolonged neuroglycopenia during hypoglycaemia as a direct consequence of inadequate glucose counterregulation. Although attenuated growth hormone and cortisol responses are less common, they are late manifestations in terms of diabetes duration.

GLYCAEMIC THRESHOLDS AND COUNTERREGULATORY FAILURE

In clinical practice it is a common experience that diabetic patients, especially when pregnant, may feel and appear "normal" despite having a blood glucose below 2.0 mmol/l, i.e. well below the usual glycaemic threshold for impairment of cognitive function. This may be a consequence of modifying the blood glucose threshold for the release of adrenaline and other hormones following sustained improvement in

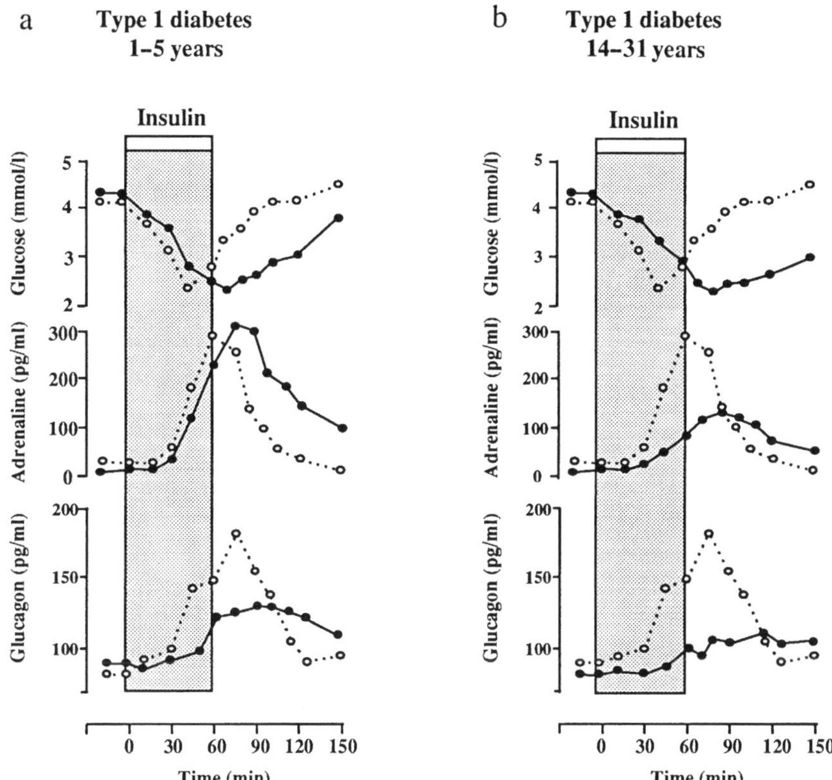

Figure 4.8 Influence of duration of diabetes on glucagon and adrenaline responses to hypoglycaemia in patients with type 1 diabetes (●) after (a) 1–5 years. Glucagon response is blunted whereas adrenaline release is preserved; (b) with long-standing diabetes, both responses become severely impaired. ○, non-diabetic controls. Reproduced from *Textbook of Diabetes*, 2nd Edition, 1997 (eds J Pickup and G Williams) by permission of Blackwell Science Ltd. Data from Bolli et al (1983) and reproduced by permission of the American Diabetes Association

glycaemic control. It has also been suggested that the lack of autonomic symptoms in these patients, such as tremor, sweating or pounding heart, is a consequence of the development of tolerance to the peripheral effects of adrenaline (Berlin et al, 1987).

The blood glucose "thresholds" for the release of individual counterregulatory hormones, the onset of symptoms and the development of cognitive impairment are not static but are influenced by the prevailing standard of glycaemic control. Strict glycaemic control alters the thresholds for hormonal release and onset of warning symptoms which commence at lower blood glucose levels, while leaving the threshold for cognitive dysfunction unchanged (Widom and Simonson, 1990). The effect of strict glycaemic control on counterregulation is discussed in Chapters 5 and 6.

Studies in animals and humans suggest that under experimental conditions the onset of the hormonal counterregulatory response (as well as the onset of cognitive dysfunction) during hypoglycaemia can be delayed by the simultaneous infusion of either ketone bodies or lactate (Veneman et al, 1994). The clinical relevance of these observations is unclear.

ANTECEDENT HYPOGLYCAEMIA AND DEFECTIVE COUNTERREGULATION

Hypoglycaemia may influence normal glucose counterregulation. A single episode of hypoglycaemia can reduce the symptomatic and neuroendocrine responses to a subsequent episode of hypoglycaemia occurring within 24 hours (Heller and Cryer, 1991). As a corollary, strict avoidance of hypoglycaemia, both asymptomatic and symptomatic, may restore warning symptoms and some of the hormonal counterregulatory responses (with the exception of glucagon) (Cranston et al, 1994) (Figure 4.9). In patients with insulin-secreting pancreatic tumours (insulinomas) who suffer repeated and severe episodes of hypoglycaemia, removal of the tumour (and thus avoidance of hypoglycaemia) also restores these defects (Mitrakou et al, 1993). The role of antecedent hypoglycaemia is discussed in more detail in Chapter 5.

AGE AND GLUCOSE COUNTERREGULATION

In children with type 1 diabetes, the glucagon response to hypoglycaemia is markedly attenuated compared to non-diabetic individuals. During hypoglycaemia the deficient glucagon response is compensated for by vigorous secretion of other counterregulatory hormones, particularly adrenaline, with the peak adrenaline response increased almost two-fold compared to adults (Amiel et al, 1987) (Figure 4.10). Non-diabetic children also have a greater rise in adrenaline than adult controls. Furthermore, it appears that the glycaemic thresholds for the secretion of adrenaline and growth hormone are set at a higher blood glucose level in non-diabetic children (3.9 mmol/l) compared to adults (3.4 mmol/l) (Jones et al, 1991). In children with type 1 diabetes, the adrenaline release in response to hypoglycaemia commences at an even higher level. In

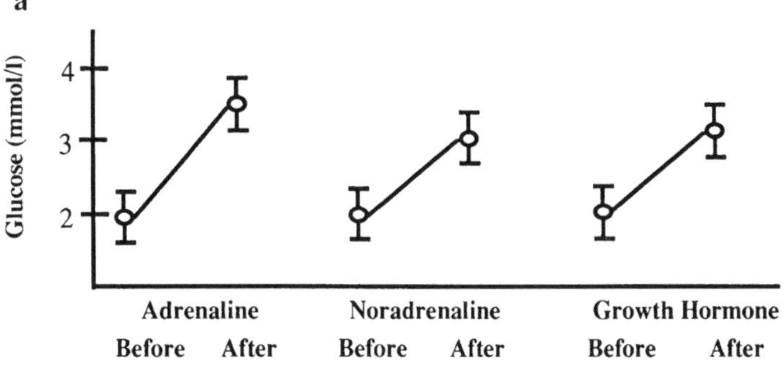

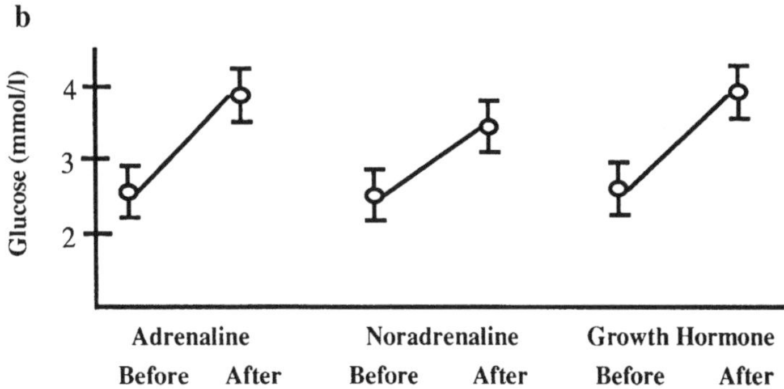

Figure 4.9 Partial restoration of glucose counterregulation by strict avoidance of hypoglycaemia in patients with type 1 diabetes. (a) Patients with good glycaemic control, HbA1c $< 7\%$; (b) patients with poor glycaemic control, HbA1c $> 8\%$. Mean plasma glucose thresholds for counterregulatory hormone responses, before and after intervention period. Adapted from Cranston et al (1994) with permission of the *Lancet*

children who have markedly elevated HBA1c values, there is a further shift upwards of the blood glucose threshold for the release of counter-regulatory hormones. Other aspects of hypoglycaemia in children with diabetes are discussed in Chapter 9.

Advanced age, in otherwise healthy people, does not appear to diminish or delay counterregulatory responses to hypoglycaemia (Brierley et al, 1995), although the magnitude of responses of adrenaline and glucagon is lower at mild hypoglycaemia (blood glucose 3.3 mmol/l) compared to younger non-diabetic subjects, but comparable with a more profound hypoglycaemic stimulus (2.8 mmol/l) (Ortiz-Alonso et al, 1994).

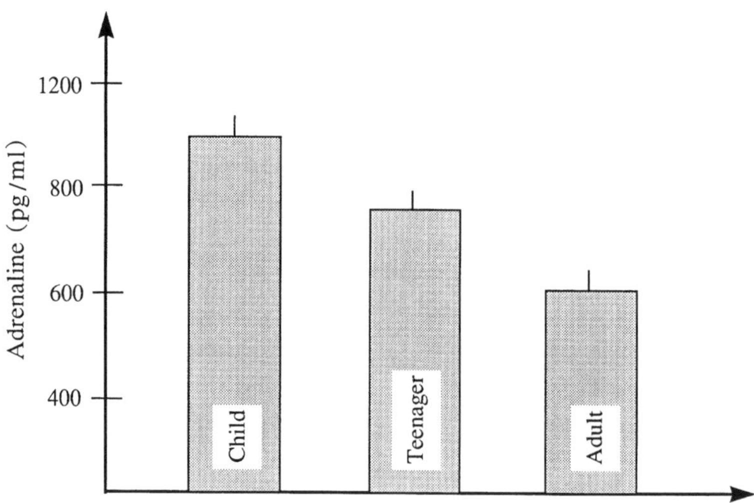

Figure 4.10 Effect of puberty on adrenaline release during hypoglycaemia. In children the response is markedly exaggerated compared to adults. Adapted from Amiel et al (1987) with permission of *Journal of Pediatrics*

HUMAN INSULIN AND COUNTERREGULATION

At present there is no consistent evidence that the species of insulin is an important determinant of the counterregulatory response to hypoglycaemia. Over 25 clinical laboratory studies have examined the effect of insulin species on the counterregulatory response to hypoglycaemia induced either by an intravenous bolus, intravenous infusion, or subcutaneous injection of insulin (Fisher and Frier, 1993; Nellemann Jorgensen et al, 1994). Most of the studies showed no significant differences between the hormonal responses. Two studies showed a reduction in the adrenaline response to hypoglycaemia, and both of these studies also reported diminished autonomic symptoms to hypoglycaemia after human insulin (Schluter et al, 1982; Heine et al, 1989).

Most studies were performed in small groups of subjects, introducing the risk of a type II statistical error. Nellemann Jorgensen et al (1994) performed a qualitative meta-analysis of the catecholamine responses to hypoglycaemia in these studies. No evidence emerged of a "hidden" lower catecholamine response with human insulin, and most patients showed a trend to greater catecholamine responses with human insulin. They concluded that the majority of studies showed no statistically significant differences between the hormonal responses to human and porcine insulins, that there was no trend of any difference, and that most studies found no differences in hypoglycaemic symptoms or in cerebral function (see Chapter 5).

DRUGS AND COUNTERREGULATION

A wide variety of pharmaceutical agents (proprietary and non-proprietary) have been implicated in causing hypoglycaemia (Box 4.2), although relatively few, apart from insulin and sulphonylureas, have been firmly established as having clinically significant glucose-lowering properties. Most reports of drug-induced hypoglycaemia are of dubious clinical relevance. In most instances they have been described in malnourished elderly patients suffering from concomitant kidney or liver disease or they have been associated with alcohol (Kerr, 1993).

Box 4.2 Drugs which can induce hypoglycaemia

Established
Insulin, sulphonylureas, alcohol, quinine, pentamidine and salicylates

Possible
Antibiotics
Ketoconazole, chloramphenicol, sulphonamides, methicillin and oxytetracycline

Cardiovascular
β-adrenoceptor antagonists, angiotensin-converting enzyme inhibitors and lignocaine

Psychological
Monoamine oxidase inhibitors, tryptophan, haloperidol, chlorpromazine, lithium, imipramine and doxepin

Rheumatological
Colchicine, azapropazone, phenylbutazone, paracetamol, indomethacin and penicillamine

Other
Ranitidine, cimetidine, bezafibrate and clofibrate

ALCOHOL AND COUNTERREGULATION

Alcohol has been implicated as a contributing factor in almost a quarter of episodes of severe hypoglycaemia, although the frequency of alcohol-associated hypoglycaemia is probably underestimated since, in the absence of blood alcohol measurement or obvious clinical signs of intoxication, it is dependent on self-reporting by the patient.

Even modest alcohol intoxication decreases awareness of hypoglycaemia and slows reaction time. Loss of awareness associated with alcohol can occur despite the presence of the usual warning symptoms (Kerr et al, 1990). By contrast, the clinical features of a low blood glucose can be mistaken for ethanol intoxication, with unfortunate social, economic and medical consequences for the patient.

Alcohol inhibits gluconeogenesis even at blood alcohol levels not usually associated with intoxication. It might be anticipated that people with type 1 diabetes are at increased risk from alcohol-induced hypoglycaemia as the contribution of gluconeogenesis to total hepatic glucose output is greater in diabetic than non-diabetic subjects (Wahren et al, 1972). Under laboratory conditions, using non-physiological intravenous insulin infusions, the effects of alcohol on glucose counterregulation have produced conflicting results. During sustained hypoglycaemia (blood glucose 2.5 mmol/l for 40 min) in a group of patients with type 1 diabetes (in six of the seven patients studied, the duration of diabetes was five years or less) levels of counterregulatory hormones were unaffected by alcohol (Kerr et al, 1990). Others have reported that alcohol attenuates glucagon and cortisol responses at blood glucose concentrations between 2.3 and 2.5 mmol/l in non-diabetic men (Kolaczynski et al, 1988). Acute and sustained use of alcohol can also suppress growth hormone release in response to hypoglycaemia and other stimuli. During the night, alcohol administration is associated with up to a 75% reduction in the usual night-time, sleep-related release of growth hormone, theoretically increasing the risk of nocturnal hypoglycaemia (Prinz et al, 1980).

PANCREATIC TRANSPLANTATION AND GLUCOSE COUNTERREGULATION

For patients with diabetes, the aim of pancreatic transplantation is freedom from insulin injections, achievement of normoglycaemia and avoidance of hypoglycaemia. Successful pancreatic transplantation for type 1 diabetes is the only treatment which restores the glucagon response to hypoglycaemia (Gerich and Bolli, 1993), although there is controversy as

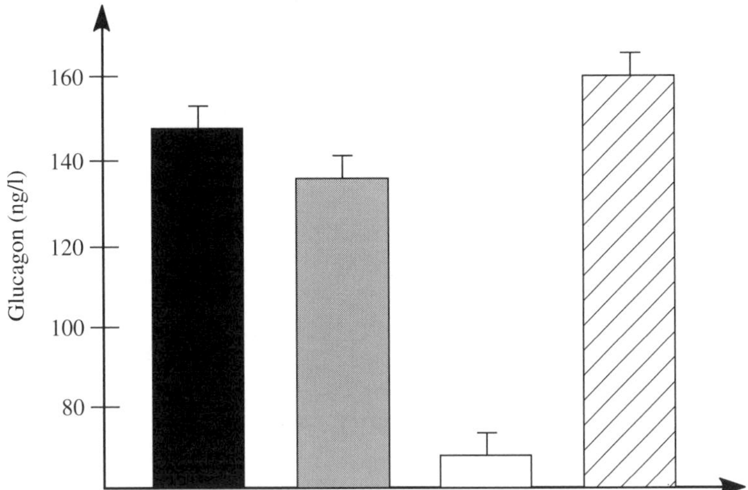

Figure 4.11 Restoration of glucagon responses to hypoglycaemia following pancreatic transplantation in patients with type 1 diabetes (■). Control groups included non-diabetic subjects with kidney transplant (▩), type 1 diabetic patients without transplantation (□), and healthy volunteers (▨). Reproduced from Kendall et al (1997) by permission of the American Diabetes Association

to whether the glucagon responses are truly "normalised" (Figure 4.11). In patients with long-standing type 1 diabetes and autonomic neuropathy, transplantation can also improve the adrenaline response to hypoglycaemia as well as symptomatic awareness of hypoglycaemia in some, but not all, cases. The effects on other counterregulatory hormonal responses and noradrenaline secretion are also variable.

CONCLUSIONS

- In non-diabetic individuals, clinically significant hypoglycaemia is an extremely rare event and glucose counterregulation has a major role in glucose homeostasis. This includes suppression of pancreatic insulin secretion, and release of glucagon which stimulates the liver to produce glucose.
- Stimulation of the sympathetic nervous system with the secretion of adrenaline also raises blood glucose by limiting peripheral glucose utilisation as well as stimulating glucose production by the liver.

continues

continued

- Growth hormone and cortisol have similar effects which only become important if hypoglycaemia is prolonged.
- Patients with diabetes almost inevitably lose their ability to release glucagon in response to a fall in blood glucose within five years of diagnosis.
- After 10 years, a significant proportion of patients also have deficient adrenaline responses and thus are at increased risk of more protracted hypoglycaemia and neuroglycopenia.
- Counterregulatory failure is also associated with improvements in glycaemic control following the use of intensive insulin therapy, recurrent hypoglycaemia *per se* and consumption of excessive alcohol.
- Treatment of counterregulatory failure is unsatisfactory although improvement in glucagon (and probably adrenaline) secretion with pancreatic transplantation appears to be a consistent finding, and avoidance of hypoglycaemia may help to reverse some of the acquired counterregulatory deficiencies.

REFERENCES

Amiel S (1991). Glucose counter-regulation in health and disease: current concepts in hypoglycaemia recognition and response. *Quarterly Journal of Medicine* **293**: 707–27.

Amiel SA, Simonson DC, Sherwin RS, Lauriano AA, Tamborlane WV (1987). Exaggerated epinephrine responses to hypoglycemia in normal and insulin-dependent diabetic children. *Journal of Pediatrics* **110**: 832–7.

Berlin I, Grimaldi A, Payan C, Sachon C, Bosquet F, Thervet F, Puech AJ (1987). Hypoglycemic symptoms and decreased β-adrenergic sensitivity in insulin-dependent diabetic patients. *Diabetes Care* **10**: 742–7.

Bolli G, De Feo P, Compagnucci P, Cartechini MG, Angeletti G, Santeusanio F, Brunetti P, Gerich JE (1983). Abnormal glucose counterregulation in insulin-dependent diabetes mellitus. Interaction of anti-insulin antibodies and impaired glucagon and epinephrine secretion. *Diabetes* **32**: 134–41.

Borg WP, During MJ, Sherwin RS, Borg MA, Brines ML, Shulman GI (1994). Ventromedial hypothalamic lesions in rats suppress counter regulatory responses to hypoglycemia. *Journal of Clinical Investigation* **93**: 1677–82.

Brierley EJ, Broughton DL, James OFW, Alberti KGMM (1995). Reduced awareness of hypoglycaemia in the elderly despite an intact counter-regulatory response. *Quarterly Journal of Medicine* **88**: 439–45.

Cox DJ, Irving GA, Gonder-Frederick L, Nowacek G, Butterfield J (1987). Fear of hypoglycemia: quantification, validation and utilization. *Diabetes Care* **10**: 617–21.

Cranston I, Lomas J, Maran A, Macdonald IA, Amiel SA (1994). Restoration of hypoglycaemia awareness in patients with long-duration insulin-dependent diabetes. *Lancet* **344**: 283–7.

Cryer PE, Gerich JE (1985). Glucose counterregulation, hypoglycemia, and intensive therapy in diabetes mellitus. *New England Journal of Medicine* **313**: 232–41.

Fisher BM, Frier BM (1993). Hypoglycaemia and human insulin. In: *Hypoglycaemia and Diabetes: Clinical and Physiological Aspects.* Frier BM and Fisher BM, eds. Edward Arnold, London, 314–27.

Flynn MD, Cundy TF, Watkins PJ (1988). Antepartum pituitary necrosis in diabetes mellitus. *Diabetic Medicine* **5**: 295–7.

Frier BM, Fisher BM, Gray CE, Beastall GH (1988). Counterregulatory hormonal responses to hypoglycaemia in type 1 (insulin-dependent) diabetes: evidence for diminished hypothalamic-pituitary hormonal secretion. *Diabetologia* **31**: 421–9.

Gerich JE, Bolli GB (1993). Counterregulatory failure. In: *Hypoglycaemia and Diabetes: Clinical and Physiological Aspects.* Frier BM and Fisher BM, eds. Edward Arnold, London, 253–67.

Gerich JE, Langlois M, Noacco C, Karam JH, Forsham PH (1973). Lack of glucagon response to hypoglycemia in diabetes: evidence for an intrinsic pancreatic alpha cell defect. *Science* **182**: 171–3.

Hardy KJ, Burge MR, Boyle P, Scarpello JHB (1994). A treatable cause of recurrent severe hypoglycemia. *Diabetes Care* **17**: 722–4.

Havel PJ, Åhren B (1997). Activation of autonomic nerves and the adrenal medulla contributes to increased glucagon secretion during moderate insulin-induced hypoglycemia in women. *Diabetes* **46**: 801–7.

Heine RJ, Van der Heyden EAP, Van der Veen EA (1989). Responses to human and porcine insulin in healthy subjects. *Lancet* **334**: 946–9.

Heller SR, Cryer PE (1991). Reduced neuroendocrine and symptomatic responses to subsequent hypoglycemia after 1 episode of hypoglycemia in nondiabetic humans. *Diabetes* **40**: 223–6.

Hilsted J (1993). Classical autonomic neuropathy and denervation. In: *Hypoglycaemia and Diabetes: Clinical and Physiological Aspects.* Frier BM, Fisher BM, eds. Edward Arnold, London, 268–74.

Hilsted J, Madsbad S, Krarup T, Tronier B, Galbo H, Sestoft L, Schwartz TW (1982). No response of pancreatic hormones to hypoglycemia in diabetic autonomic neuropathy. *Journal of Clinical Endocrinology and Metabolism* **54**: 815–9.

Hvidberg A, Juel Christensen N, Hilsted J (1998). Counterregulatory hormones in insulin-treated diabetic patients admitted to an Accident and Emergency Department with hypoglycaemia. *Diabetic Medicine* **15**: 199–204.

Jones TW, Boulware SD, Kraemer DT, Caprio S, Sherwin RS, Tamborlane WV (1991). Independent effects of youth and poor diabetes control on responses to hypoglycemia in children. *Diabetes* **40**: 358–63.

Kendall DM, Rooney DP, Smets YFC, Bolding LS, Robertson RP (1997). Pancreas transplantation restores epinephrine response and symptom recognition during hypoglycemia in patients with long-standing type 1 diabetes and autonomic neuropathy. *Diabetes* **46**: 249–57.

Kerr D, Macdonald IA, Heller SR, Tattersall RB (1990). Alcohol causes hypoglycaemic unawareness in healthy volunteers and patients with type 1 (insulin-dependent) diabetes. *Diabetologia* **33**: 216–21.

Kerr D, Reza M, Smith N, Leatherdale BA (1991). Importance of insulin in subjective, cognitive and hormonal responses to hypoglycemia in patients with IDDM. *Diabetes* **40**: 1057–62.

Kerr D, Stanley JC, Barron M, Thomas R, Leatherdale BA, Pickard J (1993a).

Symmetry of cerebral blood flow and cognitive responses to hypoglycaemia in humans. *Diabetologia* **36**: 73–8.

Kerr D, Tamborlane WV, Rife F, Sherwin RS (1993b). Effect of insulin-like growth factor-1 on the responses to and recognition of hypoglycemia in humans. *Journal of Clinical Investigation* **91**: 141–7.

Kerr D (1993). Drugs and alcohol. In: *Hypoglycaemia and Diabetes: Clinical and Physiological Aspects.* Frier BM, Fisher BM, eds. Edward Arnold, London, 328–36.

Kolaczynski JW, Ylikahri R, Härkonen M, Koivisto VA (1988). The acute effect of ethanol on counterregulatory response and recovery from insulin-induced hypoglycemia. *Journal of Clinical Endocrinology A: Metabolism* **67**: 384–8.

Mitrakou A, Ryan C, Veneman T, Mokan M Jenssen T, Kiss I, Durrant J, Cryer P, Gerich J (1991). Hierarchy of glycemic thresholds for counterregulatory hormonal secretion, symptoms, and cerebral dysfunction. *American Journal of Physiology* **260**: E67–74.

Mitrakou A, Fanelli C, Veneman T, Perriello G, Calderone S, Platanisiotis D, Rambotti A, Raptis S, Brunetti P, Cryer P, Gerich J, Bolli G (1993). Reversibility of unawareness of hypoglycemia in patients with insulinomas. *New England Journal of Medicine* **329**: 834–9.

Nellemann Jorgensen L, Dejgaard A, Parmming SK (1994). Human insulin and hypoglycaemia: a literature survey. *Diabetic Medicine* **11**: 925–34.

Ortiz-Alonso FJ, Galecki A, Herman WH, Smith MJ, Jacquez JA, Halter JB (1994). Hypoglycemia counterregulation in elderly humans: relationship to glucose levels. *American Journal of Physiology* **267**: E497–506.

Prinz PN, Roehrs TA, Vitaliano PP, Linnoila M, Wetzman A (1980). Effect of alcohol on sleep and night-time plasma growth hormone and cortisol concentrations. *Journal of Clinical Endocrinology and Metabolism* **51**: 759–64.

Schluter KJ, Petersen KG, Sontheimer K, Enzmann F, Kerp L (1982). Different counterregulatory responses to human insulin (recombinant DNA) and purified pork insulin. *Diabetes Care* **5**(suppl 2): 78–81.

Veneman T, Mitrakou A, Mokan M, Cryer P, Gerich J (1994). Effect of hyperketonemia and hyperlacticacidemia on symptoms, cognitive dysfunction, and counterregulatory hormone responses during hypoglycemia in normal humans. *Diabetes* **43**: 1311–7.

Wahren J, Felig P, Cerasi E, Luft R (1972). Splanchnic and peripheral glucose and amino acid metabolism in diabetes mellitus. *Journal of Clinical Investigation* **51**: 1870–8.

White NH, Gingerich RL, Levandoski LA, Cryer PE, Santiago JV (1985). Plasma pancreatic polypeptide response to insulin-induced hypoglycemia as a marker for defective glucose counterregulation in insulin-dependent diabetes. *Diabetes* **34**: 870–5.

Widom B, Simonson DC (1990). Glycemic control and neurophysiologic function during hypoglycemia in patients with insulin-dependent diabetes. *Annals of Internal Medicine* **112**: 904–12.

5

Impaired Hypoglycaemia Awareness

BRIAN M. FRIER and B. MILES FISHER*
Royal Infirmary, Edinburgh and *Royal Alexandra Hospital, Paisley

"Dangerous hypoglycaemia may occur without warning symptoms."
E. P. Joslin et al, 1922

INTRODUCTION

The generation of symptoms in response to a low blood glucose provides a fundamental defence for the brain, by alerting the affected individual to the imminent development of neuroglycopenia. This should provoke an appropriate response—obtaining and ingesting some form of carbohydrate to reverse the decline in blood glucose. A failure of these warning symptoms to occur, or their delay until the blood glucose has fallen to a level which causes disabling neuroglycopenia, can have serious consequences. When the normal warning mechanisms are deficient or are bypassed, no avoiding action is taken, allowing severe hypoglycaemia to occur, with progression to confusion, altered consciousness and eventually to coma. An inadequate symptomatic warning often occurs in people with insulin-treated diabetes, in various circumstances, and with differing causes and is described as *impaired awareness of hypoglycaemia* or *hypoglycaemia unawareness*. This is an acquired abnormality which is effectively a complication of insulin therapy, and should rank alongside recognised microvascular complications of dia-

Hypoglycaemia in Clinical Diabetes. Edited by B. M. Frier and B. M. Fisher.

betes such as retinopathy, neuropathy or nephropathy, as its consequences can be just as serious and disabling.

NORMAL RESPONSES TO HYPOGLYCAEMIA

Acute hypoglycaemia induces a series of changes—hormonal, neurophysiological, symptomatic and cognitive—which occur at different and defined blood glucose concentrations (Figure 5.1). The thresholds at which these changes are triggered have been described in non-diabetic humans, most occurring within a relatively narrow range of blood glucose concentrations. In diabetic individuals these glycaemic thresholds are not static and permanent, but are dynamic and plastic, altering in response to external influences such as changes in glycaemic control. Thus the blood glucose level at which symptoms are activated can be

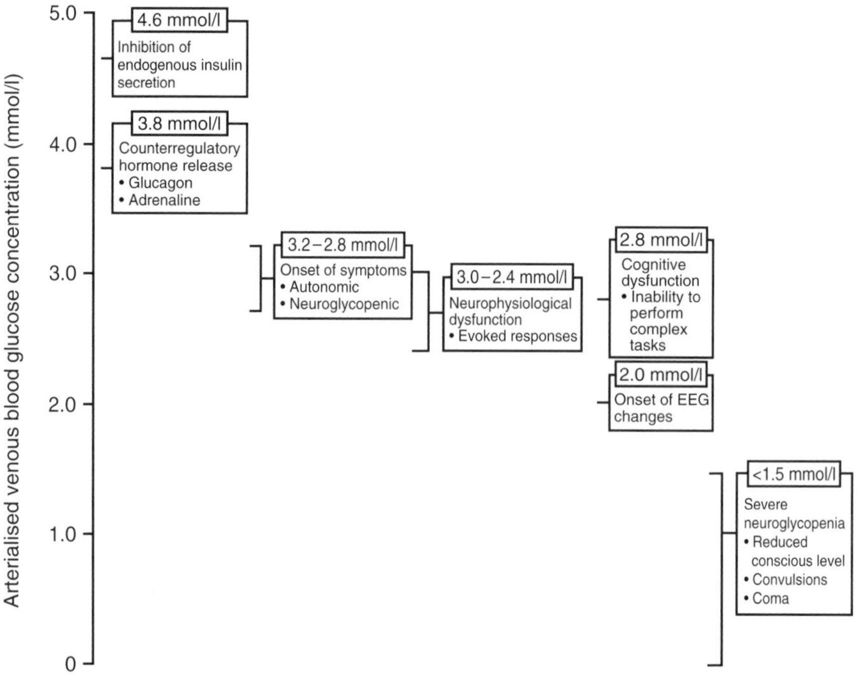

Figure 5.1 Hierarchy of endocrine, symptomatic and neurological responses to acute hypoglycaemia in non-diabetic subjects. Glycaemic thresholds are based on glucose concentrations in arterialised venous blood. Reproduced from *Textbook of Diabetes*, 2nd edition, 1997 (eds J Pickup and G Williams) by permission of Blackwell Science Ltd

modified through the ability of the brain to adapt to an environmental change, namely the prevailing blood glucose concentrations.

Depriving the brain of glucose causes it to malfunction, and cognitive impairment quickly becomes evident as an overt manifestation of neuroglycopenia. Some of these features are relatively subtle, and may not be detected immediately by the patient. A fall in blood glucose triggers activation of the peripheral autonomic nervous system via central hypothalamic autonomic centres within the brain, and stimulates the sympathoadrenal system. This promotes typical physiological responses including sweating, increased rate and contractility of the heart (sensed as a pounding heart), and tremor, these being some of the classical features of the *autonomic reaction* (Figure 5.2). Adrenaline is secreted in large quantities from the adrenal medullae and contributes to some of the symptoms, mainly by heightening the magnitude of the response. The early literature on hypoglycaemia and diabetes provides accurate descriptions of the autonomic features of acute hypoglycaemia, and patients and physicians alike commonly discussed hypoglycaemic "reactions", a term that regrettably has fallen into disuse. It emphatically describes the sudden, and often dramatic, onset of the autonomic features of hypoglycaemia, which drive the individual to seek assistance or obtain a supply of glucose to promote rapid correction of the symptoms.

"Awareness" of Hypoglycaemia

The generation of typical physiological responses to hypoglycaemia is perceived through sensory feedback to the brain, and after central processing within the brain, an appropriate motor response is made. Much has been made by some commentators of the predominant importance of autonomic symptoms in the detection of the onset of hypoglycaemia. This premise is based partly on the laboratory-based observation that in non-diabetic subjects autonomic symptoms commence at a higher blood glucose concentration (around 0.5 mmol/l) than neuroglycopenic symptoms (Mitrakou et al, 1991). In everyday experience reported by patients, a rapid decline in blood glucose does not permit any subjective distinction to be made between the different thresholds for the development of autonomic and neuroglycopenic symptoms and people treated with insulin identify both types with equal frequency as their initial warning symptoms (Hepburn et al, 1992).

It has been assumed that because neuroglycopenia may interfere with cognitive function, this will affect the individual's ability to perceive and interpret neuroglycopenic cues such as inability to concentrate, drowsiness or difficulty with mentation. This may be true when a falling blood glucose is not treated and is allowed to drop to a level associated with

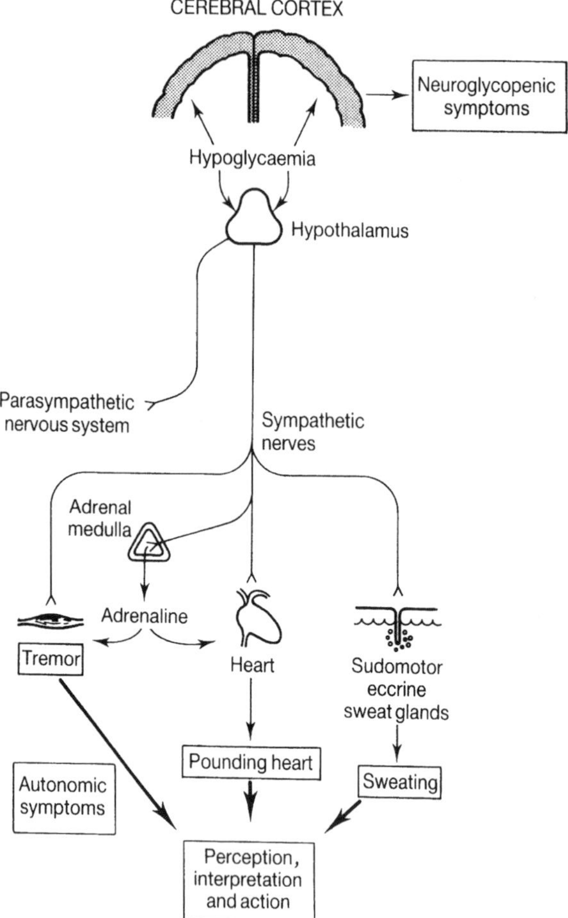

Figure 5.2 Generation of neuroglycopenic and autonomic symptoms in response to hypoglycaemia. Autonomic activation and the involvement of the sympatho-adrenal system in the stimulation of representative end-organs associated with common autonomic symptoms of hypoglycaemia. Reproduced from *Hypoglycaemia and Diabetes* (eds B M Frier and B M Fisher) by permission of Edward Arnold (Publisher) Ltd

severe neuroglycopenia, but many patients can detect (and rely upon) neuroglycopenic symptoms at an early stage of hypoglycaemia, and rate these as important as autonomic symptoms in providing a warning. It is the initial perception of *any* symptom of hypoglycaemia, irrespective of whether this is autonomic, neuroglycopenic or simply a vague sensation of apprehension or loss of well-being (a common early feature noticed by patients), that constitutes "awareness" of hypoglycaemia. Only the *initial* warning symptoms are important in this respect, and not the total spectrum or actual number of symptoms, some of which occur too late to have any value in alerting the patient to the impending risk of a fall in blood glucose. A major difference between the autonomic and the neuroglycopenic symptom response is that, once triggered, the autonomic response quickly reaches a maximum intensity which then gradually declines with time, whereas the neuroglycopenic response becomes more profound the further the blood glucose falls. This qualitative difference in response is important if early cues are ignored or are not detected, as progressive neuroglycopenia will eventually interfere with the individual's ability to identify and self-treat the low blood glucose.

When a person is fully awake, alert and on guard against possible hypoglycaemia, this symptomatic warning system generally works very effectively. However, there are many times in everyday life when the symptoms may be either diminished or disregarded, particularly during sleep when they are not detected, or they may be ignored when the individual is distracted by other activities, such as watching television or participating in sport. Circumstances can modify the value of specific warning symptoms, making them difficult to interpret as features of hypoglycaemia. Examples include sweating on a hot day, shivering when the weather is cold or feeling drowsy during a boring meeting! All of these may represent early hypoglycaemia but are attributed to other causes by the affected person. A list of the factors which influence normal awareness of hypoglycaemia is shown in Box 5.1. The intensity of

Box 5.1 Factors influencing normal awareness of hypoglycaemia

Internal	**External**
Physiological	*Drugs*
Recent glycaemic control	Beta-adrenoceptor blockers (non-selective)
Degree of neuroglycopenia	Hypnotics, tranquillisers
Symptom intensity/sensitivity	Alcohol
Psychological	*Environmental*
Arousal	Sleep
Focused attention	Posture
Congruence; denial	Distraction
Competing explanations	
Education	
Knowledge	
Symptom belief	

symptoms can vary and the value of individual symptoms as warning features may not be constant in any single individual This is often not appreciated in the assessment of research findings, and it is difficult to extrapolate the careful measurement of symptomatic responses to hypoglycaemia in studies performed in a laboratory setting, to the hurly-burly of everyday life.

Warning symptoms provide *internal* cues, but most people with insulin-dependent diabetes also rely on *external* cues based on their experience of the timing of insulin administration in relation to food, the effect of delaying meals or the amount of food ingested, the effect of exercise on blood glucose and many other factors which can influence short-term glycaemic control. These cues are supplemented by blood glucose monitoring, which gives an exact and objective measure of prevailing glycaemia. Further useful feedback may be obtained from observers such as relatives or friends, many of whom become adept at noticing early neuroglycopenia before the onset of the patient's subjective warning symptoms. "Awareness" of hypoglycaemia is therefore distilled from a combination of resources, and has to be learned by newly diagnosed patients starting insulin therapy. They have no previous experience of symptoms of hypoglycaemia and must receive appropriate education on the potential range of symptoms. Through experience they will recognise the cluster of symptoms peculiar to themselves, as symptoms are idiosyncratic in nature. "Awareness" of hypoglycaemia therefore assists in protecting the individual from the risk of an unexpected fall in blood glucose. When awareness of hypoglycaemia becomes impaired or is absent while awake, the individual becomes progressively vulnerable to the development of severe hypoglycaemia.

IMPAIRED AWARENESS OF HYPOGLYCAEMIA

Definition

No satisfactory definition of impaired hypoglycaemia awareness has been suggested to date. Many laboratory-based studies of experimental hypoglycaemia have used arbitrary definitions based on witnessed observations of subjects who fail to develop classical features of hypoglycaemia, or the failure of physiological or hormonal responses to exceed twice the standard deviation from mean basal levels. These are statistical devices, which take no account of subjective reality, require the application of sophisticated and unphysiological glucose clamp procedures, and have little application to clinical management.

Asymptomatic biochemical hypoglycaemia occurs more frequently during routine blood glucose monitoring in diabetic patients who report impaired awareness of hypoglycaemia (Clarke et al, 1995) and such a record may alert the clinician to the possibility that an individual is developing this problem. However, a careful history is essential in determining whether reduced warning symptoms of hypoglycaemia are a significant problem, and that this is occurring consistently. Patients who assert that they have a problem with perceiving the onset of symptoms of hypoglycaemia are generally correct in this belief (Clarke et al, 1995), so that the identification of impaired awareness of hypoglycaemia should be based principally on clinical history. A scoring system for symptoms relating to awareness of hypoglycaemia has been described by Gold et al (1994). Detailed questioning of the patient about their ability to detect the onset of hypoglycaemic symptoms may need to be supplemented by enquiry to their relatives to obtain their witnessed descriptions of how hypoglycaemia develops, its true frequency and severity. Patients often underestimate the frequency of severe hypoglycaemia, partly because of post-hypoglycaemia amnesia.

Classification

In one study, Hepburn et al (1990) subdivided hypoglycaemia awareness into three categories: normal, partial and absent awareness. These were defined as follows:

- *Normal awareness*: the individual is always aware of the onset of hypoglycaemia
- *Partial awareness*: the symptom profile has changed with a reduction either in the intensity or in the number of symptoms and, in addition, the individual may be aware of some episodes of some episodes of hypoglycaemia but not of others
- *Absent awareness*: the individual is no longer aware of any episode of hypoglycaemia.

Although the subdivision into partial and absent awareness is artificial, it reflects the natural history of this clinical problem with a gradual progression of this disability, and emphasises that some patients have a severe abnormality (absent awareness) although *total* absence of clinical manifestations of hypoglycaemia (particularly the neuroglycopenic features) is extremely rare (Gold et al, 1994; Clarke et al, 1995). The problem may not be simply an absence of symptoms, but that the time during which warning symptoms can be detected is extremely short, permitting the affected individual a very limited opportunity to take avoiding action. Some patients describe how the onset of hypoglycaemia appears to have become much more rapid compared with their previous experience and progresses quickly to severe neuroglycopenia. However, impaired awareness may not necessarily evolve into total unawareness of hypoglycaemia, and may vary over time, presumably because of major influences of environmental factors on the generation and perception of symptoms.

The above classification of awareness of hypoglycaemia is far from comprehensive. In addition, the state of hypoglycaemia awareness can be ascertained only when the individual is in a physical state in which recognition of the onset of hypoglycaemia is possible. Therefore, if the person is asleep, intoxicated, inebriated, anaesthetised or sedated, so that their conscious level is reduced, they are not able to perceive (as subjective symptoms) the normal physiological manifestations of hypoglycaemia. An individual's awareness of hypoglycaemia can be evaluated only if hypoglycaemia occurs while the individual is awake.

A further prerequisite is that the person must have had previous experience of hypoglycaemia at some time during treatment with insulin. In assessing the present state of hypoglycaemia awareness, it is desirable that the patient should have experienced one or more episodes of hypoglycaemia (confirmed biochemically) within a recent time interval, usually the preceding year, so that a comparison of the symptoms can be made with earlier episodes of hypoglycaemia. A diagnosis of impaired hypoglycaemia awareness cannot be entertained or surmised if a patient has either never been exposed previously to acute hypoglycaemia or has only started to experience hypoglycaemic events very recently. Because hypoglycaemia awareness and its impairment lie on a continuum ranging from normality to complete inability to detect the onset of hypoglycaemia, a classification of this condition will need to consider alterations in symptom intensity as well as detection of hypoglycaemia by any means and the ability of the patient to self-treat a low blood glucose.

PREVALENCE OF HYPOGLYCAEMIA UNAWARENESS

Impaired awareness of hypoglycaemia is common in people treated with insulin. While the chronic form of this acquired condition mainly affects those with type 1 diabetes, it appears that a similar problem does eventually emerge in patients with type 2 diabetes who have been treated with insulin for several years (Hepburn et al, 1993a). However, because few patients with type 2 diabetes who require insulin therapy survive for a sufficiently long period to permit this complication to develop, it is principally a problem associated with type 1 diabetes. It is not known whether impaired awareness of hypoglycaemia occurs in diabetic patients treated with oral hypoglycaemic agents. In these patients with type 2 diabetes, many of whom are elderly, hypoglycaemia is frequently unrecognised by the patients or their carers, or the clinical features are misinterpreted as features of cerebrovascular disease.

Impaired awareness of hypoglycaemia has been shown to be associated with strict glycaemic control (see Chapter 6), but significant modification of the symptomatic response to hypoglycaemia does not occur unless the glycated haemoglobin concentration is within the non-diabetic range (Kinsley et al, 1995; Boyle et al, 1995; Pampanelli et al, 1996). Only a small proportion of people with insulin-treated diabetes can sustain this degree of super-optimal glycaemic control indefinitely. In the Diabetes Control and Complications Trial (DCCT), with its vast resources devoted to maintaining intensive insulin therapy, more than 40% of the patients in the group with strict glycaemic control achieved a HbA1c of 6.05% or less (the upper limit of the non-diabetic range) at some time during the study, but only 5% were able to maintain this level of glycaemic control continuously (The DCCT Research Group, 1993). The proportion of any insulin-treated diabetic population that can achieve this therapeutic goal will depend on local policies regarding insulin therapy, the expertise of local diabetes specialist teams, available resources and the enthusiasm of individual patients. With the exception of a few highly motivated patients, most people treated with insulin are unable to maintain strict glycaemic control for protracted periods. In clinical practice this "acute" form of hypoglycaemia unawareness is probably relatively uncommon. None the less, the influence of strict glycaemic control on symptomatic and neuroendocrine responses to hypoglycaemia has been studied extensively, and has provided insights into the potential pathogenetic mechanisms underlying impaired awareness of hypoglycaemia.

Reduced warning symptoms of hypoglycaemia (of varying severity) occur in approximately one-quarter of all insulin-treated patients. These cross-sectional population surveys in different European and North American populations of insulin-treated diabetic patients are remarkably consistent (Table 5.1). Impaired awareness of hypoglycaemia becomes more common with increasing duration of insulin-treated diabetes (Hep-

Table 5.1 Prevalence of hypoglycaemia unawareness in population studies of insulin-treated diabetes

Country	Number of patients	Impaired awareness of hypoglycaemia (%)	Reference
Scotland	302	23	Hepburn et al (1990)
Germany	523	25	Muhlhauser et al (1991)
Denmark	411	27	Pramming et al (1991)
USA	628	20	Orchard et al (1991)

burn et al, 1990), with almost 50% of patients experiencing hypoglycaemia without warning symptoms after 25 years or more of treatment (Pramming et al, 1991) (Figure 5.3). It appears therefore to be an acquired abnormality associated with insulin therapy.

Frequency of Associated Severe Hypoglycaemia

It is apparent that impaired awareness of hypoglycaemia is a major risk factor for severe hypoglycaemia. In the DCCT, 36% of all episodes of severe hypoglycaemia occurred with no warning symptoms in patients who were awake (The DCCT Research Group, 1991). In a population study in Edinburgh, retrospective assessment of the frequency of severe hypoglycaemia revealed that 90% of patients with impaired awareness of symptoms experienced severe hypoglycaemia in the preceding year, compared to 18% in a comparable group who had retained normal awareness (Hepburn et al, 1990). Prospective studies have confirmed the increase in frequency of mild and severe hypoglycaemia associated with impaired awareness of hypoglycaemia (Gold et al, 1994; Clarke et al, 1995), with a six-fold higher frequency of severe hypoglycaemia being documented in people with impaired awareness (Gold et al, 1994) (Figure 5.4).

PATHOGENESIS OF IMPAIRED AWARENESS OF HYPOGLYCAEMIA

The mechanisms underlying impaired awareness of hypoglycaemia are not known and may be multifactorial Possible mechanisms are listed in Box 5.2.

Altered Glycaemic Threshold for Initiation of Symptoms

Symptoms of hypoglycaemia commence when the blood glucose reaches a specific level, and although this threshold may differ between individuals, it is usually constant in the non-diabetic state (Vea et al, 1992). This blood glucose threshold for symptoms can be modified by protracted hypoglycaemia (Boyle et al, 1994) and is not fixed in people with diabetes who are treated with insulin, with its dynamic nature being demonstrated in various situations. In clinical practice, it has long been recognised that insulin-treated diabetic patients who have poor glycaemic control experience symptoms of hypoglycaemia when their blood glucose declines within a *hyperglycaemic* range (Maddock and Krall, 1953), and

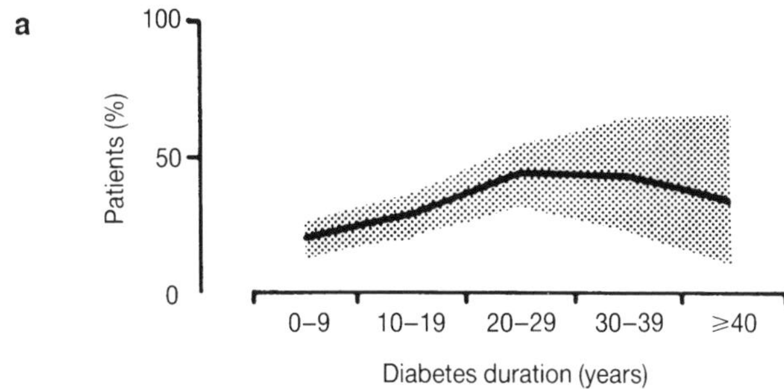

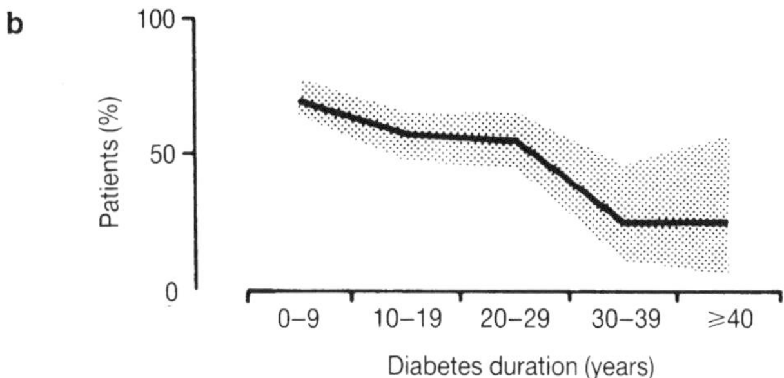

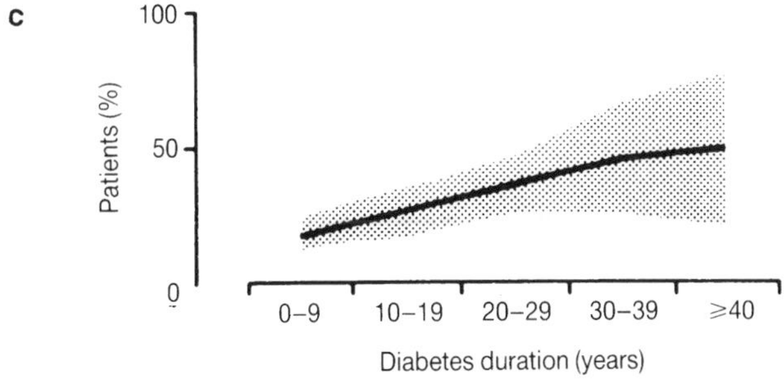

Figure 5.3 Comparisons between the duration of diabetes and the percentage of 411 type 1 diabetic patients reporting (a) changes in symptoms of hypoglycaemia, (b) sweating and/or tremor as one of the two cardinal autonomic symptoms of hypoglycaemia, and (c) severe hypoglycaemic episodes without warning symptoms. Values are medians; shaded areas show 95% confidence limits. Reproduced from Pramming et al (1991). Reproduced with permission of John Wiley & Sons

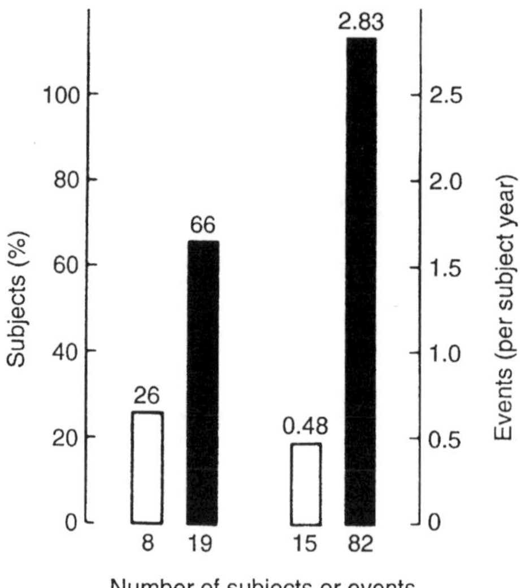

Figure 5.4 Proportion of patients affected and event rates for severe hypoglycaemia in patients with type 1 diabetes with normal (□, $n = 31$) or impaired (■, $n = 29$) awareness of hypoglycaemia. Derived from Gold et al (1994) and published by permission of the American Diabetes Association

Box 5.2 Impaired awareness of hypoglycaemia: possible mechanisms

CNS adaptation

Chronic exposure to low blood glucose

- glucose clamp (2.9 mmol/l) for 56 h in non-diabetic subjects
- insulinoma in non-diabetic patients
- strict glycaemic control in diabetic patients

Recurrent transient exposure to low blood glucose

- antecedent hypoglycaemia

CNS glucoregulatory failure

- counterregulatory deficiency (hypothalamic defect?)
- hypoglycaemia-associated central autonomic failure

Peripheral nervous system dysfunction

- peripheral autonomic neuropathy
- reduced peripheral adrenoceptor sensitivity

this has been shown to be associated with the onset of hypoglycaemic symptoms at a significantly higher blood glucose (4.3 mmol/l) compared to non-diabetic subjects (2.9 mmol/l) (Boyle et al, 1988). Conversely, strict glycaemic control modifies the glycaemic threshold for the onset of symptoms, which do not commence until blood glucose has declined to a lower level than that required in less well controlled patients to initiate a symptomatic response (see Chapter 6).

The terminology which is used in relation to a change in the glycaemic threshold is potentially confusing. When a *lower* blood glucose is required to initiate a response, whether symptomatic, physiological or neuroendocrine, the glycaemic threshold is said to be *raised* or elevated, i.e. a more profound hypoglycaemic stimulus is necessary to trigger the relevant response. Thus, strict glycaemic control raises the glycaemic threshold for the onset of symptoms, which do not occur until blood glucose has declined to a much lower concentration than would be observed in non-diabetic subjects.

For many years, clinicians have recognised that the glycaemic threshold for the onset of hypoglycaemic symptoms is higher in patients with a long duration of type 1 diabetes, who require a much lower blood glucose to provoke a symptomatic response. Lawrence (1941) wrote that "as years of insulin life go on, sometimes only after 5–10 years, I find it almost the rule that the type of insulin reactions change, the premonitory autonomic symptoms are missed out and the patient proceeds directly to the more serious manifestations affecting the central nervous system." He astutely suggested that "the tissues may become attuned to a lower sugar concentration". Recent studies in animals and in humans have shown that the brain does adapt to chronic exposure to a low blood glucose (see below) but this may not be beneficial to the individual with diabetes who is treated with insulin, i.e. it is a maladaptive response.

An early study by Sussman et al (1963) which was revisited and extended by Hepburn et al (1991) showed that diabetic patients who had self-reported unawareness of hypoglycaemia did mount a sympatho-adrenal response to acute hypoglycaemia, but that this occurred at a lower blood glucose concentration than comparable diabetic subjects who had normal symptomatic awareness (Figure 5.5). However, the autonomic response was preceded by the development of overt neuroglycopenia, which interfered with perception of the autonomic warning symptoms when they did eventually occur. This sequence of responses disrupts the ability of the individual subject to take appropriate action to self-treat a low blood glucose. Similar findings have been reported by others (Grimaldi et al, 1990; Mokan et al, 1994; Bacatselos et al, 1995).

In these studies, the counterregulatory hormonal responses to hypoglycaemia were delayed (Grimaldi et al, 1990; Hepburn et al, 1991) and their

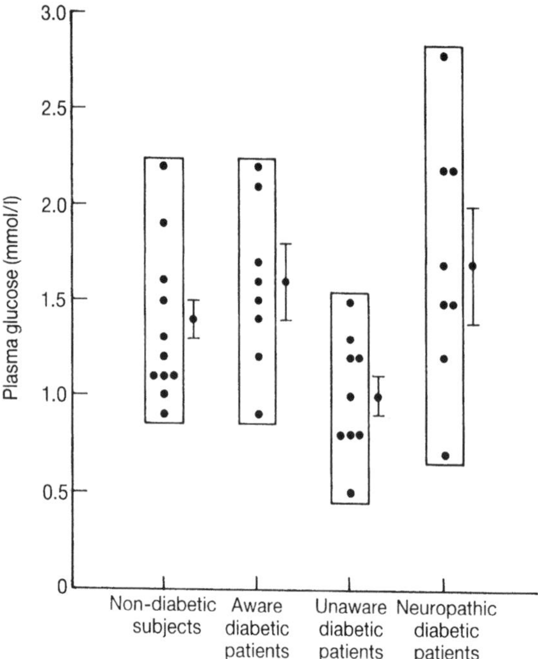

Figure 5.5 Venous blood glucose concentrations for onset of autonomic reaction in response to insulin-induced hypoglycaemia in individual non-diabetic control subjects, and in type 1 diabetic patients with normal and impaired awareness of hypoglycaemia and with autonomic neuropathy. Mean + SEM is shown for each group. Data derived from Hepburn et al, 1991 and reproduced from *Hypoglycaemia and Diabetes* (eds B M Frier and B M Fisher) by permission of Edward Arnold (Publishers) Ltd

glycaemic thresholds had also shifted to occur at lower blood glucose concentrations (Mokan et al, 1994). This is consistent with the reported observation that hypoglycaemia unawareness co-segregates with counterregulatory hormonal deficiency in people with longstanding insulin-treated diabetes (Ryder et al, 1990). In addition, Mokan et al (1994) reported that cognitive dysfunction and neuroglycopenic symptoms also occurred at a lower blood glucose than in aware diabetic patients. This suggests that those with impaired awareness can continue to function at very low blood glucose concentrations, which, in non-diabetic and aware diabetic subjects, would usually provoke symptoms and cognitive impairment. The potential risk of this situation is apparent. This is akin to walking along the edge of a cliff on a dark night. With such a narrow glycaemic warning zone the propensity rapidly to develop severe neuroglycopenia is high and the margin for error is dangerously narrow.

The results of these laboratory-based experimental studies of diabetic patients with established hypoglycaemia unawareness are very consistent with clinical observations of people with this acquired problem. At one moment they appear to be cerebrating normally (despite a low blood glucose) then rapidly they become confused or drowsy and may have a dazed appearance, with an accompanying inertia to seek some form of carbohydrate to reverse the neuroglycopenia. They may have to rely on relatives, friends or colleagues to identify the hypoglycaemia and quickly provide treatment. This becomes a serious emergency if the patient is alone or if the insidious, but often rapid, development of neuroglycopenia goes unobserved. This explains the increased risk of progression to severe hypoglycaemia, and the higher rates reported in people with hypoglycaemia unawareness.

Studies examining the effects of strict glycaemic control on symptomatic and neuroendocrine responses to hypoglycaemia have also demonstrated a similar shift in glycaemic threshold for autonomic symptoms and an acute sympatho-adrenal response. However, the effect on neuroglycopenic symptoms and cognitive dysfunction remains unresolved and is an area of controversy (see Chapter 6).

Peripheral Autonomic Neuropathy

For many years, peripheral autonomic neuropathy was considered to be the principal cause of impaired awareness of hypoglycaemia (Hoeldtke et al, 1982). This was based on the assumption that the diminished secretion of adrenaline in response to hypoglycaemia (Hilsted et al, 1981; Bottini et al, 1997) would either prevent the generation of autonomic symptoms (such as sweating or a pounding heart) or reduce their intensity, resulting in an inability to perceive the onset of hypoglycaemia. Thus, autonomic neuropathy would interfere with the normal physiological responses stimulated by autonomic activation.

There are various reasons why this hypothesis is unlikely:

- Adrenaline has a limited role in generating hypoglycaemic symptoms, and the reduced secretory response of adrenaline in autonomic neuropathy is compensated by increased sensitivity of peripheral beta-adrenoceptors (Hilsted et al, 1987).
- Diabetic subjects with autonomic neuropathy have normal physiological responses and experience typical autonomic symptoms during hypoglycaemia (Hilsted et al, 1981; Hepburn et al, 1993b), and no relationship has been found between autonomic dysfunction and hypoglycaemic symptoms (Berlin et al, 1987).
- Impaired awareness of hypoglycaemia co-segregates with deficient

counterregulatory hormonal responses and not with autonomic neuropathy (Ryder et al, 1990).

- The prevalence of autonomic neuropathy is similar in patients with type 1 diabetes of long duration (more than 15 years), whether or not they have impaired awareness of hypoglycaemia (Hepburn et al, 1990).
- Although impaired awareness of hypoglycaemia is a major risk factor for severe hypoglycaemia, the latter is either no more common in type 1 diabetic patients with autonomic neuropathy (Bjork et al, 1990; The DCCT Research Group, 1991), or is only modestly increased (Stephenson et al, 1996).
- Autonomic neuropathy is not a determinant of whether glycaemic thresholds for autonomic (including symptomatic) responses to hypoglycaemia are affected by antecedent hypoglycaemia (Dagogo-Jack et al, 1993).

Both impaired awareness of hypoglycaemia and peripheral autonomic neuropathy are common in people with type 1 diabetes of long duration, and frequently co-exist. This does not prove a causal relationship, and it appears that peripheral autonomic dysfunction does not have a prominent role in the pathogenesis of this syndrome.

However, reduced sensitivity of cardiac beta-adrenoceptors to catecholamines has been observed in patients with type 1 diabetes who have impaired awareness of hypoglycaemia (Berlin et al, 1987), and hypoglycaemia *per se* reduces beta-adrenergic sensitivity in type 1 diabetes (Fritsche et al, 1998). Maladaptation of tissue sensitivity to catecholamines may therefore contribute to the development of hypoglycaemia unawareness although autonomic neuropathy is not present.

Hypoglycaemia-associated Autonomic Failure

The co-segregation of impaired hypoglycaemia awareness with counterregulatory deficiency suggests that they share a common underlying pathogenetic mechanism. These acquired abnormalities associated with hypoglycaemia in type 1 diabetes (Box 5.3) are characterised by a high frequency of severe hypoglycaemia and a common pathophysiological feature, namely the elevated glycaemic thresholds (or lower blood glucose concentrations) that are required to trigger symptomatic and hormonal secretory responses. In other words, more profound hypoglycaemia is necessary to produce the usual symptomatic and neuroendocrine responses to acute hypoglycaemia. Cryer (1992) has designated this group of abnormalities as a form of "hypoglycaemia-associated autonomic failure", and has speculated that recurrent severe hypoglycaemia

Box 5.3 Acquired syndromes associated with hypoglycaemia in type 1 diabetes

- Counterregulatory deficiency
- Impaired hypoglycaemia awareness
- Altered glycaemic thresholds for neuroendocrine and symptomatic responses

may be the primary problem which establishes a vicious circle (Figure 5.6). It seems likely that this defect resides within the central nervous system.

Central Nervous System Adaptation to Hypoglycaemia

Some people with insulin-treated diabetes remain lucid, with no evidence of impaired cognitive function, when their blood glucose is low (often well below 3.5 mmol/l). Biochemical hypoglycaemia which is asymptomatic is commonly recorded by patients who have impaired awareness

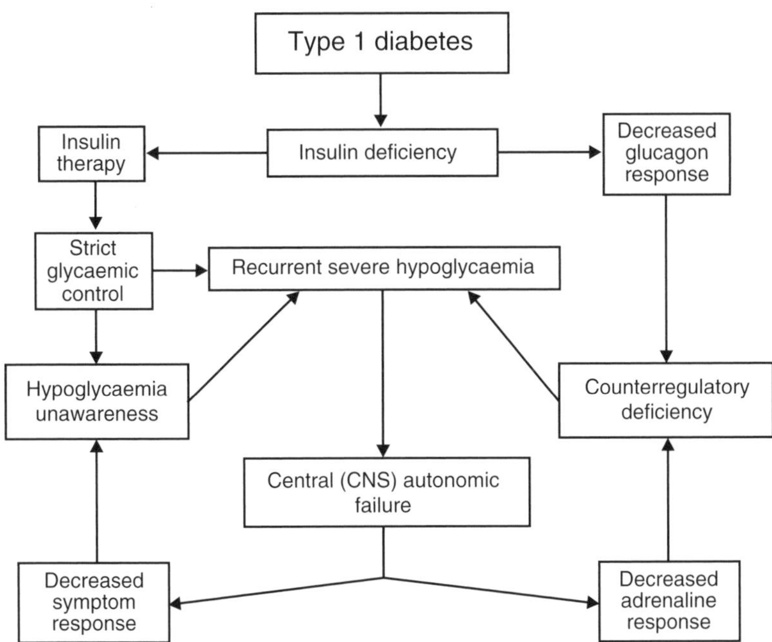

Figure 5.6 Schematic diagram of the concept of hypoglycaemia-associated autonomic failure, based on Cryer (1992)

of hypoglycaemia, and they appear to have developed a neurological adaptation to chronic neuroglycopenia. The altered glycaemic threshold prevents the onset of warning symptoms and cognitive dysfunction until the blood glucose falls to a dangerously low level, which is extremely undesirable when striving for safe clinical management of insulin-treated diabetes.

Although the human brain is dependent on a continuous supply of glucose for normal function, it can adapt to prolonged exposure to hypoglycaemia. This adaptation process takes at least several hours and possibly a few days to occur. Short-term exposure to acute hypoglycaemia (blood glucose 2.5 mmol/l) for 60 minutes in non-diabetic subjects showed no improvement in cognitive function and no reduction in symptom scores during this brief time interval (Gold et al, 1995a). However, when non-diabetic volunteers were subjected to chronic hypoglycaemia (blood glucose 2.9 mmol/l) for 56 hours, using a glucose clamp, significant cerebral adaptation did occur (Boyle et al, 1994). The responses to acute hypoglycaemia (blood glucose 2.5 mmol/l) were compared before and after the period of chronic hypoglycaemia. Brain glucose uptake was initially reduced at a blood glucose of 3.6 mmol/l, but after chronic hypoglycaemia this was preserved and cerebral function was maintained (Figure 5.7), demonstrating the effect of cerebral adaptation to chronic neuroglycopenia. The glycaemic thresholds for the onset of symptoms, counterregulatory hormonal secretion and cognitive dysfunction, were all modified and occurred at much lower blood glucose concentrations. A similar phenomenon has been observed in non-diabetic patients who had chronic hypoglycaemia caused by an insulinoma, in whom symptomatic responses to acute hypoglycaemia were blunted, and counterregulatory hormonal responses were impaired (Mitrakou et al, 1993); compared to normal controls, cognitive function was unaffected. Surgical removal of the insulinomas reversed these abnormalities, indicating that they had resulted from cerebral adaptation to chronic hypoglycaemia.

Strict glycaemic control in people with insulin-treated diabetes also alters the glycaemic thresholds for the development of counterregulatory hormones and symptoms (Chapter 6), so that a lower blood glucose concentration is required to trigger these responses. The observation that this requires a reduction in HbA1c to within the non-diabetic range (Kinsley et al, 1995) suggests that the median daily blood glucose in these individuals is relatively low, and the frequency of biochemical (and symptomatic) hypoglycaemia will be greater than in insulin-treated diabetic patients who are not as well controlled (Thorsteinsson et al, 1986). Boyle et al (1995) have shown that those patients who had near normal HbA1c values, maintained normal uptake of glucose by the brain

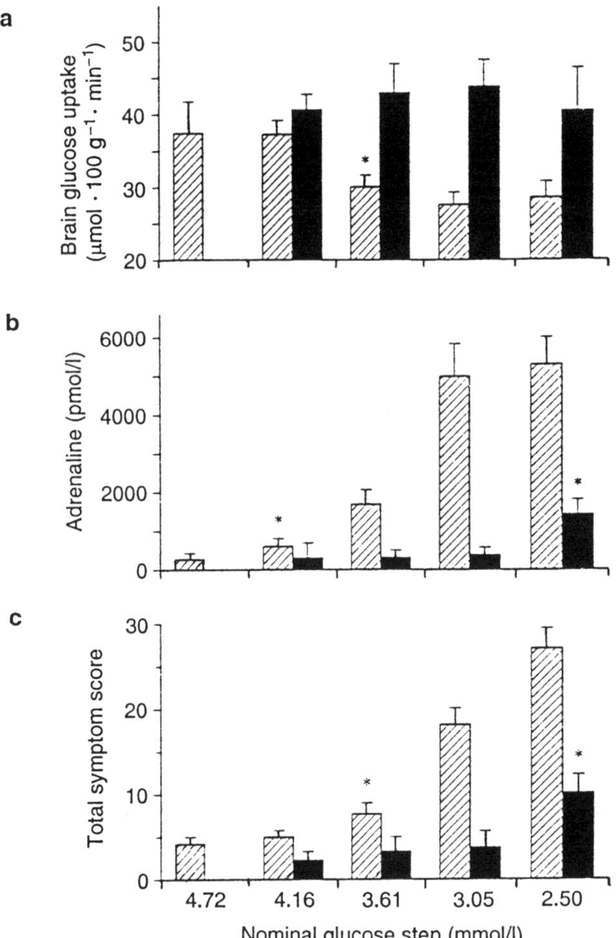

Figure 5.7 Rates of (a) brain glucose uptake, (b) adrenaline (epinephrine) concentration and (c) total symptoms of hypoglycaemia in non-diabetic subjects before and after prolonged hypoglycaemia. Initial day of investigation (hatched); after 56 hours of hypoglycaemia (solid). *Significant difference from baseline for each of the two days. Data derived from Boyle et al, 1994, and figure taken from *Diabetologia* 1997; **40**: S69–74, by permission of Springer-Verlag

during hypoglycaemia, so preserving cerebral metabolism, reducing the neuroendocrine responses to hypoglycaemia, and diminishing symptomatic awareness. Although this capacity to maintain, and even increase, cerebral blood glucose uptake during hypoglycaemia is a protective response for the brain in these patients with strict glycaemic control, it is considered to be maladaptive, as it suppresses the normal symptomatic warning of responses and so risks the development of much more profound neuroglycopenia.

During hypoglycaemia, glucose transport into the brain becomes rate-limiting, and brain energy metabolism deteriorates. The adaptive response results from an increased utilisation of glucose by the brain. In rodents, the transport of glucose across the blood–brain barrier is increased after several days of chronic hypoglycaemia (McCall et al, 1986). Further elegant studies in rats of glucose transport activity across the blood–brain barrier have shown that changes in expression of the glucose transporter, GLUT-1, in brain microvasculature occur in response to chronic hypoglycaemia, i.e. blood glucose less than 2.0 mmol/l for several days (Kumagai et al, 1995). The increase in GLUT-1 activity is responsible for the compensatory increase in glucose transport across the blood–brain barrier.

Antecedent (Episodic) Hypoglycaemia

It has been recognised for many years that severe hypoglycaemia begets more episodes of severe hypoglycaemia, and one episode may influence the clinical manifestations of another occurring soon afterwards (Severinghaus, 1926). In recent years, several studies have shown that the symptomatic and neuroendocrine responses to an episode of acute hypoglycaemia are diminished if a preceding (or *antecedent*) episode of hypoglycaemia has occurred within the previous 24 hours. Several studies have been performed in non-diabetic human subjects (Table 5.2) and in subjects with insulin-treated diabetes (Table 5.3). Although these studies differ considerably in design and methods of inducing hypoglycaemia, in general it appears that antecedent hypoglycaemia of between one and two hours' duration has a significant influence on the magnitude of the symptomatic and neuroendocrine responses to subsequent hypoglycaemia occurring within the following 24 to 48 hours (Figure 5.8).

The glycaemic thresholds for symptomatic and counterregulatory hormonal responses are altered by antecedent hypoglycaemia, and the degree to which subsequent responses are blunted is determined by the duration and depth of antecedent hypoglycaemia (Davis et al, 1997). Some of the physiological responses (e.g. sweating) may be blunted for longer than other responses following antecedent hypoglycaemia (George et al, 1995). Recurrent, short-lived (15 minutes) episodes of hypoglycaemia on four consecutive days, had no effect on neuroendocrine and symptomatic responses in non-diabetic subjects (Peters et al, 1995), so transient reduction in blood glucose may not produce this effect. Some studies have examined the effect of antecedent hypoglycaemia on cognitive function, but in many the methods of assessment were inade-

Table 5.2 Studies of antecedent hypoglycaemia (AH) in non-diabetic humans

References	No. of subjects	Method of induction, nadir BG (mmol/l) and duration of AH	Interval before test hypoglycaemia	Test hypo: method and BG nadir (mmol/l)	Effect of AH on subsequent responses to hypoglycaemia
Heller & Cryer (1991)	9	Clamp (3.0) 2 h	18 h	Clamp (2.8)	Reduced symptoms and CR responses
Widom and Simonson (1992)	10	Clamp (2.2–2.8) 1 h	Four consecutive daily hypos	Stepped clamp (2.2)	Elevated BG thresholds for symptoms and CR responses
Veneman et al (1993)	10	iv infusion (2.2–2.5) 2 h	7 h	Stepped clamp (2.3)	Nocturnal hypo: BG thresholds for symptoms and CR responses elevated
Mellman et al (1994)	9	Clamp (3.2) 2 h	1.5 h	Stepped clamp (2.8)	Elevated BG thresholds for symptoms and CR responses
Robinson et al (1995)	10	Clamp (3.0) 2 h	24 h and 6 days	Clamp (2.5)	Reduced adrenaline and sweating at 6 days
Peters et al (1995)	10	iv bolus injection of insulin (<2.8) <15 min	Four consecutive daily hypos	iv bolus (<2.8) × 4	No effect on symptoms or CR responses
George et al (1995)	8	Clamp (2.9) 2 h	2 and 5 days	Clamp (2.5)	Physiological responses still reduced after 1 week
Davis et al (1997)	8	Stepped clamp (2.9) 2 h	<24 h	Clamp (2.9)	Magnitude of reduced CR response related to depth of AH

BG = blood glucose; AH = antecedent hypoglycaemia; CR = counterregulatory (hormonal); iv = intravenous

Table 5.3 Studies on antecedent hypoglycaemia in people with insulin-treated diabetes

Reference	No. of subjects	Method of induction, nadir BG (mmol/l), and duration of AH	Interval before test hypoglycaemia	Test hypo: method and BG nadir (mmol/l)	Effect of AH on subsequent responses to hypoglycaemia
Davis et al (1992)	13	Clamp (3.0) 2 h	60 min	Clamp (3.0)	Reduced CR responses and hepatic glucose output
Dagogo-Jack et al (1993)	26 (+AN) 12 (non-diabetic)	Clamp (2.7) 2 h	15 h	Stepped clamp (2.6)	Elevated BG thresholds for symptoms and autonomic responses
Lingenfelser et al (1993)	18	iv bolus injection of insulin (<2.2) mins × 3	3 days	Stepped clamp (1.7)	Reduced symptoms, CR and neurophysiological responses
George et al (1997)	8	Clamp (2.8) 2 h	2 days	Stepped clamp (2.2)	Physiological responses diminished for 2 days
Ovalle et al (1998)	6	Clamp (2.8) 2 h, twice weekly for 1 month	48 h	Stepped clamp (2.5)	Reduced symptoms, CR and cognitive dysfunction. Fewer symptomatic episodes of clinical hypoglycaemia.
Fanelli et al (1998)	15	Clamp (2.6) $3\frac{1}{2}$ h, nocturnal	5–10 h	Stepped clamp (2.5)	Less deterioration in cognitive function after nocturnal hypoglycaemia (vs euglycaemia) Elevated BG threshold for cognitive dysfunction.

AH = antecedent hypoglycaemia; AN = autonomic neuropathy; iv = intravenous; CR = counterregulatory (hormonal)

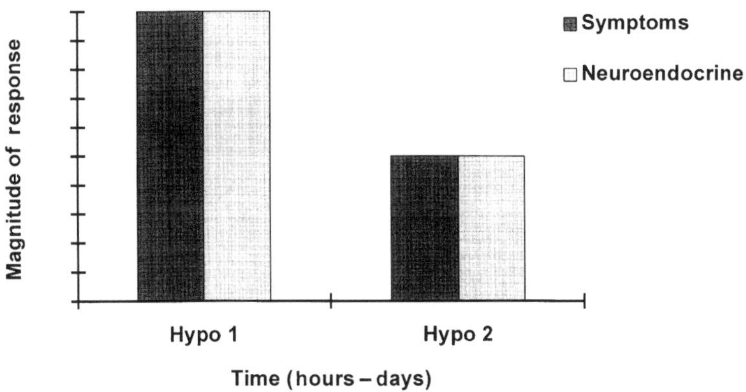

Figure 5.8 Schematic representation of the effect of antecedent hypoglycaemia on the neuroendocrine and symptomatic responses to subsequent hypoglycaemia

quate and insufficient to provide definitive evidence of a change in cognitive response. While one view maintains that the glycaemic threshold for cognitive dysfunction is not altered by hypoglycaemia (see Chapter 6), an increasing number of studies have suggested that this does shift to a lower blood glucose concentration in the same manner as autonomic and neuroendocrine responses (Veneman et al, 1993; Ovalle et al, 1998; Fanelli et al, 1998). Nocturnal (episodic) hypoglycaemia, which is frequently not identified by patients, has been proposed as a mechanism for the induction of hypoglycaemia unawareness in people who give no history of recurrent hypoglycaemia (Veneman et al, 1993). The mechanisms of cerebral adaptation causing impaired awareness of hypoglycaemia are summarised in Box 5.4.

Although antecedent hypoglycaemia may induce transient impairment of awareness of hypoglycaemia, it is unclear how this mechanism would

Box 5.4 Mechanisms of cerebral adaptation causing impaired awareness of hypoglycaemia

Symptomatic and **neuroendocrine** responses to hypoglycaemia in insulin-treated diabetes are diminished in association with:

- strict glycaemic control (HbA1c in non-diabetic range)
- antecedent (episodic) hypoglycaemia
- chronic (protracted) hypoglycaemia

and may be restored by:

- relaxation of glycaemic control
- scrupulous avoidance of hypoglycaemia

induce chronic or prolonged loss of symptomatic perception. While frequent, recurrent hypoglycaemia may have a contributory effect to inducing hypoglycaemia unawareness, presumably the hypoglycaemia has to be relatively protracted to induce cerebral adaptation, and the phenomenon is not limited solely to patients who have strict glycaemic control. The problem remains of explaining the induction of protracted or chronic hypoglycaemia unawareness, which often appears to be a permanent defect. Presumably repetitive hypoglycaemic insults to the brain (which are not necessarily severe) eventually "downregulate" the central mechanisms which sense a low blood glucose and activate the glucoregulatory responses within the hypothalamus. There is evidence of a permanent redistribution of regional cerebral blood flow in diabetic patients with a history of recurrent severe hypoglycaemia (MacLeod et al, 1994a) with, in particular, a relative increase in blood flow to the frontal lobes. This may represent a chronic adaptive response to protect vulnerable areas of the brain from recurrent, severe neuroglycopenia. However, a further study showed that the changes in regional cerebral blood flow in response to controlled hypoglycaemia in patients with type 1 diabetes occurred independently of the state of awareness of hypoglycaemia (MacLeod et al, 1996). The EEG changes associated with modest hypoglycaemia are more pronounced in patients with type 1 diabetes who have impaired awareness of hypoglycaemia (Tribl et al, 1996). Most studies suggest that a diffuse functional abnormality is present in the anterior part of the brain in diabetes, and this may be implicated in the impaired perception of hypoglycaemia. The pre-frontal areas of the cortex are closely connected to sub-cortical areas, and localised dysfunction could theoretically reduce the ability of the brain to perceive symptomatic hypoglycaemia.

COGNITIVE FUNCTION AND HYPOGLYCAEMIA UNAWARENESS

Impaired hypoglycaemia unawareness is a major risk factor for severe hypoglycaemia, and patients with the chronic form of this condition have a six-fold higher frequency (Gold et al, 1994). It is possible therefore that impaired hypoglycaemia awareness may be associated with evidence of a decline in cognitive function. Hepburn et al (1991) noted that diabetic patients with a history of impaired hypoglycaemia awareness performed more poorly on limited cognitive function testing, than those with normal awareness of hypoglycaemia, both at a normal blood glucose and during hypoglycaemia. This suggested that an acquired cognitive impairment may have been superimposed upon an increased susceptibility to neuroglycopenia.

A modest, but insignificant, decline in intellectual function was noted with progressive loss of hypoglycaemia awareness in a population study (MacLeod et al, 1994b) and formal measurement of cognitive function during controlled hypoglycaemia (blood glucose 2.5 mmol/l) showed that patients with type 1 diabetes who had impaired hypoglycaemia awareness exhibited more profound cognitive dysfunction during acute hypoglycaemia than patients with normal awareness, and that this persisted for longer following recovery of blood glucose (Gold et al, 1995b). This observation may have practical importance for diabetic management. Patients with insulin-treated diabetes who have impaired awareness of hypoglycaemia should be instructed that cognitive function may remain affected for a considerable time (up to an hour) after the recovery of blood glucose following an episode of moderate hypoglycaemia. Intellectual activity is likely to be affected and cause sub-optimal performance during this recovery period. This has implications for skilled tasks such as driving or operating machinery and equipment.

HUMAN INSULIN

For 60 years after its discovery, insulin for therapeutic use was obtained from the pancreata of cattle and pigs. With the development of recombinant DNA technology it was possible to "genetically engineer" molecules, and insulin was the first protein to be made in this way, becoming available for the treatment of humans in the 1980s. Several of the existing animal insulin formulations were withdrawn, principally for commercial reasons, and human insulin rapidly became the most commonly prescribed form of insulin, so that nowadays more than 90% of patients who require insulin are treated with human insulin. The structure of human insulin differs from porcine insulin by a single amino acid, and from bovine insulin by three amino acids. In initial trials it was not expected that human insulin would differ substantially in potency from animal insulin, but because human insulin was slightly purer than some of the animal insulins, patients were advised to reduce the dose by around 10% when converting from animal to human insulin.

Detailed pharmacokinetic studies comparing human and animal insulins have not demonstrated any major differences, but human insulin has a slightly faster onset of action, a slightly shorter duration of action, and is less immunogenic than equivalent animal insulins. Most clinical studies, conducted on a worldwide scale, showed no significant differences between human and animal insulins in their clinical application.

In Switzerland, one group of research workers reported serious clinical problems which they associated with the use of human insulin in diabetic patients (Teuscher and Berger, 1987). In particular, they claimed that patients were experiencing more frequent hypoglycaemia with human insulin, and that warning symptoms were altered with human insulin, as a result of which many patients were unable to detect the onset of hypoglycaemia (Box 5.5). Around this time a pathologist in the United Kingdom claimed that the numbers of patients dying from severe hypoglycaemia had increased since the introduction of human insulin (see Chapter 7).

In the UK many anecdotal reports emerged of problems experienced by patients with human insulin, and solicitors acting on behalf of over 400 UK patients tried to bring a legal action against the insulin manufacturers, alleging that human insulin gave less warning of hypoglycaemia. Additional claims included allegations that human insulin may have caused personality changes in individuals and even other disease states such as multiple sclerosis. This group action was abandoned in 1993 because the scientific evidence for the claims was considered to be insufficient.

This issue has generated much controversy and heated debate and promoted several studies comparing human with animal insulins. With recent advances in the understanding of the mechanisms of impaired awareness of hypoglycaemia it may be possible to offer, in retrospect, explanations for the observations of the Swiss doctors (Fisher and Frier, 1993).

Counterregulation and Human Insulin

The hormonal responses to human insulin are described in Chapter 4. In summary, most clinical laboratory studies in which hypoglycaemia was induced by intravenous insulin showed no statistically significant differences between the hormonal responses to hypoglycaemia, whether induced by human or porcine insulins. This has included studies which were performed in patients who specifically claimed to have developed

Box 5.5 Possible problems with human insulin

- More hypoglycaemic episodes
- Reduced hormonal responses
- Different symptoms of hypoglycaemia
- Impaired hypoglycaemia awareness
- More deaths from hypoglycaemia

impaired awareness of hypoglycaemia after being changed to human insulin (Patrick et al, 1991; Maran et al, 1993). None of these studies showed any differences between the insulin species in the hormonal or symptomatic responses to hypoglycaemia. One laboratory study in elderly diabetic patients, who had not been treated previously with insulin, showed similar counterregulatory hormonal responses to human and animal insulins, but a lower score was obtained for both the autonomic and the neuroglycopenic symptoms of hypoglycaemia with human insulin (Meneilly et al, 1995). The interpretation of this investigation is unclear, as symptom responses alter with age, and the investigators examined a symptom profile that had been derived from studies of young non-diabetic subjects.

Epidemiological Studies of Human Insulin

At least nine retrospective observational studies have examined the incidence and symptomatology of hypoglycaemia in diabetic patients treated with human insulin (Nelleman Jorgensen et al, 1994). The results must be treated with caution, however, because of the weaknesses inherent with retrospective studies. With the exception of the Swiss group (Teuscher and Berger, 1987) none of the studies was able to show any differences in the incidence, symptoms or awareness of hypoglycaemia.

A smaller number of case studies have been performed. In two studies no difference was found (Jick et al, 1990a, 1990b), and the only study to show a significant difference was from the Swiss group (Egger et al, 1991a), where the risk of severe hypoglycaemia appeared to be three-fold higher with human insulin. Detailed analysis of that study revealed that the group on human insulin had better glycaemic control and a higher frequency of previous hypoglycaemic coma, both of which are associated with an increased risk of hypoglycaemia (Fisher and Frier, 1993).

Clinical Trials of Human Insulin

Hypoglycaemia induced in a clinical laboratory may have limited relevance to the everyday life of a person with insulin-treated diabetes. Of more relevance are prospective clinical trials examining any differences in incidence and symptomatology of hypoglycaemia over a longer period of time. Over 16 studies have been reported, and none, including two double-blind studies from Switzerland (Berger et al, 1989; Egger et al, 1991b), was able to demonstrate any difference in the incidence of hypoglycaemia. Few studies examined the symptoms of hypoglycaemia and only two studies from Switzerland have described a difference in the symptom profile induced by human and animal insulins. These authors showed that the symptom of "anxiety" was less evident with human insulin. As noted previously, the separation of symptoms into autonomic and neuroglycopenic groups is of little value when considering awareness of hypoglycaemia. It is the initial perception of any symptom of hypoglycaemia, irrespective of whether this is autonomic or neuroglycopenic, that promotes awareness of hypoglycaemia. In addition, the intensity of one or more cardinal symptoms of hypoglycaemia is more important in the perception of symptoms, than the total number that are generated. It is therefore fallacious to presume that a reduction in the number of autonomic symptoms equates with reduced awareness, and a more accurate interpretation of the Swiss studies is that awareness of hypoglycaemia may be altered but not impaired with human insulin. It should be emphasised, however, that this conclusion was not confirmed by others using a detailed, validated scoring system for the symptoms of hypoglycaemia (MacLeod et al, 1995).

Despite an extensive research effort, the question of whether human insulin does affect the awareness of hypoglycaemia remains unproven. In clinical practice there are undoubtedly a small number of people with insulin-treated diabetes in whom the use of human insulin has been very unsatisfactory, being associated with frequent and unpredictable hypoglycaemia and a diminished sense of well-being. Whether this is related to the different pharmacokinetics of human insulin or is an idiosyncratic response in affected individuals, is unknown, but there is clearly a need for insulin manufacturers to maintain the availability of animal insulins for such patients.

TREATMENT STRATEGIES

When impaired awareness of hypoglycaemia is therapy-related, i.e. resulting from strict glycaemic control, the approach to management is relatively simple. The total insulin dose should be reduced, attention paid to the appropriateness of the insulin regimen, and overall glycaemic control should be relaxed. Liu et al (1996) have reported an improvement in symptomatic and counterregulatory hormonal responses to hypoglycaemia after three months of less strict glycaemic control in a small group of insulin-treated patients, in whom the mean HbA1c rose from 6.9% to 8.0%.

It has been claimed that impaired awareness of hypoglycaemia (and to some extent counterregulatory hormonal deficiency) can be reversed by scrupulous avoidance of hypoglycaemia through meticulous attention to diabetic management (Cranston et al, 1994; Fanelli et al, 1994; Dagogo-

Jack et al, 1994). The effect which this had on glycaemic thresholds for cognitive dysfunction and the recovery of counterregulatory hormonal secretion to hypoglycaemia, differed between these studies, but all demonstrated an improved symptomatic response following avoidance of hypoglycaemia for periods varying from three weeks to one year. However, the studies can be criticised because:

- Only a small number of patients were studied.
- The definition of hypoglycaemia unawareness was based on an increased frequency of asymptomatic biochemical hypoglycaemia, and with the exception of the study by Dagogo-Jack et al (1994), was not based on having a *history* of hypoglycaemia unawareness.
- In all studies there was a small but definite rise in glycated haemoglobin, suggesting that the improved symptomatic awareness was related primarily to relaxation of glycaemic control.

Although the scrupulous avoidance of hypoglycaemia is clearly desirable, and may be beneficial to reducing the severity of hypoglycaemia unawareness, it is very difficult to achieve as it is extremely time-consuming both for patients and health professionals. The use of continuous subcutaneous insulin infusion overnight instead of isophane insulin at bedtime has been shown to be beneficial in diabetic patients with impaired awareness of hypoglycaemia, improving warning symptoms and counterregulatory responses to hypoglycaemia, presumably by reducing the frequency of nocturnal hypoglycaemia (Kanc et al, 1998).

The ingestion of caffeine uncouples the relationship between cerebral blood flow and glucose metabolism, and it has been observed that the prior consumption of caffeine augments the symptomatic and counterregulatory hormonal responses to a modest reduction of blood glucose in non-diabetic subjects (Kerr et al, 1993). A similar phenomenon occurs in people with type 1 diabetes following the ingestion of a dose of caffeine equivalent to two or three cups of coffee, with a sustained reduction in cerebral blood flow, an augmented counterregulatory response (Figure 5.9) and greater awareness of hypoglycaemia (Debrah et al, 1996). How this could be of practical benefit in patients with type 1 diabetes to improve their symptomatic awareness of hypoglycaemia is not clear, but it raises the prospect of identifying some form of therapeutic intervention which utilises a similar mechanism, to heighten the residual symptomatic response.

It is clearly desirable to avoid severe hypoglycaemia at all costs, and treatment strategies should be adopted to achieve this aim (Box 5.6). Frequent blood glucose monitoring is essential in affected patients, and may require occasional nocturnal measurements to detect a low blood

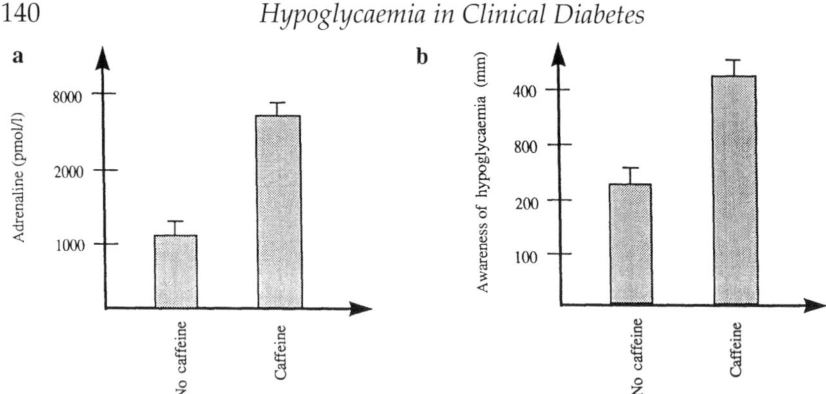

Figure 5.9 (a) Augmentation of the normal secretory response of adrenaline to, and (b) awareness of, acute hypoglycaemia (blood glucose 2.8 mmol/l) by the prior ingestion of caffeine in insulin-treated diabetic patients. Derived from data in Debrah et al (1996)

> **Box 5.6** Treatment strategies for patients with impaired awareness of hypoglycaemia
>
> - Frequent blood glucose monitoring (including nocturnal measurements)
> - Avoid blood glucose values < 4.0 mmol/l
> - Set target range of blood glucose higher than for "aware" patients (e.g. preprandial between 6.0 and 12.0 mmol/l; bedtime > 8.0 mmol/l)
> - Avoid HbA1c in non-diabetic range
> - Use predominantly short-acting insulins (e.g. basal-bolus regimen; insulin analogues)
> - Consume regular snacks between meals and at bedtime, containing unrefined carbohydrate
> - Ensure appropriate carbohydrate consumption and/or insulin dose adjustment for premeditated exercise
> - Learn to identify subtle neuroglycopenic cues to low blood glucose

glucose during the night. Blood glucose awareness training has been developed in the USA, with re-education of affected patients to recognise neuroglycopenic cues (Cox et al, 1995), but this also requires facilities and resources which are not available in most centres. Intensive insulin therapy is contraindicated in patients who have impaired awareness of hypoglycaemia, and treatment goals have to be considered individually.

The avoidance of severe hypoglycaemia is paramount as this may exacerbate the problem, and the use of mostly short-acting insulin (and possibly insulin analogues) in basal-bolus regimens may be particularly useful in avoiding biochemical and symptomatic hypoglycaemia without compromising overall glycaemic control.

CONCLUSIONS

- An inadequate symptomatic warning can occur in people with insulin-treated diabetes and is described as impaired awareness of hypoglycaemia or hypoglycaemia unawareness.
- In diabetic patients who report impaired awareness of hypoglycaemia, asymptomatic hypoglycaemia occurs more frequently during routine blood glucose monitoring and should alert the clinician to the possibility that an individual is developing this problem.
- Impaired awareness of hypoglycaemia has been shown to be associated with strict glycaemic control, but significant modification of the symptomatic response does not occur unless the glycated haemoglobin concentration is within the non-diabetic range.
- The mechanisms underlying impaired awareness of hypoglycaemia are unknown and may be multifactorial. Possible mechanisms include chronic exposure to a low blood glucose, antecedent hypoglycaemia, and glucoregulatory failure.
- Antecedent hypoglycaemia of short duration has a significant influence on the magnitude of the symptomatic and neuroendocrine responses to subsequent hypoglycaemia occurring within the following 48 hours.
- When impaired awareness of hypoglycaemia results from strict glycaemic control, the total insulin dose should be reduced, attention paid to the suitability of the insulin regimen, and overall glycaemic control should be relaxed.
- Impaired awareness of hypoglycaemia and to some extent counterregulatory hormonal deficiency can probably be reversed by scrupulous avoidance of hypoglycaemia through meticulous attention to diabetic management.
- Intensive insulin therapy is contraindicated in patients who have impaired awareness of hypoglycaemia. The use of mostly short-acting insulin (and possibly insulin analogues) in basal-bolus regimens may be particularly useful in avoiding biochemical and symptomatic hypoglycaemia without compromising overall glycaemic control.

REFERENCES

Bacatselos SO, Karamitsos DT, Kourtoglou GI, Zambulis CX, Yovos JG, Vyzantiadis AT (1995). Hypoglycaemia unawareness in type 1 diabetic patients under conventional insulin treatment. *Diabetes, Nutrition and Metabolism* **8**: 267–75.

Berger W, Keller U, Honegger B, Jaeggi E (1989). Warning symptoms of hypoglycaemia during treatment with human and porcine insulin in diabetes mellitus. *Lancet* **333**: 1041–4.

Berlin I, Grimaldi A, Payan C, Sachon C, Bosquet F, Thervet F, Puech AJ (1987). Hypoglycemic symptoms and decreased *B*-adrenergic sensitivity in insulin-dependent diabetic patients. *Diabetes Care* **10**: 742–7.

Bjork E, Palmer M, Schvarcz E, Berne C (1990). Incidence of severe hypoglycaemia in an unselected population of patients with insulin-treated diabetes mellitus, with special reference to autonomic neuropathy. *Diabetes, Nutrition and Metabolism* **4**: 303–9.

Bottini P, Boschetti E, Pampanelli S, Ciofetta M, Del Sindaco P, Scionti L, Brunetti P, Bolli GB (1997). Contribution of autonomic neuropathy to reduced plasma adrenaline responses to hypoglycemia in IDDM. Evidence for a nonselective defect. *Diabetes* **46**: 814–23.

Boyle PJ, Schwartz NS, Shah SD, Clutter WE, Cryer PE (1988). Plasma glucose concentrations at the onset of hypoglycemic symptoms in patients with poorly controlled diabetes and in nondiabetics. *New England Journal of Medicine* **318**: 1487–92.

Boyle PJ, Nagy RJ, O'Connor AM, Kempers SF, Yeo RA, Qualls C (1994). Adaptation in brain glucose uptake following recurrent hypoglycemia. *Proceedings of National Academy of Science, USA* **91**: 9352–6.

Boyle PJ, Kempers SF, O'Connor AM, Nagy RJ (1995). Brain glucose uptake and unawareness of hypoglycemia in patients with insulin-dependent diabetes mellitus. *New England Journal of Medicine* **333**: 1726–31.

Clarke WL, Cox DJ, Gonder-Frederick LA, Julian D, Schlundt D, Polonsky W (1995). Reduced awareness of hypoglycemia in adults with IDDM. A prospective study of hypoglycemic frequency and associated symptoms. *Diabetes Care* **18**: 517–22.

Cox D, Gonder-Frederick L, Polonsky W, Schlundt D, Julian D, Clarke W (1995). A multicenter evaluation of blood glucose awareness training – II. *Diabetes Care* **18**: 523–8.

Cranston I, Lomas J, Maran A, Macdonald I, Amiel SA (1994). Restoration of hypoglycaemia awareness in patients with long-duration insulin-dependent diabetes. *Lancet* **344**: 283–7.

Cryer PE (1992). Iatrogenic hypoglycemia as a cause of hypoglycemia-associated autonomic failure in IDDM. A vicious circle. *Diabetes* **41**: 255–60.

Dagogo-Jack SE, Craft S, Cryer PE (1993). Hypoglycemia-associated autonomic failure in insulin-dependent diabetes mellitus. *Journal of Clinical Investigation* **91**: 819–28.

Dagogo-Jack S, Rattarasarn C, Cryer PE (1994). Reversal of hypoglycemia unawareness, but not defective glucose counterregulation, in IDDM. *Diabetes* **43**: 1426–34.

Davis MR, Mellman M, Shamoon H (1992). Further defects in counterregulatory responses induced by recurrent hypoglycemia in IDDM. *Diabetes* **41**: 1335–40.

Davis SN, Shevers C, Mosqueda-Garcia R, Costa F (1997). Effects of differing antecedent hypoglycemia on subsequent counterregulation in normal humans. *Diabetes* **46**: 1328–35.

Debrah K, Sherwin RS, Murphy J, Kerr D (1996). Effect of caffeine on recognition of and physiological responses to hypoglycaemia in insulin dependent diabetes. *Lancet* **347**: 19–24.

Egger M, Smith GD, Imhoof H, Teuscher A (1991a). Risk of severe hypoglycaemia in insulin-treated diabetic patients transferred to human insulin: a case control study. *British Medical Journal* **303**: 617–21.

Egger M, Smith GD, Teuscher AU, Teuscher A (1991b). Influence of human insulin on symptoms and awareness of hypoglycaemia: a randomised double blind crossover trial. *British Medical Journal* **303**: 622–6.

Fanelli C, Pampanelli S, Epifano L et al (1994). Long-term recovery from unawareness, deficient counterregulation and lack of cognitive dysfunction during hypoglycaemia, following institution of rational, intensive insulin therapy in IDDM. *Diabetologia* **37**: 1265–76.

Fanelli CG, Paramore DS, Hershey T, Terkamp C, Ovalle F, Craft S, Cryer PE (1998). Impact of nocturnal hypoglycemia on hypoglycemic cognitive dysfunction in type 1 diabetes. *Diabetes* **47**: 1920–7.

Fisher BM, Frier BM (1993). Hypoglycaemia and human insulin. In: *Hypoglycaemia and Diabetes: Clinical and Physiological Aspects.* Frier BM, Fisher BM, eds. Edward Arnold, London: 314–27.

Fritsche A, Renn W, Stumvoll M et al (1998). Effect of hypoglycaemia on β-adrenergic sensitivity in normal and type 1 diabetic subjects. *Diabetes Care* **21**: 1505–10.

George E, Harris N, Bedford C, Macdonald IA, Hardisty CA, Heller SR (1995). Prolonged but partial impairment of the hypoglycaemic physiological response following short-term hypoglycaemia in normal subjects. *Diabetologia* **38**: 1183–90.

George E, Marques JL, Harris ND, Macdonald IA, Hardisty CA, Heller SR (1997). Preservation of physiological responses to hypoglycemia 2 days after antecedent hypoglycemia in patients with IDDM. *Diabetes Care* **20**: 1293–8.

Gold AE, MacLeod KM, Frier BM (1994). Frequency of severe hypoglycemia in patients with type 1 diabetes with impaired awareness of hypoglycemia. *Diabetes Care* **17**: 697–703.

Gold AE, Deary IJ, MacLeod KM, Thomson KJ, Frier BM (1995a). Cognitive function during insulin-induced hypoglycemia in humans: short-term cerebral adaptation does not occur. *Psychopharmacology* **119**: 325–33.

Gold AE, MacLeod KM, Deary IJ, Frier BM (1995b). Hypoglycemia-induced cognitive dysfunction in diabetes mellitus: effect of hypoglycemia unawareness. *Physiology and Behavior* **58**: 501–11.

Grimaldi A, Bosquet F, Davidoff P et al (1990). Unawareness of hypoglycemia by insulin-dependent diabetics. *Hormone and Metabolic Research* **22**: 90–5.

Heller SR, Cryer PE (1991). Reduced neuroendocrine and symptomatic responses to subsequent hypoglycemia after 1 episode of hypoglycemia in nondiabetic humans. *Diabetes* **40**: 223–6.

Hepburn DA, Patrick AW, Eadington DW, Ewing DJ, Frier BM (1990). Unawareness of hypoglycaemia in insulin-treated diabetic patients: prevalence and relationship to autonomic neuropathy. *Diabetic Medicine* **7**: 711–7.

Hepburn DA, Patrick AW, Brash HM, Thomson I, Frier BM (1991). Hypoglycaemia unawareness in type 1 diabetes: a lower plasma glucose is required to stimulate sympatho-adrenal activation. *Diabetic Medicine* **8**: 934–45.

Hepburn DA, Deary IJ, Frier BM (1992). Classification of symptoms of hypoglycaemia in insulin-treated diabetic patients using factor analysis: relationship to hypoglycaemia unawareness. *Diabetic Medicine* **9**: 70–5.

Hepburn DA, MacLeod KM, Pell ACH, Scougal IJ, Frier BM (1993a). Frequency and symptoms of hypoglycaemia experienced by patients with type 2 diabetes treated with insulin. *Diabetic Medicine* **10**: 231–7.

Hepburn DA, MacLeod KM, Frier BM (1993b). Physiological symptomatic and hormonal responses to acute hypoglycaemia in type 1 diabetic patients with autonomic neuropathy. *Diabetic Medicine* **10**: 940–9.

Hilsted J, Madsbad S, Krarup T, Sestoft L, Christensen NJ, Tronier B, Galbo H (1981). Hormonal metabolic, and cardiovascular responses to hypoglycemia in diabetic autonomic neuropathy. *Diabetes* **30**: 626–33.

Hilsted J, Richter E, Madsbad S, Tronier B, Christensen NJ, Hildebrandt P, Damkjaer M, Galbo H (1987). Metabolic and cardiovascular responses to epinephrine in diabetic autonomic neuropathy. *New England Journal of Medicine* **317**: 421–6.

Hoeldtke RD, Boden G, Shuman CR, Owen OE (1982). Reduced epinephrine secretion and hypoglycemia unawareness in diabetic autonomic neuropathy. *Annals of Internal Medicine* **96**: 459–62.

Jick H, Hall GC, Dean AD, Jick SS, Derby LE (1990a). A comparison of the risk of hypoglycemia between users of human and animal insulins. 1. Experience in the United Kingdom. *Pharmacotherapy* **10**: 395–7.

Jick SS, Derby LE, Gross KM, Jick H (1990b). Hospitalizations because of hypoglycemia in users of animal and human insulins. 2. Experiences in the United States. *Pharmacotherapy* **10**: 398–9.

Joslin EP, Gray H, Root HF (1922). Insulin in hospital and home. *Journal of Metabolic Research* **2**: 651–99.

Kanc K, Janssen MMJ, Keulen ETP, Jacobs MAJM, Popp-Snijders C, Snoek FJ, Heine RJ (1998). Substitution of night-time continuous subcutaneous insulin infusion therapy for bedtime NPH insulin in a multiple injection regimen improves counterregulatory hormonal responses and warning symptoms of hypoglycaemia in IDDM. *Diabetologia* **41**: 322–9.

Kerr D, Sherwin RS, Pavalkis F, Fayad P, Sikorski L, Rife F, Tamborlane WV, During M (1993). Effect of caffeine on the recognition of and responses to hypoglycemia in humans. *Annals of Internal Medicine* **119**: 799–804.

Kinsley BT, Widom B, Simonson DC (1995). Differential regulation of counterregulatory hormone secretion and symptoms during hypoglycemia in IDDM. Effect of glycemic control. *Diabetes Care* **18**: 17–26.

Kumagai AK, Kang Y-S, Boado RJ, Pardridge WM (1995). Upregulation of blood–brain barrier GLUT 1 glucose transporter protein and mRNA in experimental chronic hypoglycemia. *Diabetes* **44**: 1399–1404.

Lawrence RD (1941). Insulin hypoglycaemia. Changes in nervous manifestations. *Lancet* **ii**: 602.

Lingenfelser T, Renn W, Sommerwerck U, Jung MF, Buettner UW, Zaiser-Kaschel H, Kaschel R, Eggstein M, Jakober B (1993). Compromised hormonal counterregulation, symptom awareness, and neurophysiological function after recurrent short-term episodes of insulin-induced hypoglycemia in IDDM patients. *Diabetes* **42**: 610–8.

Liu D, McManus RM, Ryan EA (1996). Improved counter-regulatory hormonal and symptomatic responses to hypoglycemia in patients with insulin-dependent diabetes mellitus after 3 months of less strict glycemic control. *Clinical and Investigative Medicine* **19**: 71–82.

MacLeod KM, Hepburn DA, Deary IJ, Goodwin GM, Dougall N, Ebmeier KP, Frier BM (1994a). Regional cerebral blood flow in IDDM patients: effects of diabetes and of recurrent severe hypoglycaemia. *Diabetologia* **37**: 257–63.

MacLeod KM, Deary IJ, Graham KS, Hepburn DA, Frier BM (1994b). Hypoglycaemia unawareness in adult patients with type 1 diabetes: relationship to severe hypoglycaemia and cognitive impairment. *Diabetes, Nutrition and Metabolism* **7**: 205–12.

MacLeod KM, Gold AE, Frier BM (1995). Frequency, severity and symptomatology of hypoglycaemia: a comparative trial of human and porcine insulins in type 1 diabetic patients. *Diabetic Medicine* **12**: 134–41.

MacLeod KM, Gold AE, Ebmeier KP, Hepburn DA, Deary, IJ, Goodwin GM, Frier BM (1996). The effects of acute hypoglycemia on relative cerebral blood flow distribution in patients with type 1 (insulin-dependent) diabetes and impaired hypoglycemia awareness. *Metabolism* **45**: 974–80.

McCall AL, Fixman LB, Fleming N, Tornheim K, Chick W, Ruderman NB (1986). Chronic hypoglycemia increases brain glucose transport. *American Journal of Physiology* **251**: E442–7.

Maddock RK, Krall LP (1953). Insulin reactions. Manifestations and need for recognition of long-acting insulin reactions. *Archives of Internal Medicine* **91**: 695–703.

Maran A, Lomas J, Archibald H, Macdonald IA, Gale EAM, Amiel SA (1993). Double blind clinical and laboratory study of hypoglycaemia with human and porcine insulin in diabetic patients reporting hypoglycaemia unawareness after transferring to human insulin. *British Medical Journal* **306**: 167–71.

Mellman MJ, Davis MR, Brisman M, Shamoon H (1994). Effect of antecedent hypoglycemia on cognitive function and on glycemic thresholds for counterregulatory hormone secretion in healthy humans. *Diabetes Care* **17**: 183–8.

Meneilly GS, Milberg WP, Tuokko H (1995). Differential effects of human and animal insulin on the responses to hypoglycemia in elderly patients with NIDDM. *Diabetes* **44**: 272–7.

Mitrakou A, Ryan C, Veneman T, Mokan M, Jenssen T, Kiss I, Durrant J, Cryer P, Gerich J (1991). Hierarchy of glycemic thresholds for counterregulatory hormone secretion, symptoms and cerebral dysfunction. *American Journal of Physiology* **260**: E67–74.

Mitrakou A, Fanelli C, Veneman T, Perriello G, Calderone S, Platanisiotis D, Rambotti A, Raptis S, Brunetti P, Cryer P, Gerich J, Bolli G (1993). Reversibility of unawareness of hypoglycemia in patients with insulinomas. *New England Journal of Medicine* **329**: 834–9.

Mokan M, Mitrakou A, Veneman T, Ryan C, Korytkowski M, Cryer P, Gerich J (1994). Hypoglycemia unawareness in IDDM. *Diabetes Care* **17**: 1397–403.

Muhlhauser I, Heinemann L, Fritsche E, von Lennep K, Berger M (1991). Hypoglycemic symptoms and frequency of severe hypoglycemia in patients treated with human and animal insulin preparations. *Diabetes Care* **14**: 745–9.

Nellemann Jorgensen L, Dejgaard A, Pramming SK (1994). Human insulin and hypoglycaemia: a literature survey. *Diabetic Medicine* **11**: 925–34.

Orchard TJ, Maser RE, Becker DJ, Dorman JS, Drash AL (1991). Human insulin use and hypoglycaemia: insights from the Pittsburgh Epidemiology of Diabetes Complications Study. *Diabetic Medicine* **8**: 469–74.

Ovalle F, Fanelli CG, Paramore DS, Hersley T, Craft S, Cryer PE (1998). Brief twice-weekly episodes of hypoglycemia reduce detection of clinical hypoglycemia in type 1 diabetes Mellitus. *Diabetes* **47**: 1472–9.

Pampanelli S, Fanelli C, Lalli C et al (1996). Long-term intensive insulin therapy in

IDDM: effects on HbA_{1c}, risk for severe and mild hypoglycaemia, status of counterregulation and awareness of hypoglycaemia. *Diabetologia* **39**: 677–86.

Patrick AW, Bodmer CW, Tieszen KL, White MC, Williams G (1991). Human insulin and awareness of acute hypoglycaemic symptoms in insulin-dependent diabetes. *Lancet* **338**: 528–32.

Peters A, Rohloff F, Kerner W (1995). Preserved counterregulatory hormone release and symptoms after short term hypoglycemic episodes in normal men. *Journal of Clinical Endocrinology and Metabolism* **80**: 2894–8.

Pramming S, Thorsteinsson B, Bendtson I, Binder C (1991). Symptomatic hypoglycaemia in 411 type 1 diabetic patients. *Diabetic Medicine* **8**: 217–22.

Robinson AM, Parkin HM, Macdonald IA, Tattersall RB (1995). Antecedent hypoglycaemia in non-diabetic subjects reduces the adrenaline response for 6 days but does not affect the catecholamine response to other stimuli. *Clinical Science* **89**: 359–66.

Ryder REJ, Owens DR, Hayes TM, Ghatei MA, Bloom SR (1990). Unawareness of hypoglycaemia and inadequate hypoglycaemic counterregulation: no causal relation with diabetic autonomic neuropathy. *British Medical Journal* **301**: 783–7.

Severinghaus EL (1926). Hypoglycemic coma due to repeated insulin overdosage. *American Journal of Medical Sciences* **172**: 573–80.

Stephenson JM, Kempler P, Cavallo Peria P, Fuller JH and the EURODIAB IDDM Complications Study Group (1996). Is autonomic neuropathy a risk factor for severe hypoglycaemia? The EURODIAB IDDM Complications Study. *Diabetologia* **39**: 1372–6.

Sussman KE, Crout JR, Marble A (1963). Failure of warning in insulin-induced hypoglycemic reactions. *Diabetes* **12**: 38–45.

Teuscher A, Berger WG (1987). Hypoglycaemia unawareness in diabetics transferred from beef/porcine insulin to human insulin. *Lancet* **330**: 382–5.

The DCCT Research Group (1991). Epidemiology of severe hypoglycemia in the Diabetes Control and Complications Trial. *American Journal of Medicine* **90**: 450–9.

The Diabetes Control and Complications Trial Research Group (1993). The effect of intensive treatment of diabetes on the development and progression of long-term complications in insulin-dependent diabetes mellitus. *The New England Journal of Medicine* **329**: 977–86.

Thorsteinsson B, Pramming S, Lauritzen T, Binder C (1986). Frequency of daytime biochemical hypoglycaemia in insulin-treated diabetic patients: relation to daily median blood glucose concentrations. *Diabetic Medicine* **3**: 147–51.

Tribl G, Howorka K, Heger G, Anderer P, Thoma H, Zeitlhofer J (1996). EEG topography during insulin-induced hypoglycemia in patients with insulin-dependent diabetes mellitus. *European Neurology* **36**: 303–9.

Vea H, Jorde R, Sager G, Vaaler S, Sundsfjord J (1992). Reproducibility of glycaemic thresholds for activation of counterregulatory hormones and hypoglycaemic symptoms in healthy subjects. *Diabetologia* **35**: 958–61.

Veneman T, Mitrakou A, Mokan M, Cryer P, Gerich J (1993). Induction of hypoglycemia unawareness by asymptomatic nocturnal hypoglycemia. *Diabetes* **42**: 1233–7.

Widom B, Simonson DC (1992). Intermittent hypoglycemia impairs glucose counterregulation. *Diabetes* **41**: 1335–40.

6

Risks of Strict Glycaemic Control

STEPHANIE A. AMIEL
King's College School of Medicine and Dentistry, London

INTRODUCTION

The benefit of strict glycaemic control in diminishing the risks of the development of long-term complications of diabetes is beyond doubt, but the negative aspects of such therapies need to be considered, and their risks identified, understood and minimised. As a result of continuing research, some of the acute morbidity of hypoglycaemia associated with current insulin regimens for strict glycaemic control has been reduced (Jorgens et al, 1993; The Diabetes Control and Complications Trial Research Group, 1997) but more can still be done. The residual risk needs to be explained carefully to each patient, who can then make their individual, informed choice about the degree of glycaemic control that they consider to be acceptable.

The risks of intensified insulin therapy are those of insulin therapy itself, intensified. Thus the major side-effects are *weight gain* (The DCCT Research Group, 1988), resulting mainly from the elimination of the loss of calories through glycosuria and therefore (theoretically) responsive to dietary strategies, and *hypoglycaemia* (The Diabetes Control and Complications Trial Research Group, 1993; 1995a; 1997). When cohorts of patients are studied rather than individuals, other potential risks of the demands of intensified insulin therapies, and in particular the inherent psychosocial strains, do not appear to be a major problem (The Diabetes

Hypoglycaemia in Clinical Diabetes. Edited by B. M. Frier and B. M. Fisher.

Control and Complications Trial Research Group, 1996a). The data in the Diabetes Control and Complication Trial (DCCT) showed that patients in the intensive treatment arm of the study had an overall improvement in their subjective feelings of control and well-being that were offset by an increased fear of hypoglycaemia (The Diabetes Control and Complications Trial Research Group, 1996a). This balance may be particularly positive in people who actively choose to use intensified therapies, and benefits to the individual may be less apparent in the context of a large trial. This chapter examines the problem of hypoglycaemia associated with strict glycaemic control, an area that has aroused much concern and controversy.

DEFINITION OF HYPOGLYCAEMIA

It is difficult to determine a frequency of hypoglycaemia without first defining what is meant by "hypoglycaemia". In many studies, hypoglycaemia is documented by self-reporting, which may be very unreliable (Heller et al, 1995). Retrospective analyses suffer from problems of recall, and accurate documentation of hypoglycaemia is obtained only in prospective research studies that require biochemical verification of low blood glucose concentrations.

Hypoglycaemia can be categorised by its symptomatology and its severity, but even here there is no real consensus (see Chapter 3). "Mild" hypoglycaemia is usually defined as an episode that is recognised by and treated by the patient and does not significantly disrupt daily living; "severe" hypoglycaemia may employ the DCCT definition as an episode where blood glucose has fallen to a level where the patient has become so disabled that assistance is required from another person (The Diabetes Control and Complications Trial Research Group, 1991). Alternatively, "severe" hypoglycaemia may be defined by the requirement for parenteral treatment (intramuscular glucagon or intravenous dextrose), with or without hospital admission, or by the development of coma (The Diabetes Control and Complications Trial Research Group, 1987). A category of "moderate" hypoglycaemia, in which an individual requires external assistance but which falls short of requiring parenteral therapy or developing a coma, or the division of hypoglycaemia into grades of severity can also be used (Limbert et al, 1993). Obviously the definition used will affect the estimate of incidence, and if severe hypoglycaemia is defined solely as coma, rates will be lower than if all episodes requiring assistance are included.

Various levels of blood glucose concentration have been used to define mild and moderate hypoglycaemia, but increasingly there is an awareness that the blood glucose concentrations which are used arbitrarily to define pathological spontaneous hypoglycaemia (e.g. < 2.2 mmol/l) are unsuitable for defining hypoglycaemia in people with diabetes. Arterialised plasma glucose concentration of around 3.6 mmol/l is sufficient to cause physiological autonomic responses in healthy volunteers (Chapter 1). Subtle changes in cognitive function can initially be detected by formal testing below 4.0 mmol/l, although clinically relevant cognitive impairment does not occur until the arterialised plasma glucose concentration has fallen to approximately 3.0 mmol/l (Chapter 2). There is evidence that if plasma glucose falls below 3.0 mmol/l for a period of time, this can reduce the symptomatic responses to a further episode of hypoglycaemia occurring within the following 24 hours (Heller and Cryer, 1991), so-called *antecedent hypoglycaemia* (Chapter 5). The continuous avoidance of low plasma glucose concentrations (below 3.0 mmol/l) can restore impaired hormonal and symptomatic responses to hypoglycaemia (Fanelli et al, 1993; Cranston et al, 1994), and it follows that values below 3.0 mmol/l can be considered to be hypoglycaemic. The British Diabetic Association have coined the phrase "make four the floor" to protect against potentially dangerous hypoglycaemia so that blood glucose concentrations of 3.3 (Kaufman and Devgan, 1996), or even 3.9 mmol/l (Clarke et al, 1995), may be considered to be "hypoglycaemia" with respect to optimising treatment regimens.

ALTERED COUNTERREGULATION AND SYMPTOMATIC AWARENESS IN RESPONSE TO HYPOGLYCAEMIA

Several studies have confirmed that impaired symptomatic awareness of hypoglycaemia is associated with an increased rate of severe hypoglycaemia (Hepburn et al, 1990; Gold et al, 1994; Clarke et al, 1995), although affected patients in these studies were not subject to strict glycaemic control. It is very important to appreciate that neither asymptomatic nor severe hypoglycaemia are restricted to people using intensified insulin therapy. However, patients using intensified insulin therapy may be three times more likely to record blood glucose concentrations of less than 2.8 mmol/l at times when they are asymptomatic but are routinely performing home blood glucose monitoring, than patients on conventional therapy (Lager et al, 1986). This is consistent with the three-fold higher rate of severe hypoglycaemia that was experienced by the intensively treated patients in the DCCT, when compared with that recorded by those on conventional therapy (The Diabetes Control and Complications Trial Research Group, 1991; 1993; 1997).

Patients describe symptoms of hypoglycaemia at a wide range of blood glucose concentrations. In an individual patient the main determinant of the blood glucose concentration at which protective responses start, is probably the prevailing range of blood glucose concentration to which the patient has been exposed in the recent past. For example, when patients with poorly controlled type 2 diabetes were studied with a controlled hypoglycaemic challenge after blood glucose had been normalised overnight, their adrenaline responses to hypoglycaemia started at a higher blood glucose than in well controlled patients (Korzon-Burakowska et al, 1998).

The first indication that strict glycaemic control might cause abnormal responses to hypoglycaemia was observed when controlled hypoglycaemia was induced in a small group of patients with type 1 diabetes before, and after, they had been treated with intensified insulin therapy (Simonson et al, 1985a). Following the improvement in glycaemic control, the magnitude of the counterregulatory hormonal response to an abrupt lowering of blood glucose to 2.8 mmol/l was significantly less than observed previously. This study had been planned to investigate the potential of better glycaemic control to restore some of the defects of normal counterregulation that develop in people with type 1 diabetes (see Chapter 4), so these results were unexpected. The importance of these preliminary observations was underlined by a subsequent study in which patients with type 1 diabetes receiving intensified insulin treatment were found to have impaired glucose counterregulation (Amiel et al, 1987). During an intravenous infusion of insulin, most patients were unable to maintain an arterialised plasma glucose above 3.0 mmol/l, in contrast to conventionally treated diabetic subjects who were less well controlled and had higher glycated haemoglobin concentrations, or to non-diabetic volunteers. The intensively treated diabetic patients were less symptomatic, and although the rise in their plasma adrenaline was of similar magnitude to the other groups, this occurred when the hypoglycaemia was more profound. Further studies of hypoglycaemia, using a stepped glucose clamp to produce controlled reduction of blood glucose, confirmed that the symptomatic and hormonal responses started at lower plasma glucose concentrations in patients with strict glycaemic control, and were delayed in onset and diminished in magnitude, for any given plasma glucose concentration (Amiel et al, 1988) (Figure 6.1).

Many subsequent studies have confirmed that the onset of symptomatic and hormonal responses to hypoglycaemia is both delayed and diminished in intensively treated diabetic subjects who have strict glycaemic control. This offers a partial explanation for the increased occurrence of asymptomatic biochemical hypoglycaemia. The risk may be particularly manifest when the glycated haemoglobin concentration is

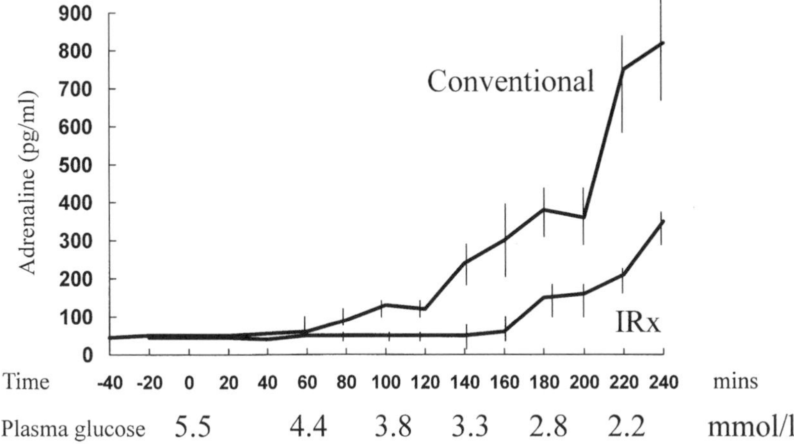

Figure 6.1 The effect of intensified diabetes therapy (IRx) on adrenaline responses to a slow reduction in plasma glucose over four hours. Adapted from Amiel et al (1988) with permission of The American Diabetes Association

reduced to within, or just above, the non-diabetic range (Box 6.1). This was shown in a study of 34 subjects with type 1 diabetes who had a wide range of total HbA1 values (Kinsley et al, 1995). They were subjected to a stepped glucose clamp to lower arterialised blood glucose to 2.2 mmol/l and the responses were compared with a non-diabetic control group. Symptomatic responses (particularly autonomic) and some counterregulatory hormonal responses were diminished in the seven diabetic subjects who had a total HbA1 of 7.85% or less, i.e. glycaemic control that was

Box 6.1 Effects of strict glycaemic control in type 1 diabetes

- Reduction in microvascular and macrovascular complications
- Increased risk of severe hypoglycaemia
- Diminished neuroendocrine and symptomatic responses to hypoglycaemia
- Altered glycaemic thresholds for activation of responses (i.e. lower blood glucose required)
- Promotion of increased frequency of exposure to hypoglycaemia which exacerbates impaired awareness of hypoglycaemia
- Tendency to weight gain

within their local non-diabetic range of total HbA1. A very similar study by Pampanelli et al (1996) produced identical observations in 10 of 33 subjects, whose HbA1c was within the local non-diabetic range, and in whom it was also noted that the onset of some aspects of cognitive dysfunction was delayed. Current evidence would suggest that it is the increased exposure to episodic hypoglycaemia associated with the treatment strategy that is promoting the problem (Fanelli et al, 1993; Cranston et al, 1994).

A study of 24 subjects with type 1 diabetes and 15 non-diabetic control subjects compared glucose uptake in the brain, symptoms of hypoglycaemia and counterregulatory hormonal responses at blood glucose values of 5.8 and 3.0 mmol/l (Boyle et al, 1995). The patients were stratified into three subject groups on the basis of their prevailing glycaemic control (estimated by total HbA1). In the group with the lowest glycated haemoglobin (equivalent to the upper end of the non-diabetic range) hypoglycaemic symptoms were absent and the patients had impaired awareness of hypoglycaemia (Figure 6.2). Counterregulatory hormonal responses were also diminished. This group also maintained their intake of glucose into the brain during hypoglycaemia, while this fell in other groups (Figure 6.2). The ability of the brain to maintain the supply of glucose during hypoglycaemia in strictly controlled patients may be a maladaptive response as it occurs at the expense of losing the normal warning signs of hypoglycaemia. This study by Boyle et al (1995) is consistent with the other studies demonstrating the risks of achieving strict glycaemic control in people with diabetes who have glycated haemoglobin values that are within the non-diabetic range. While this level of control does not by itself cause acute hypoglycaemia, the normal symptomatic warning and counterregulatory mechanisms may be compromised if hypoglycaemia does occur.

Although relatively few patients can achieve this level of glycaemic control, or sustain it for long, in clinical practice impaired awareness of hypoglycaemia is a major problem, and the risk is clearly associated with intensive insulin therapy. This may influence the level of glycaemic control that is recommended for individual patients. The problem is reversible, at least in the setting of carefully controlled research studies, by scrupulous avoidance of even modest hypoglycaemia in daily life (Fanelli et al, 1993; Cranston et al, 1994). Although this may result in a deterioration of glycaemic control, with a rise in mean HbA1c from 6.9% to 8.0% in one small study of seven patients with impaired awareness of hypoglycaemia as the problem was reversed (Liu et al, 1996), this is not inevitable (Cranston et al, 1994). It is possible for avoidance of hypoglycaemia to result in an improvement of glycated haemoglobin, as post-hypoglycaemia hyperglycaemia is eradicated.

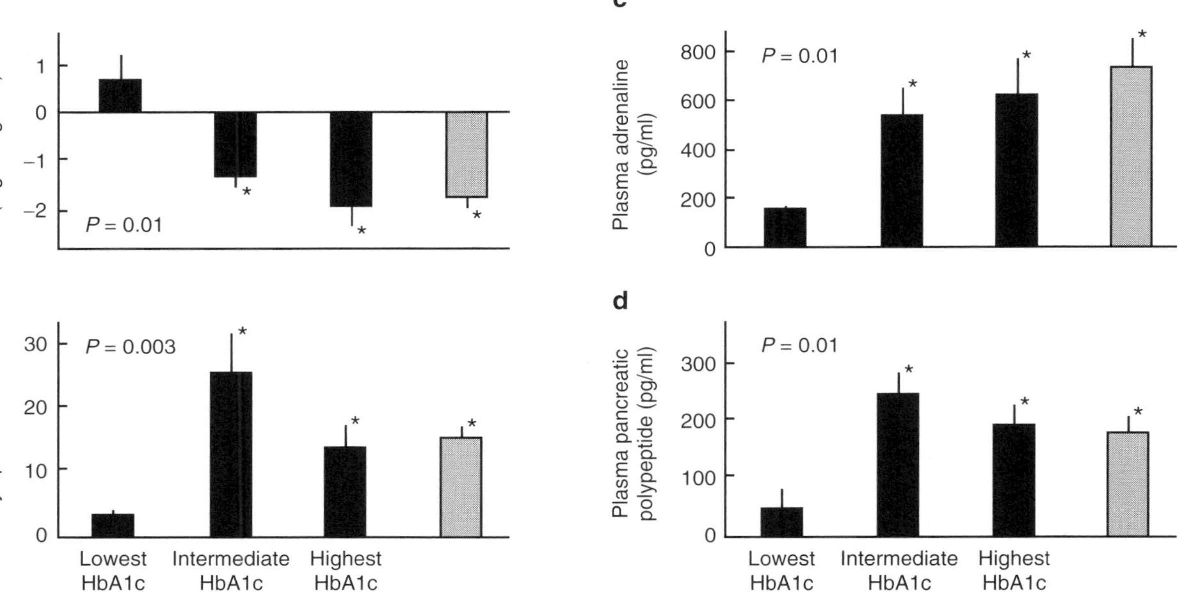

Figure 6.2 Changes from baseline (mean ± SD) in (a) glucose uptake in the brain, (b) hypoglycaemia symptom scores and plasma concentrations of (c) adrenaline and (d) pancreatic polypeptide during hypoglycaemia in patients with type 1 (insulin dependent) diabetes mellitus with differing degrees of glycaemic control (black bars), and in non-diabetic subjects (grey bars). From Boyle et al (1995) with permission of the *New England Journal of Medicine*

CEREBRAL ADAPTATION

When hypoglycaemia occurs, the stimulus for counterregulation appears to be a fall in the cerebral metabolic rate. Boyle et al (1994) measured arteriovenous differences in glucose concentration in the human brain during hypoglycaemia to show that the rate of uptake of glucose (and by implication of metabolism) falls before most of the counterregulatory responses and cognitive changes occur. They also demonstrated that this fall in metabolic rate of the brain was reduced in healthy volunteers who were made acutely hypoglycaemic following a period of 56 hours of protracted moderate hypoglycaemia, suggesting that the metabolism of the human brain can adapt to prolonged exposure to a low blood glucose. This enables the brain to maintain its metabolism and continue to function in response to subsequent hypoglycaemia. These findings are consistent with the observation described above, that diabetic patients with strict glycaemic control and impaired awareness of hypoglycaemia, were able to maintain the rate of cerebral uptake of glucose during experimental hypoglycaemia, while others with normal symptomatic awareness exhibited a marked fall in cerebral uptake of glucose, associated with symptomatic and counterregulatory hormonal responses (Boyle et al, 1995). Impaired awareness of hypoglycaemia and defective glucose counterregulation may therefore result from an adaptation in the sensitivity of the cerebral glucose sensor, which allows it to sustain its metabolic rate (and so not trigger counterregulation) during subsequent hypoglycaemia. This adaptation may be a consequence of previous recurrent exposure to hypoglycaemia and is therefore a particular risk to patients who are treated with intensive insulin therapy (Lager et al, 1986). Observations that the secretory response of cortisol to an initial hypoglycaemic challenge may blunt subsequent sympatho-adrenal responsiveness remain to be explained (Davis et al, 1997a).

Controversy has arisen over the extent to which adaptations of brain glucose metabolism to antecedent hypoglycaemia can occur. The cerebral cortex may be able to adapt to antecedent hypoglycaemia in a similar way to the putative cerebral glucose sensor. Some aspects of cognitive function are better preserved during hypoglycaemia in subjects who have previous experience of hypoglycaemia than in hypoglycaemia-naive subjects who have normal counterregulation (Fanelli et al, 1993; Boyle et al, 1995). This does not entirely fit the clinical picture of patients becoming significantly confused during hypoglycaemia while remaining asymptomatic. One measure of cognitive function, the choice reaction time, does not appear to adapt, and during slowly induced hypoglycaemia, deteriorates at similar levels of blood glucose in most subjects, irrespective of their previous glycaemic experience and their state of hypoglycaemia awareness (Maran et al, 1995). Other measures of cognitive function also deteriorate at similar levels of blood glucose in diabetic subjects who have had very disparate experiences of preceding glycaemia (Widom and Simonson, 1990; Amiel et al, 1991; Hvidberg et al, 1996).

These apparent discrepancies have led to suggestions that the ability of the brain to adapt its glucose metabolic capacity according to previous glycaemic experience may vary across different regions of the brain. It is possible that the regions of the brain that detect hypoglycaemia, and some parts of the cerebral cortex, may be able to adapt more effectively than other areas to sustain glucose metabolism during hypoglycaemia. As blood glucose falls this would effectively destroy the normal protective hierarchy of corrective and symptomatic responses that precede cognitive impairment, replacing it with the dangerous situation whereby cognitive impairment is the initial response to hypoglycaemia, with autonomic responses not occurring until the blood glucose reaches a lower level. In this situation the patient becomes too confused and unable to recognise the warning symptoms and so take appropriate corrective action (Figure 6.3).

The magnitude of the change in glycaemic thresholds for various functions of the brain in response to strict control of diabetes, is variable. Where glucose thresholds for cognitive dysfunction do alter in people with impaired awareness of hypoglycaemia, the differences between the blood glucose thresholds for the symptomatic and autonomic responses and those for the onset of cognitive impairment are much smaller. As a result, the window of opportunity for the patient to recognise that hypoglycaemia is developing is much narrower, giving less time for corrective action to be taken.

Intermittent antecedent hypoglycaemia appears to play a prominent role in the pathogenesis of impaired hypoglycaemia awareness and counterregulatory failure, and a high risk of severe hypoglycaemia is a major consequence (see Chapter 5). This causes an acute and transient impairment of the generation of symptoms and of hormonal responses to subsequent hypoglycaemia induced in an experimental setting, an effect that lasts for between 24 and 72 hours (George et al, 1995; 1997). It is surmised that possibly two episodes, each lasting one hour, with a blood glucose around 3.0 mmol/l, may be enough to induce significant defects in counterregulation to subsequent hypoglycaemia (Heller and Cryer 1991; Davis et al, 1997b).

OTHER RISKS OF INTENSIFIED INSULIN THERAPY: HYPERGLYCAEMIA AND HYPERINSULINAEMIA

While severe hypoglycaemia was indisputably the major metabolic side-

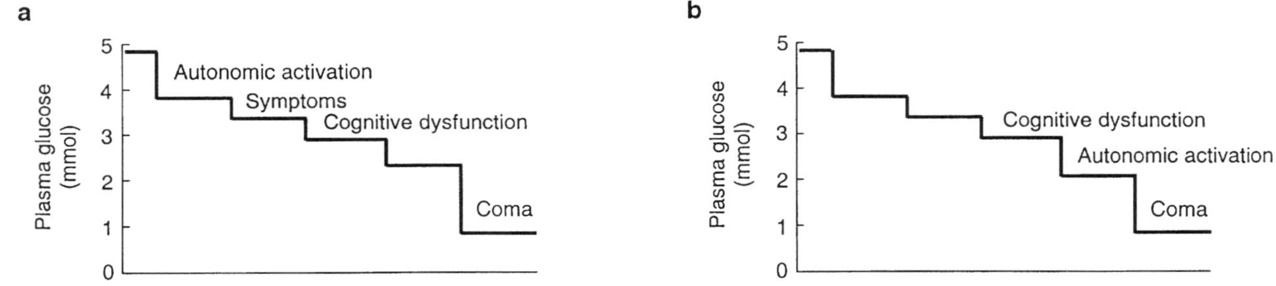

Figure 6.3 The change in hierarchy of responses to hypoglycaemia (a) before and (b) after intensified insulin therapy in type 1 diabetes mellitus

effect of intensive insulin therapy in the DCCT, concerns have been expressed that some intensive treatment regimens may also increase the risk of developing hyperglycaemia and ketosis. This relates mostly to the use of continuous subcutaneous insulin infusion (CSII) or insulin pump therapy, in which soluble insulin in low dosage is delivered steadily by a slow infusion throughout the day, and is accelerated before meals to deliver boluses, akin to giving intermittent subcutaneous injections of short-acting insulin. Because the basal insulin is delivered in a very low volume and there is no depot of intermediate-acting insulin in the subcutaneous tissues to act as a reservoir, an interruption in the delivery of insulin can rapidly lead to hyperglycaemia and even ketosis, especially if the patient's blood glucose is already elevated (Castilloa et al, 1996). This may occur as a result of disconnection of the pump, air in the delivery system, blockage in the tubing or more rarely, mechanical failure of the pump. Whether diabetic ketoacidosis (DKA) is more common with CSII remains controversial, but a meta-analysis of trials of CSII has indicated that the rate of DKA is significantly increased (Egger et al, 1997). The rate of development of DKA was slightly higher in intensively treated patients in the DCCT, although many of those patients used multiple injections of insulin to improve their glycaemic control (The Diabetes Control and Complications Trial Research Group, 1995b). It is thought that the learning experiences obtained in the early years of the DCCT, helped to reduce the risk of DKA in patients on intensive therapy in the later years of the study. This certainly appeared to be the case for severe hypoglycaemia, which became progressively less common as time progressed, both in intensively and conventionally treated subjects in the DCCT. However, the 3:1 incidence ratio of severe hypoglycaemia persisted between the two groups (The Diabetes Control and Complications Trial Research Group, 1997).

Intensive insulin therapy often leads to a redistribution of the times of administration of insulin rather than a straightforward increase in dosage, and there are concerns that continuous peripheral hyperinsulinaemia may be deleterious. This anxiety may be more theoretical than real, as improved glycaemic control in type 1 diabetes improves insulin sensitivity (Simonson et al, 1985b) which ultimately should reduce hyperinsulinaemia. However, achieving adequate plasma concentrations of insulin in the hepatic circulation is always likely to be at the cost of promoting hyperinsulinaemia in the systemic circulation, as insulin has to be delivered by subcutaneous injection. This potential overinsulinisation may contribute to the risk of hypoglycaemia, and when insulin is delivered portally, as in intraperitoneal infusion systems, hypoglycaemia is less frequent at any given blood glucose level (Lassmann-Vague et al, 1996; Dunn et al, 1997). However, one study (Figure 6.4) has demon-

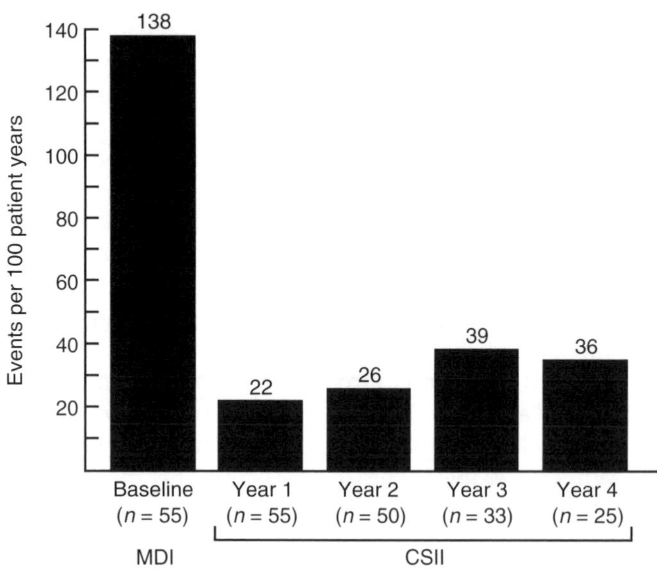

Figure 6.4 Severe hypoglycaemia (events per 100 patient-years) at baseline with multiple daily injections (MDI) and by year on continuous subcutaneous insulin infusion (CSII). From Bode et al (1996) with permission of the The American Diabetes Association

strated a pronounced and sustained reduction in the frequency of severe hypoglycaemia following the transfer of patients from multiple injections of insulin to CSII (Bode et al, 1996) so appropriate temporal distribution of the action of insulin may be the critical factor in preventing hypoglycaemia. A further concern is that hyperinsulinaemia is the link between insulin resistance and an increased risk of macrovascular disease. In the DCCT, surrogate markers of macrovascular disease either showed no change, or demonstrated a lower frequency of macrovascular events in the intensively treated group, but as the frequency of such events was very low in this young population, this is difficult to evaluate (The Diabetes Control and Complications Trial Research Group, 1995c).

THERAPEUTIC MANIPULATION: AVOIDANCE OF HYPOGLYCAEMIA

It is important to stress that management of the potentially devastating syndrome of impaired awareness of hypoglycaemia and deficient counterregulation, with its high risk of severe hypoglycaemia, should not be an excuse for encouraging poor glycaemic control. However, patients with this acquired syndrome are not suitable for intensive insulin therapy and very strict glycaemic control, and blood glucose targets may have to be higher when faced with these problems. Frequent blood glucose monitoring is essential to identify biochemical hypoglycaemia, and the use of basal-bolus insulin regimens (which use predominantly short-acting insulins) may be beneficial in avoiding recurrent hypoglycaemia. However, the restoration of defences to hypoglycaemia is dependent upon the avoidance of hypoglycaemia in daily life, and not on the overall elevation of blood glucose and tolerance of a high glycated haemoglobin. As discussed above, the studies which have attempted to restore awareness of hypoglycaemia by avoidance of hypoglycaemia did not induce any major loss of glycaemic control, although a modest increase in HbA1c of around 0.5–1.0% occurred (Fanelli et al, 1993; Dagogo-Jack et al, 1994). Anecdotally, average blood glucose concentrations and HbA1c may even improve with strategies for avoiding hypoglycaemia, as the patient's blood glucose stops fluctuating from too high to too low.

Strategies to avoid hypoglycaemia are very time-consuming and labour-intensive, for the patient as well as for the physician, and require several supportive measures, such as having to maintain daily telephone contact between the patient and the medical and nursing staff (Fanelli et al, 1993). It took Cranston et al (1994) up to 12 months for the subjects taking part in their study to achieve three consecutive weeks when the home blood glucose readings did not fall below 3.0 mmol/l. Two of three studies have demonstrated partial recovery of the counterregulatory responses to hypoglycaemia (Fanelli et al, 1993; Cranston et al, 1994), but one has not (Dagogo-Jack et al, 1994), although the symptoms of hypoglycaemia were restored. The number of subjects was small in all of the studies. The practical application of strategies to avoid daily hypoglycaemia requires resources which at present are probably beyond those of most diabetes centres.

PATIENT EDUCATION

Given the labour-intensive nature of attempts to avoid hypoglycaemia and to treat impaired awareness of hypoglycaemia, and the undesirable development of patient dependency on the staff of the diabetes clinic, is it possible to apply these strategies in routine clinical care? Patient education remains the mainstay of such efforts, and it is the patient who must control their treatment regimen and daily activities to try to avoid recurrent hypoglycaemia coexisting with strict glycaemic control. Conventional patient education may not be able to equip patients adequately when intensive insulin therapy is utilised to achieve satisfactory levels of glycated haemoglobin without also inducing undesirable hypoglycaemia. A German group has claimed remarkable success with such treatment using a structured programme of education (Jorgens et al, 1993). Similarly, an American study used an eight-week, structured programme of group education to achieve a similar reduction in glycated haemoglobin with less exposure to significant hypoglycaemia (Kinsley et al, 1997), applying the technique of blood glucose awareness training (Cox et al, 1989). However, this also required considerable resources and will have to be tested outside North America to assess its universal applicability.

The main defence against recurrent hypoglycaemia with its consequent blunting of subjective symptomatic awareness, remains the establishment of therapeutic goals that are realistic for individual patients. The physician's tendency to concentrate on eliminating hyperglycaemia has led to subnormal blood glucose values being ignored, a practice worsened by the belief of some physicians and patients that, because an episode of biochemical hypoglycaemia is asymptomatic, it is not important. There is no doubt that a clinically detectable deterioration in performance of some aspects of cognitive function occurs in human subjects at arterialised blood glucose concentrations of 3.0 mmol/l (see Chapter 2), and an absence of symptoms at that level should ring alarm bells with the patient's physician. Given that healthy non-diabetic subjects do not commonly exhibit fasting blood glucose concentrations under 4.0 mmol/l, it seems wholly unnecessary to encourage or even permit such subnormality in patients with diabetes (one exception to this maxim being during diabetic pregnancy where healthy pregnant women do exhibit lower blood glucose levels—see Chapter 10). With intensive insulin therapy the therapeutic target should be near-normal blood glucose levels: before meals 4.0 to 7.0 mmol/l, after meals 4.0 to 9.0 mmol/l (depending on time of testing), with a slightly higher than normal glucose at bedtime (7.0 to 9.0 mmol/l) to reduce the risk of hypoglycaemia occurring during the night. Blood glucose measured during the night may be a little lower ($\geqslant$ 3.6 mmol/l) but in view of the evidence presented above, patients should avoid being any lower than this.

PATIENTS UNSUITABLE FOR STRICT CONTROL

The DCCT has demonstrated that any reduction in glycated haemoglobin is associated with a reduced risk of microvascular complications over time, and the benefits are greater with higher glycated haemoglobin concentrations (The Diabetes Control and Complications Trial Research Group, 1996b). A cross-sectional study which suggested that the risk reduction for nephropathy is near-maximal at a glycated haemoglobin of

8% (Krolewski et al, 1995) cannot be extrapolated to other microvascular complications, as in the DCCT no glycaemic threshold (estimated by glycated haemoglobin) for the development of retinopathy was demonstrated in a patient group whose average HbA1c was 7%. Thus, unless an individual already has a normal glycated haemoglobin with no problematical hypoglycaemia, no patient who has diabetes is unsuitable for attempts to improve their glycaemic control.

Realistically, there are patients in whom attempts to achieve a near normal glycated haemoglobin are not appropriate (Box 6.2). Patients with advanced complications, especially retinopathy, have not been shown to benefit and a sudden improvement in glycaemic control may cause an acceleration in severity of pre-proliferative or early proliferative retinopathy (Hanssen et al, 1986). Although some authorities claim that this should not be a contraindication to improving glycaemic control (Chantelau and Kohner, 1997), as yet there is no real evidence for benefit in advanced cases and the retinopathy should be stabilised with appropriate laser treatment before glycaemic control is tightened. Similarly, in patients with established renal impairment and severe macrovascular disease, attempts to treat elevated blood pressure and plasma lipids and to encourage patients to stop smoking may be more beneficial than targeting glycaemic control. As intensive insulin therapy is aimed at achieving benefit over a period of 10 to 15 years or more, patients with a lower life expectancy should not be exposed to the risks and rigours associated with this treatment regimen. This applies also to elderly patients, many of whom are frail and physically inactive.

Box 6.2 Application of strict glycaemic control in type 1 diabetes

Caution required:

- Long duration of insulin-treated diabetes (counterregulatory deficiences)
- Previous history of severe hypoglycaemia
- Established impaired awareness of hypoglycaemia
- History of epilepsy
- Patient unwilling to do home blood glucose monitoring

Contraindicated:

- Extremes of age
- Ischaemic heart disease
- Advanced diabetic complications
- Limited life expectancy (e.g. serious co-existing disease)

Very young patients may not be good candidates for very strict glycaemic control. Poor control should not be encouraged in children, as growth may be jeopardised, and there is some evidence that prepubertal glycaemic control may influence the later risk of complications (Donaghue et al, 1997; Holl et al, 1998). However, very small children, who are very insulin-sensitive, may be at risk of intellectual damage if exposed to recurrent severe hypoglycaemia (see Chapter 8).

It is the patient who determines the degree of glycaemic control that they feel is worth the effort. Patients with very erratic life styles, and those who are not prepared to commit themselves to regular self-monitoring of blood glucose, with frequent attention to the timing of injection and adjustment of dosage of insulin, cannot safely undertake measures to achieve near-normoglycaemia. A compromise must be reached after a full discussion of the risks. Patients currently experiencing problematical hypoglycaemia may not wish to aim for glycaemic targets near the normal range, although the regimens of intensive insulin therapy may still be appropriate for them if they can eliminate hypoglycaemia from their daily lives. This may also be true of people undertaking dangerous or physically demanding jobs, who may deliberately set higher blood glucose targets to protect against hypoglycaemia, but who should be encouraged to practice regular self-monitoring and adjustment of insulin doses. It is the informed patient who must determine their therapeutic aims at any given time. The doctor's role is to try to ensure that the patient has the knowledge to make appropriate decisions and to provide the tools to achieve these.

CONCLUSIONS

- The principal risks of intensive insulin therapy are hypoglycaemia and weight gain.
- Patients using intensive insulin regimens may be three times more likely to have an episode of severe hypoglycaemia than those on conventional insulin regimens.
- The counterregulatory responses to hypoglycaemia and symptomatic awareness are reduced in patients on intensive insulin therapy, particularly if glycated haemoglobin is within the non-diabetic range.
- Total avoidance of hypoglycaemia can restore the symptomatic response to hypoglycaemia, but achieving this is de-

continues

continued

manding and time-consuming, both for patients and health-care professionals.

- Few patients are unsuitable for attempts to improve glycaemic control, but the increased risk of severe hypoglycaemia for patients on intensive insulin regimens may make strict control of diabetes difficult to achieve and may limit what is possible or even desirable in some patients.

REFERENCES

Amiel SA, Tamborlane WV, Simonson DC, Sherwin RS (1987). Defective glucose counterregulation after strict glycemic control of insulin-dependent diabetes mellitus. *N Engl J Med* **316**: 1376–83.

Amiel SA, Sherwin RS, Simonson DC, Tamborlane WV (1988). Effect of intensive insulin therapy on glycemic thresholds for counterregulatory hormone release. *Diabetes* **37**: 901–7.

Amiel SA, Pottinger RC, Archibald HR, Chusney G, Cunnah DTF, Prior PF, Gale EAM (1991). Effect of antecedent glucose control on cerebral function during hypoglycemia. *Diabetes Care* **14**: 109–18.

Bode BW, Steed RD, Davidson PC (1996). Reduction in severe hypoglycemia with long-term continuous subcutaneous insulin infusion in type 1 diabetes. *Diabetes Care* **19**: 324–7.

Boyle PJ, Nagy RJ, O'Connor AM, Kempers SF, Yeo RA, Qualls C (1994). Adaptation in brain glucose uptake following recurrent hypoglycemia. *Proc Natl Acad Sci USA* **91**: 9352–6.

Boyle PJ, Kempers SF, O'Connor AM, Nagy RJ (1995). Brain glucose uptake and unawareness of hypoglycemia in patients with insulin-dependent diabetes mellitus. *N Engl J Med* **333**: 1726–31.

Castilloa MJ, Sheen AJ, Lefebvre PJ (1996). The degree/rapidity of the metabolic deterioration following interruption of a continuous subcutaneous insulin infusion is influenced by the prevailing blood glucose level. *J Clin Endocrinol Metab* **81**: 1975–8.

Chantelau E, Kohner EM (1997). Why some cases of retinopathy worsen when diabetic control improves. *BMJ* **315**: 1105–6.

Clarke WL, Cox DJ, Gonder-Frederick LA, Julian D, Schlundt D, Polonsky W (1995). Reduced awareness of hypoglycemia in adults with IDDM. A prospective study of hypoglycemic frequency and associated symptoms. *Diabetes Care* **18**: 517–22.

Cox DJ, Gonder-Frederick LA, Lee JH, Julian DM, Carter WR, Clarke WL (1989). Effects and correlates of blood glucose awareness training among patients with IDDM. *Diabetes Care* **12**: 313–8.

Cranston I, Lomas J, Maran A, Macdonald IA, Amiel SA (1994). Restoration of hypoglycaemia awareness in patients with long-duration insulin-dependent diabetes. *Lancet* **344**: 283–7.

Dagogo-Jack S, Rattarasarn C, Cryer PE (1994). Reversal of hypoglycemia unawareness, but not defective glucose counterregulation, in IDDM. *Diabetes* **43**: 1426–34.

Davis SN, Shavers C, Davis B, Costa F (1997a). Prevention of an increase in plasma cortisol during hypoglycemia prevents subsequent counterregulatory responses. *J Clin Invest* **100**: 429–38.

Davis SN, Shavers C, Mosqueda-Garcia R, Costa F (1997b). Effects of differing antecedent hypoglycemia on subsequent counterregulation in normal humans. *Diabetes* **46**: 1328–35.

Donaghue KC, Fung AT, Hing S, Fairchild J, King J, Chan A, Howard NJ, Silink M (1997). The effect of prepubertal diabetes duration on diabetes microvascular complications in early and late adolescence. *Diabetes Care* **20**: 77–80.

Dunn FL, Nathan DM, Scavini M, Selam JL, Wingrove TG (1997). Long term therapy of IDDM with an implantable insulin pump. The implantable insulin pump trial study group. *Diabetes Care* **20**: 59–63.

Egger M, Davey Smith G, Stettler C, Diem P (1997). Risk of adverse effects of intensified treatment in insulin-dependent diabetes mellitus: a meta-analysis. *Diabet Med* **14**: 919–28.

Fanelli CG, Epifano L, Rambotti AM et al (1993). Meticulous prevention of hypoglycemia normalizes the glycemic thresholds and magnitude of most of neuroendocrine responses to, symptoms of, and cognitive function during hypoglycemia in intensively treated patients with short-term IDDM. *Diabetes* **42**: 1683–9.

George E, Harris N, Bedford C, Macdonald IA, Hardisty CA, Heller SR (1995). Prolonged but partial impairment of the hypoglycaemic physiological response following short-term hypoglycaemia in normal subjects. *Diabetologia* **38**: 1183–90.

George E, Marques JL, Harris ND, Macdonald IA, Hardisty CA, Heller SR (1997). Preservation of physiological responses to hypoglycemia 2 days after antecedent hypoglycemia in patients with IDDM. *Diabetes Care* **20**: 1293–8.

Gold AE, MacLeod KM, Frier BM (1994). Frequency of severe hypoglycemia in patients with type 1 diabetes with impaired awareness of hypoglycemia. *Diabetes Care* **17**: 697–703.

Hanssen KF, Dahl-Jorgensen K, Lauritzen T, Feldt-Rasmussen B, Brinchmann-Hansen O, Deckert T (1986). Diabetic control and microvascular complications: the near-normoglycaemic experience. *Diabetologia* **29**: 677–84.

Heller SR, Cryer PE (1991). Reduced neuroendocrine and symptomatic responses to subsequent hypoglycemia after 1 episode of hypoglycemia in nondiabetic humans. *Diabetes* **40**: 223–6.

Heller S, Chapman J, McLoud J, Ward J (1995). Unreliability of reports of hypoglycaemia by diabetic patients. *BMJ* **310**: 440.

Hepburn DA, Patrick AW, Eadington DW, Ewing DJ, Frier BM (1990). Unawareness of hypoglycaemia in insulin-treated diabetic patients: prevalence and relationship to autonomic neuropathy. *Diabet Med* **7**: 711–7.

Holl RW, Lang GE, Grabert M, Heinze E, Lang GK, Debatin KM (1998). Diabetic retinopathy in pediatric patients with type 1 diabetes: effect of diabetes duration, prepubertal and pubertal onset of diabetes, and metabolic control. *J Pediatr* **132**: 790–4.

Hvidberg A, Fanelli CG, Hershey T, Terkamp C, Craft S, Cryer PE (1996). Impact of recent antecedent hypoglycemia on hypoglycemic cognitive dysfunction in nondiabetic humans. *Diabetes* **45**: 1030–6.

Jorgens V, Gruber M, Bott U, Mulhauser I, Berger M (1993). Effective and safe translation of intensified insulin therapy to general internal medicine departments. *Diabetologia* **36**: 99–105.

Kaufman FR, Devgan S (1996). Use of uncooked cornstarch to avert nocturnal hypoglycemia in children and adolescents with type 1 diabetes mellitus. *J Diabetes Complications* **10**: 84–7.

Kinsley BT, Widom B, Simonson DC (1995). Differential regulation of counterregulatory hormone secretion and symptoms during hypoglycemia in IDDM. Effect of glycemic control. *Diabetes Care* **18**; 17–26.

Kinsley BT, Weinger K, Bajaj M, Levy CJ, Waters M, Simonson DC, Cox D, Jacobson AM (1997). Blood Glucose Awareness Training preserves epinephrine responses to hypoglycemia during intensive treatment in IDDM. *Diabetes* **46** (suppl 1): 42A (abstract).

Korzon-Burakowska A, Hopkins D, Matyka K, Lomas J, Pernet A, Macdonald I, Amiel S (1998). Effects of glycemic control on protective responses against hypoglycemia in type 2 diabetes. *Diabetes Care* **21**: 283–90.

Krolewski AS, Laffel LM, Krolewski M, Quinn M, Warram JH (1995). Glycosylated hemoglobin and the risk of microalbuminuria in patients with insulin-dependent diabetes mellitus. *N Engl J Med* **332**: 1251–5.

Lager I, Atvall S, Blohme G, Smith U (1986). Altered recognition of hypoglycaemic symptoms in type 1 diabetes during intensified control with continuous subcutaneous insulin infusion. *Diabet Med* **3**: 322–5.

Lassmann-Vague V, Belicar P, Alessis C, Raccah D, Vialettes B, Vague P (1996). Insulin kinetics in type I diabetic patients treated by continuous intraperitoneal insulin infusion: influence of anti-insulin antibodies. *Diabet Med* **13**: 1051–5.

Limbert C, Schwingshandl J, Haas J, Roth R, Borkenstein M (1993). Severe hypoglycemia in children and adolescents with IDDM: frequency and associated factors. *J Diabetes Complications* **7**: 216–20.

Liu D, McManus RM, Ryan EA (1996). Improved counter-regulatory hormonal and symptomatic responses to hypoglycemia in patients with insulin-dependent diabetes mellitus after 3 months of less strict glycemic control. *Clin Invest Med* **19**: 71–82.

Maran A, Lomas J, Macdonald IA, Amiel SA (1995). Lack of preservation of higher brain function during hypoglycaemia in patients with intensively-treated IDDM. *Diabetologia* **38**: 1412–18.

Pampanelli S, Fanelli C, Lalli C et al (1996). Long-term intensive therapy in IDDM: effects on HbA1c, risk for severe and mild hypoglycaemia, status of counterregulation and awareness of hypoglycaemia. *Diabetologia* **39**: 677–86.

Simonson DC, Tamborlane WV, DeFronzo RA, Sherwin RS (1985a). Intensive insulin therapy reduces counterregulatory hormone responses to hypoglycemia in patients with type 1 diabetes. *Ann Intern Med* **103**: 184–90.

Simonson DC, Tamborlane WV, Sherwin RS, Smith JD, DeFronzo RA (1985b). Improved insulin sensitivity in patients with type 1 diabetes mellitus after CSII. *Diabetes* **34**(suppl 3): 80–6.

The Diabetes Control and Complications Trial Research Group (1987). The Diabetes Control and Complications Trial (DCCT). Results of a feasibility study. *Diabetes Care* **10**: 1–19.

The Diabetes Control and Complications Trial Research Group (1988). Weight gain associated with intensive therapy in the Diabetes Control and Complications Trial. *Diabetes Care* **11**: 567–73.

The Diabetes Control and Complications Trial Research Group (1991). Epidemiol-

ogy of severe hypoglycemia in the Diabetes Control and Complications Trial. *Am J Med* **90**: 450–9.
The Diabetes Control and Complications Trial Research Group (1993). The effect of intensive treatment of diabetes on the development and progression of long-term complications in insulin-dependent diabetes mellitus. *N Engl J Med* **329**: 977–86.
The Diabetes Control and Complications Trial Research Group (1995a). Adverse events and their association with treatment regimens in the Diabetes Control and Complications Trial. *Diabetes Care* **18**: 1415–27.
The Diabetes Control and Complications Trial Research Group (1995b). Implementation of treatment protocols in the Diabetes Control and Complications Trial. *Diabetes Care* **18**: 361–76.
The Diabetes Control and Complications Trial Research Group (1995c). Effect of intensive diabetes management on macrovascular events and risk factors during the Diabetes Control and Complications Trial. *Am J Cardiol* **75**: 894–903.
The Diabetes Control and Complications Trial Research Group (1996a). Influence of intensive diabetes treatment on quality-of-life outcomes in the Diabetes Control and Complications Trial. *Diabetes Care* **19**: 195–203.
The Diabetes Control and Complications Trial Research Group (1996b). The absence of a glycemic threshold for the development of long-term complications: the perspective of the Diabetes Control and Complications Trial. *Diabetes* **45**: 1289–98.
The Diabetes Control and Complications Trial Research Group (1997). Hypoglycemia in the Diabetes Control and Complications Trial. *Diabetes* **46**: 271–86.
Widom B, Simonson DC (1990). Glycemic control and neuropsychologic function during hypoglycemia in patients with insulin-dependent diabetes mellitus. *Annals of Internal Medicine* **112**: 904–12.

7

Mortality, Cardiovascular Morbidity and Possible Effects of Hypoglycaemia on Diabetic Complications

B. MILES FISHER and SIMON R. HELLER*
Royal Alexandra Hospital, Paisley and *Department of Medicine, University of Sheffield

INTRODUCTION

For patients with type 1 diabetes, insulin-induced hypoglycaemia is one of the most feared consequences of the disorder (Pramming et al, 1991). It is perhaps the major factor which prevents most patients from attempting intensive insulin therapy and achieving the level of strict glycaemic control which is necessary to prevent the development of diabetic complications. Some fear the immediate lack of self-control which can accompany the impairment of cognitive function during acute hypoglycaemia. Others are embarrassed by the dependence on other people for assistance during an episode of severe hypoglycaemia. Many share the worries expressed by some diabetes healthcare professionals about the possible long-term effects of recurrent hypoglycaemia on the brain (see Chapter 8).

An additional factor which may prevent many patients from improving their glycaemic control is the fear of dying during an episode of hypoglycaemia, especially when this occurs during sleep. These anxieties

Hypoglycaemia in Clinical Diabetes. Edited by B. M. Frier and B. M. Fisher.

may be shared by the patient's relatives who may have witnessed previous episodes of nocturnal hypoglycaemia or convulsions, about which the patient has no recollection. Fear of hypoglycaemia has been increased by the publicity which surrounded the possible adverse effects of human insulin, and in particular the knowledge that some young people with type 1 (insulin-dependent) diabetes have died suddenly and unexpectedly, the so-called "dead in bed syndrome" (Campbell, 1991).

It would be wrong for healthcare professionals to dismiss such fears as irrational. Many professionals will have first- or second-hand experience of the sudden death of a patient with type 1 diabetes in circumstances which have implicated acute hypoglycaemia. This chapter examines the epidemiology and causes of death from hypoglycaemia in patients with diabetes, including those risk factors which appear to be associated with sudden death. The "dead in bed syndrome" is explored in detail, and comparisons drawn with other syndromes of sudden death in people who do not have diabetes. Putative mechanisms and risk factors for sudden death are described. Hypoglycaemia may also cause significant cardiovascular morbidity in people with diabetes, and the effects on heart disease and cardiovascular disease are examined. Finally, the hypothesis that hypoglycaemia may worsen the chronic microvascular complications of diabetes is discussed briefly.

DEATHS ATTRIBUTABLE TO HYPOGLYCAEMIA

Epidemiological Problems

Until recently it has been difficult to estimate the total number of patients in any one area who have diabetes, but this information is now becoming available, prompted by the response to the Saint Vincent Declaration by the World Health Organisation (Europe). Hypoglycaemia and its avoidance is not one of the stated goals for people with diabetes so that information on the epidemiology of hypoglycaemia has to be collected separately from the Saint Vincent data set. However, data on hypoglycaemia have now been included in the enlarged data set as proposed by the British Diabetic Association (Vaughan and Home, 1995).

The cause of death is often recorded inaccurately on the death certificate, even to the extent of omitting "diabetes" altogether. Subsequent problems with analysis of death certificates can be compounded in the United Kingdom by the fact that "hypoglycaemia" is not coded under one single heading. Furthermore, the exact coding of the cause of death is often left to the discretion of individual coding clerks who usually have no knowledge of the clinical details (Tattersall and Gale, 1993).

These factors make it impossible to obtain any precise estimates of the frequency of sudden death, in addition to the inaccuracy of records of the frequency of severe hypoglycaemia. Many episodes of hypoglycaemia, including nocturnal hypoglycaemia, are not recognised by patients or carers. If we add the difficulty of confirming hypoglycaemia at post-mortem, it is not surprising that there is considerable uncertainty and variation in the estimated number of deaths which are attributed to hypoglycaemia in people with diabetes. However, since hypoglycaemia is extremely common, we can conclude that the risk of death from an individual episode is probably extremely low.

Problems in Establishing the Cause of Death at Post-mortem

In attempting to establish a post-mortem diagnosis of hypoglycaemia, the pathologist needs to perform biochemical tests, examine the brain for evidence of hypoglycaemic brain damage, and exclude any other possible cause of death (Tattersall and Gale, 1993). Carbohydrate metabolism continues after death, and post-mortem changes in blood glucose can cause difficulties in confirming a hypoglycaemic death forensically. The continuing breakdown of glycogen (glycogenolysis) increases the blood glucose concentration in the inferior vena cava, so that the presence of a normal or high blood glucose concentration on the right side of the heart does not exclude ante-mortem hypoglycaemia (a false negative result for a diagnosis of hypoglycaemia). In the peripheral circulation glucose continues to be utilised by red blood cells, so that the presence of a low glucose concentration does not necessarily indicate ante-mortem hypoglycaemia. Indeed a low blood glucose is often found after death in those without diabetes (a false positive result for a diagnosis of hypoglycaemia).

The measurement of the glucose concentration in the vitreous humour presents similar problems because of continued post-mortem glucose utilisation, and so this cannot be used to confirm ante-mortem hypoglycaemia (false positive). A normal or raised glucose concentration in the vitreous humour after death, however, excludes hypoglycaemia at the time of death (true negative). Thus, the sensitivities and specificities of blood and vitreous humour measurements of glucose in diagnosing ante-mortem hypoglycaemia are unknown.

In addition to the biochemical problems in diagnosing hypoglycaemia after death, errors may be introduced by an attribution bias of the pathologist performing the post-mortem. Death may be attributed to minor degrees of coronary heart disease, since it is so common in the diabetic population (false negative result for a diagnosis of hypoglycaemia). Alternatively, the pathologist, even when unsure, may attribute death to hypoglycaemia rather than indicating no cause on a certificate (false positive).

CRUDE ESTIMATES OF HYPOGLYCAEMIA MORTALITY

Because of the problems detailed above, any estimate of mortality from hypoglycaemia will be crude. Published reports range from no deaths attributable to hypoglycaemia at one extreme to between 20 and 25% in reports from some Scandinavian centres. Most studies suggest that the proportion of deaths caused by hypoglycaemia is between 2% and 6%, a lower frequency than those associated with ketoacidosis, and is higher in younger age groups (Laing et al, 1999). For a more detailed analysis the reader is referred to the review by Tattersall and Gale (1993).

If deaths caused by renal failure or coronary heart disease in people with diabetes continue to decline as diabetes care improves, then the relative proportion of deaths caused by hypoglycaemia may increase. This is particularly likely if intensive insulin therapy is adopted more widely in an attempt to prevent or reduce microvascular disease (The DCCT Research Group, 1991; The Diabetes Control and Complications Trial Research Group, 1993).

RISKS OF DEATH FROM HYPOGLYCAEMIA

The risk factors which are commonly cited as increasing the risk of death from hypoglycaemia are often based on anecdote, and may owe more to the prejudices of individual clinicians than scientific evidence. Those suggested are detailed in Box 7.1 and include alcohol abuse and/or inebriation (Arky et al, 1968; Kalimo and Olsson, 1980; Critchley et al, 1984; MacCuish, 1993), psychiatric illness or personality disorder (Shenfield et al, 1980; Tunbridge, 1981), self-neglect (Tunbridge, 1981), resis-

Box 7.1 Possible risk factors for death from hypoglycaemia

- Alcoholism and/or inebriation
- Psychiatric illness or personality disorder
- Self-neglect; inanition
- Fecklessness/resistance to education
- Diabetes secondary to pancreatic disease
- Hypopituitarism following pituitary ablation

tance to education (Shenfield et al, 1980), hypopituitarism following pituitary ablation therapy for proliferative retinopathy (Nabarro et al, 1979; Shenfield et al, 1980), and patients who have diabetes secondary to pancreatic disease (MacCuish, 1993).

SUDDEN DEATH

The sudden and unexpected death of a young person is an infrequent event, and a series of deaths either from accidents or from natural causes creates considerable media interest. At a British inquest in 1989 it was suggested that the frequency of sudden death in people with type 1 diabetes was increasing, that these deaths were caused by hypoglycaemia, and that there might be a link with the clinical use of human insulin preparations. These comments received widespread coverage in the British media, and fuelled the controversy about hypoglycaemia associated with human insulin (see Chapter 5).

Sudden death does occur, albeit very infrequently, in young people who do not have diabetes (Box 7.2), and examination of the recognised causes may give some insight into possible mechanisms of sudden death in those with type 1 diabetes (Box 7.3). Indeed, even the phenomenon of unexplained death in diabetes is not a new one. In the 1960s Malins described 14 patients who had been attending his diabetes outpatient clinic who died in circumstances implicating hypoglycaemia and in whom no alternative cause of death was identified at autopsy (Malins, 1968). Eight were over 60 years of age, and the clinical records revealed a history of poor nutrition, treatment with a large dose of long-acting insulin, nocturnal hypoglycaemia, and the absence of an alert family member. This description is strikingly similar to the circumstances

Box 7.2 Syndromes of sudden death in non-diabetic young people

- Hypertrophic obstructive cardiomyopathy (HOCM)
- Coronary heart disease (severe coronary artery occlusion or myocardial infarction)
- Other cardiac anatomical abnormalities (congenital anomalies of the coronary arteries, right ventricular dysplasia)
- Syndromes of QT prolongation
- Epilepsy
- Phaeochromocytoma
- Sudden death in water
- Toxic substance abuse

Box 7.3 Possible mechanisms contributing to sudden death

- Ventricular arrhythmias/fibrillation (HOCM, coronary artery occlusion)
- Increased adrenaline (sport, phaeochromocytoma, sudden death in water)
- Decreased potassium (sport, phaeochromocytoma)
- Autonomic stimulation/bradycardia (cold water immersion)
- Severe hyperkalaemia and red cell lysis (fresh water drowning)
- Respiratory arrest (autonomic neuropathy)
- Unknown (epilepsy)

described by Tattersall and Gill more than 20 years later (Tattersall and Gill, 1991), although, since Malin's patients were much older, their deaths are more likely to have been related to established cardiovascular disease. Sudden, unexpected death has also been described in type 1 diabetic patients with advanced diabetic autonomic neuropathy (Ewing et al, 1991).

Unexplained Deaths of Type 1 Diabetic Patients

Following the publicity generated by the assertion that there had been an increase in sudden deaths from acute hypoglycaemia, the British Diabetic Association requested notification of sudden, unexpected deaths of young people with type 1 diabetes. Cases were referred by the forensic chemist who had publicised the issue, relatives or friends who had heard of the television coverage, and physicians with an interest in diabetes who reported recent sudden deaths of patients under their care. Detailed analysis was published by Tattersall and Gill (1991) on behalf of the British Diabetic Association.

A total of 53 cases were referred, but the analysis was confined to the 50 cases who were under 50 years of age. Five cases were excluded because a definite cause of death was identified at post-mortem, and in 11, death was the result of suicide or self-poisoning.

Six patients were thought to have died from ketoacidosis, two from hypoglycaemic brain damage, and in four cases the death was totally unexplained. The largest group comprised 22 patients who were classified as "dead in bed", and in an accompanying editorial the term "dead in bed syndrome" was used (Campbell, 1991) (Figure 7.1).

Analysis of the 22 "dead in bed" patients showed that they were aged between 12 and 43 years, with a duration of diabetes from 3 to 27 years.

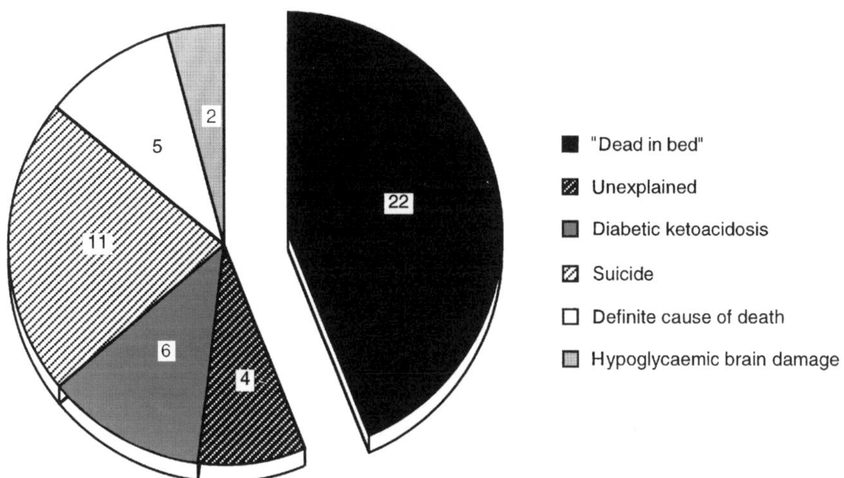

Figure 7.1 Sudden deaths of 50 young type 1 diabetic patients (data from Tattersall and Gill, 1991)

All had been treated with human insulin, and three were taking four injections a day, 18 twice-daily insulin and one was injecting insulin once a day. Information on diabetic complications was not available for all cases, but 13 had none and only four had severe complications, suggesting that undiagnosed autonomic neuropathy was not a factor. All died outside hospital, 19 were sleeping alone at the time of death, and 15 died during the night. Twenty patients were found lying in an undisturbed bed.

Because 14 patients had a history of severe nocturnal hypoglycaemia, and most were apparently well on retiring to bed but were found dead in the morning, the scenario was consistent with an episode of severe or protracted nocturnal hypoglycaemia having precipitated sudden death. Although all had been taking human insulin at the time of death, most had been transferred from animal insulin between six months and two years earlier, and the authors concluded that no temporal relationship between the change in insulin species and the fatal event could be demonstrated. They proposed that "circumstantial evidence implicates nocturnal hypoglycaemia in many cases". Neuropathological evidence of hypoglycaemia was rare, however, suggesting that protracted neuroglycopenia had not occurred in most patients, and implicating sudden cardiac or respiratory arrest as a direct consequence of hypoglycaemia.

A study in Sweden of over 4000 patients with type 1 diabetes diagnosed before the age of 14 and followed up for 13 years showed a threefold increase in the standardised mortality rate in comparison to a non-diabetic population (Sartor and Dahlquist, 1995). In nine of the 33 deaths the subjects were found "dead in bed", eight of whom had gone to bed apparently in good health but subsequently were found dead. One subject had a cardiac arrest after her morning injection of insulin, and at autopsy one had lacerations inside the mouth, suggesting preceding convulsions. The authors suggested that hypoglycaemia was the most likely cause of death in all patients. Very little additional information was provided, and because glycated haemoglobin values could not be standardised it was not possible to ascertain whether an association existed between strict glycaemic control and sudden death.

Another study from Norway of patients under the age of 40 identified 240 deaths from all causes, and 16 cases which fulfilled the criteria of "dead in bed syndrome" (Thordarson and Sovik, 1995). This represented 6.7% of all deaths in this age group. All were found in an undisturbed bed, and nine had been on regimens requiring multiple injections of insulin (eight were taking five injections a day, with one taking a total of seven injections a day). Frequent episodes of hypoglycaemia were documented in 12 cases, in 10 of whom nocturnal hypoglycaemia had occurred. Although autopsy had been performed in 13 patients, a cause of death was not evident in any case. Again, the authors concluded that hypoglycaemia was the most likely precipitant of death.

A similar study from Denmark showed an association between chronic alcohol abuse or acute alcohol intoxication and subjects who were found dead in bed (Borch-Johnsen and Helweg-Larsen, 1993). The number of subjects who were found dead in bed remained remarkably constant over a seven-year period, and no association was observed with an increasing usage of human insulin in Denmark during that time (Figures 7.2 and 7.3).

Deaths of Young People Without Typical Cardiac Disease

When assessing the risk of sudden death in people with diabetes the risks have to be compared with people without diabetes. Sudden unexpected death can occur in any young person irrespective of whether they have diabetes or not. The critical issue is whether sudden death occurs *more frequently* in individuals with type 1 diabetes. Studies which have measured the frequency of sudden death in young people have reported rates around 1.3 to 8.5 per 100 000 patient-years. Since they are based on large numbers of subjects, these estimates are probably more accurate than data reporting the risks in patients with type 1 diabetes. However, the figures suggest that the risk of sudden death is considerably greater in those with diabetes. While it is difficult to be precise, the risk in patients with diabetes seems to be around three times higher.

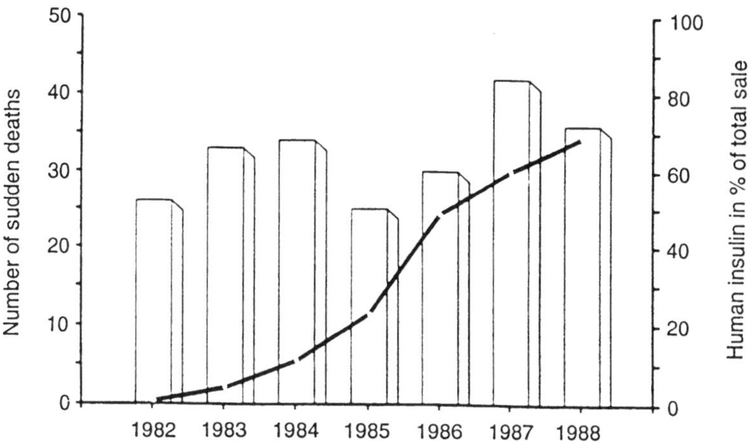

Figure 7.2 Number of sudden deaths and human insulin in percentage of total sale in Denmark from 1982 to 1988. Reproduced from Borch-Johnsen and Helweg-Larsen (1993) by permission of *Diabetic Medicine*

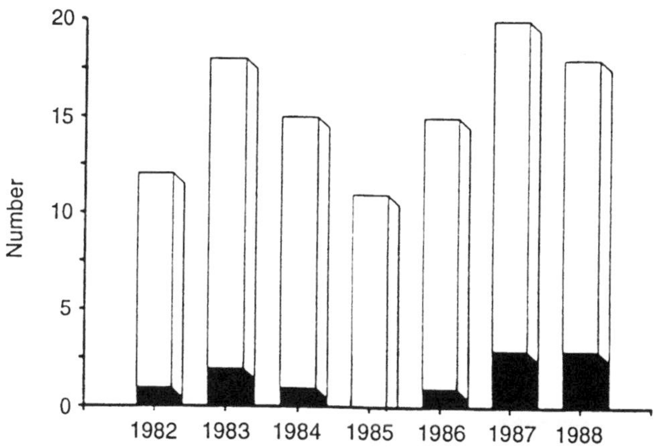

Figure 7.3 Number of deaths due to definite (closed bars) and possible (open bars) hypoglycaemia from 1982 to 1988. Reproduced from Borch-Johnsen and Helweg-Larsen (1993) by permission of *Diabetic Medicine*

RISK FACTORS FOR SUDDEN DEATH

In the general population, the most frequent cause of sudden death is a cardiac arrhythmia, largely related to coronary heart disease; it is likely that the same problem occurs in people with diabetes. Nevertheless, if sudden death is occurring more frequently in diabetic patients, then additional factors are probably responsible. Some of this increase may be a consequence of the more advanced or premature ischaemic heart disease which is associated with diabetes. In some patients the development of hypoglycaemic convulsions may impose an additional insult, although the fact that most subjects were found with their bedclothes undisturbed is against the pre-terminal development of tonic-clonic convulsions. This scenario does not exclude other forms of seizure activity, and a striking similarity exists between the syndromes of sudden death in epilepsy and diabetes (Brown et al, 1990; Nashef and Brown, 1996). When considering other factors, the strongest candidates are probably coexisting autonomic neuropathy and hypoglycaemia.

Autonomic Neuropathy

Autonomic neuropathy increases the risk of sudden death in patients with diabetes in some (Ewing et al, 1980) but not all studies. The exact cause of death remains uncertain, although most groups that have reported increased risk of death have suggested that a cardiac arrhythmia is responsible. Some groups have reported lengthened QT intervals in patients with autonomic neuropathy (Ewing and Neilson, 1990), highlighting the association between prolonged QT intervals and the risk of sudden death in other conditions such as the congenital long QT syndrome (Ewing et al, 1991). However, it seems unlikely that autonomic neuropathy alone could account for the greater risk of sudden death in young patients with diabetes. In those who died suddenly, autonomic function had seldom been formally tested. Some subjects had advanced diabetic complications and would probably have had some degree of autonomic neuropathy, but a significant proportion of those who died had a relatively short duration of diabetes with no evidence of microvascular disease. However, other indicators of autonomic dysfunction, such as reduced heart rate variability and diminished baroceptor sensitivity, are often present in patients with type 1 diabetes even when formal cardiovascular tests of autonomic function are normal (Weston et al, 1996).

Hypoglycaemia

All of the investigators who have reported sudden death in patients with type 1 diabetes have implicated hypoglycaemia as a contributing factor. Death had occurred during the night when hypoglycaemia is a common problem, and some had strict glycaemic control and had experienced nocturnal hypoglycaemia in the past (Box 7.4). The crucial question is whether any mechanism exists through which hypoglycaemia could

> **Box 7.4** Possible risk factors for "dead in bed syndrome"
>
> - Previous nocturnal hypoglycaemia
> - Living/sleeping alone
> - Intensive therapy
> - Multiple injections of insulin
> - Alcohol ingestion

cause sudden death. Hypoglycaemia can cause irreversible brain damage but those who suffer this complication require prolonged exposure to a low blood glucose and are unlikely to die suddenly. Previous authors have emphasised the likelihood of an arrhythmic death and have pointed out that the demonstration of a plausible mechanism by which hypoglycaemia caused cardiac arrhythmias would strongly implicate hypoglycaemia (Tattersall and Gale, 1993). How then does hypoglycaemia affect electrical activity in the heart?

The evidence concerning the effects of hypoglycaemia on the electrocardiogram (ECG) has been obtained from different sources. First, there is anecdotal clinical evidence where arrhythmias have been detected during episodes of hypoglycaemia and resolved when blood glucose recovered. Second, there are experimental data where the electrocardiogram has been measured both in diabetic and non-diabetic subjects during controlled hypoglycaemia induced in the laboratory.

Hypoglycaemia causes an increase in autonomic neural activity affecting both parasympathetic and sympathetic nerves, an increase in plasma adrenaline, and a fall in potassium. Simple electrocardiographic techniques have demonstrated flattening or inversion of the T wave and some studies have also reported prolongation of the QT interval (Fisher and Frier, 1993). A less consistent effect has been ST segment depression. In the presence of ischaemic heart disease it is not difficult to see how some of these changes might lead to malignant cardiac tachydysrhythmias and sudden death (see below). It is less easy to explain how even these profound but brief physiological changes could precipitate a fatal cardiac event in those whose heart is otherwise healthy.

Lengthening of the QT interval is associated with sudden death in other conditions, both congenital and acquired. The congenital long QT syndrome is an inherited disorder in which mutations within the genes coding for the membrane ion channels which contribute to the cardiac action potential cause profound lengthening of the QT interval (Jackman et al, 1988). Those affected have a considerable risk of sudden death caused by ventricular tachycardia which can be precipitated by acute increases in circulating catecholamines. However, although the lifetime risk of death in the congenital long QT syndrome is around 70% without treatment, patients can clearly survive with a long QT interval for many years. At first sight it therefore seems unlikely that a short period of hypoglycaemia lasting for an hour or so could cause a malignant arrhythmia. Yet, under other conditions, shorter periods of altered depolarisation can precipitate ventricular tachycardia. A variety of prescription drugs, including antiarrhythmics and antifungal agents, can also prolong myocardial repolarisation and in certain circumstances trigger dangerous tachydysrhythmias (Botstein, 1993). One can therefore hypothesise that during clinical episodes of hypoglycaemia, alterations in cardiac repolarisation may be sufficient to precipitate a fatal period of ventricular tachycardia. It has been demonstrated that the QT interval can lengthen during experimental hypoglycaemia both in diabetic and non-diabetic subjects (Marques et al, 1997) (Figure 7.4). Some subjects had quite pronounced increments in QT interval and a strong relationship was observed between the increase in QT interval and the rise in plasma adrenaline.

The major problem with the hypothesis is that since sudden death occurs so rarely, it is very difficult to test directly. Isolated case reports of

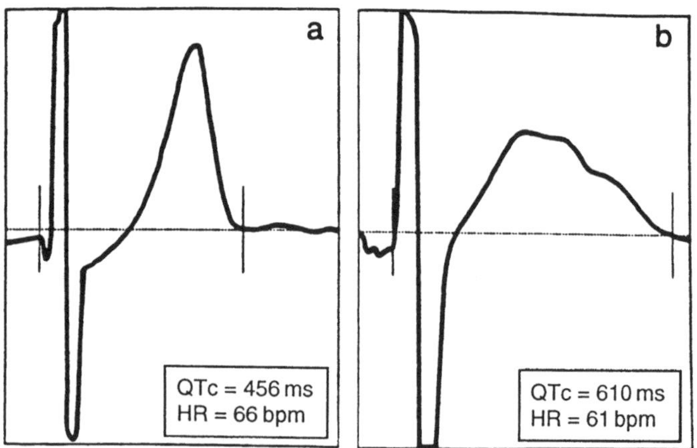

Figure 7.4 Typical QT measurement with a screen cursor placement from one subject (a) during euglycaemia showing a clearly defined T wave, and (b) during hypoglycaemia showing prolonged repolarisation and prominent U wave. Horizontal: 700 ms epoch, vertical 1.33 mV full scale. Reproduced from Marques et al (1997) by permission of *Diabetic Medicine*

transient cardiac dysrhythmias have not provided much additional useful information. There are reports of atrial fibrillation and supraventricular tachycardia during clinical episodes of hypoglycaemia but there is no direct evidence that profound hypoglycaemia can cause a life-threatening disturbance in cardiac rhythm. The evidence presented above is necessarily indirect and therefore more uncertain, although it is worth noting that the pharmaceutical industry takes a similar approach when testing the potential arrhythmogenic effect of their products (Botstein, 1993).

In summary, the majority of sudden deaths in young patients with diabetes remain unexplained and we have hypothesised that these were deaths due to ventricular arrhythmia. These might have resulted from an increase in plasma adrenaline and fall in potassium which accompany hypoglycaemia so producing prolongation of the QT interval. It is possible that this occurs on a background of autonomic instability caused by early autonomic neuropathy.

What Do We Say to Patients?

It is clear that the frequency of deaths resulting from hypoglycaemia is underestimated, and some deaths related to hypoglycaemia may be attributed to other causes at the time of certification. Nevertheless, when we consider that nocturnal hypoglycaemia is very common, affecting between 30% and 56% of patients every night, we can reassure patients that sudden death as a consequence of acute hypoglycaemia is very rare. However, the available evidence prevents us stating that there is *no risk* of death from hypoglycaemia during sleep, or at other vulnerable times when treatment is not rendered promptly.

EFFECT OF HYPOGLYCAEMIA ON CARDIOVASCULAR DISEASE

Acute hypoglycaemia provokes an intense haemodynamic response secondary to activation of the autonomic nervous system with the secretion of adrenaline. The heart rate increases over a period of 15 to 20 minutes, but rarely rises above 100 beats/minute. There is a modest but significant increase in systolic blood pressure, and a slight but significant fall in diastolic blood pressure. The pulse pressure widens, with a substantial increase in cardiac output and a fall in total peripheral vascular resistance (Figure 7.5). These haemodynamic changes are relatively short-lived, and exert no significant after-effects on the 24-hour heart rate or blood pressure (Avogaro et al, 1994). In a person with a normal heart

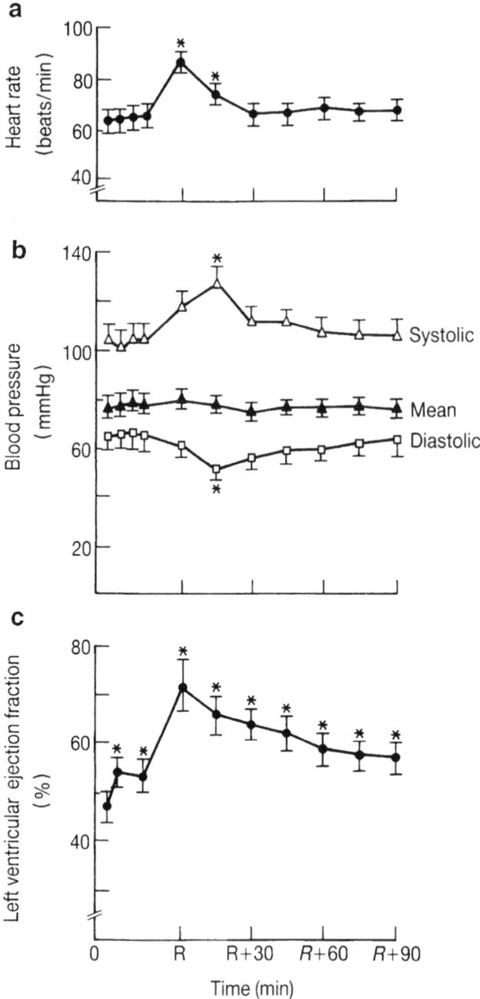

Figure 7.5 Mean response of (a) heart rate, (b) systolic blood pressure and mean arterial blood pressure, and (c) left ventricular ejection fraction following intravenous injection of insulin at time 0. R = autonomic reaction. Reproduced from Fisher et al (1987) by permission of Springer-Verlag

these haemodynamic changes are probably of no great significance, but in a patient who has underlying coronary heart disease the profound increase in cardiac workload may provoke a cardiac arrhythmia, myocardial ischaemia and even myocardial infarction (Box 7.5).

Box 7.5 Cardiac effects of acute hypoglycaemia

- Increased heart rate
- Widening of pulse pressure
- Arrhythmias
- Silent myocardial ischaemia
- Angina
- Myocardial infarction

Arrhythmias and Coronary Heart Disease

Occasional cardiac arrhythmias have been demonstrated in normal subjects during experimental hypoglycaemia studies. It would now be considered unethical to perform hypoglycaemia studies in patients with known heart disease, but many studies were performed in an earlier era both in diabetic and non-diabetic patients with coronary heart disease to examine the effects of acute hypoglycaemia (Fisher and Frier, 1993). Atrial fibrillation has been described in some patients and in addition there are several case reports of atrial fibrillation following hypoglycaemia in insulin-treated patients who had no overt evidence of heart disease (Collier et al, 1987; Baxter et al, 1990; Odeh et al, 1990).

There is a single report of a transient ventricular tachycardia during experimental hypoglycaemia in a non-diabetic patient with coronary heart disease, but ECG evidence of sustained ventricular tachycardia or ventricular fibrillation has not been documented during hypoglycaemia in diabetic patients. Obviously this does not exclude the possibility of these arrhythmias occurring in clinical practice, as these arrhythmias will be fatal if uncorrected. In most instances it is unlikely that any precipitating cause of the arrhythmia would be sought, hypoglycaemia may not have been recognised and the difficulties in establishing a putative diagnosis of hypoglycaemia at post-mortem have already been alluded to.

Angina and Myocardial Ischaemia

The provocation of angina and myocardial ischaemia by exercise is well documented in clinical practice. By contrast, acute hypoglycaemia which provokes a more intense haemodynamic response, and in particular a greater increase in plasma adrenaline, has rarely been documented as provoking anginal chest pain, either in the experimental situation or in anecdotal case reports. A literature search of over 6000 insulin tolerance tests recorded only two episodes of angina. This may reflect the fact that coronary heart disease would be considered a contraindication to insulin tolerance testing, and in clinical practice clinicians may accept higher ambient blood glucose concentrations in diabetic patients with known coronary heart disease to avoid hypoglycaemia. It is also possible that the haemodynamic changes of hypoglycaemia are so profound that they are frequently fatal in patients with coronary heart disease, and hypoglycaemia is probably overlooked as a provoking cause when determining cause of death.

It is now well established that many episodes of ST segment depression on the ECG are not associated with angina, and constitute "silent ischaemia". One case of hypoglycaemia provoking silent ischaemia has been described during 24-hour ECG monitoring in a diabetic patient with suspected coronary heart disease (Pladziewicz and Nesto, 1989).

Myocardial Infarction

Myocardial infarction has rarely been documented as a consequence of hypoglycaemia (Fisher and Frier, 1993). In a series of non-diabetic patients with schizophrenia who were treated with hypoglycaemic shock therapy in the 1930s, 12 of 90 deaths were ascribed to cardiac causes, with the majority of deaths being caused by cerebral damage. It should be emphasised that this long-abandoned form of treatment of psychiatric disease necessitated prolonged and profound hypoglycaemia.

Only a few cases have been published of myocardial infarction and hypoglycaemia in diabetic patients, mostly originating from the Joslin Clinic in the USA. This possible association is very difficult to establish because of the problems described above. In addition, the release of stress hormones such as glucagon, cortisol and adrenaline will raise blood glucose and make the contribution of preceding hypoglycaemia almost impossible to confirm.

WORSENING OF MICROVASCULAR COMPLICATIONS

Precipitation of acute vascular events (such as myocardial infarction or stroke) as a result of hypoglycaemia affecting macrovascular disease is relatively infrequent, considering how commonly episodes of hypoglycaemia occur in everyday life. It has been suggested that acute hypoglycaemia, by releasing vasoactive hormones and provoking changes in regional and capillary blood flow, might worsen established microvascular complications of diabetes (Frier and Hilsted, 1985). While microvascular complications are recognised to be the consequence of chronic hyperglycaemia and can be prevented or delayed by strict glycaemic control, the effect of recurrent hypoglycaemia on an already compromised microvasculature may be deleterious and cause further damage (Box 7.6).

Exposure to recurrent hypoglycaemia may precipitate capillary closure, inducing localised tissue ischaemia and producing a deterioration in retinopathy. A sudden fall in intraocular pressure occurs during hypoglycaemia, and could precipitate vitreous haemorrhage in patients with proliferative retinopathy, as friable new vessels are vulnerable to sudden changes in perfusion pressure or mechanical stresses. This could explain the occasional anecdotal reports of vitreous haemorrhage described by individual patients, often following nocturnal hypoglycaemia.

Acute hypoglycaemia reduces renal plasma flow and glomerular filtration in normal subjects and diabetic patients without significant complications. In patients who have established nephropathy with glomerular sclerosis and arteriolar narrowing, the reduction in renal plasma flow may precipitate further closure of arterioles and progression in renal impairment.

Box 7.6 Postulated effects of acute hypoglycaemia in the microcirculation

- Changes in capillary blood flow
- Increased coagulation factors
- Platelet activation
- Neutrophil activation
- Increased free-radical activity

CONCLUSIONS

- Biochemical and mild symptomatic hypoglycaemia occur commonly in the treatment of those with type 1 diabetes. Even severe episodes are not infrequent, but sudden and unexpected deaths from hypoglycaemia are rare.
- There does appear to be an increased risk of sudden death in people with diabetes compared to those who do not have diabetes, which may become greater as more strenuous attempts are made to control blood glucose more tightly. These deaths, referred to as the "dead in bed syndrome", are probably related to hypoglycaemia through hypoglycaemia-induced tachydysrhythmias.
- Experimental hypoglycaemia can provoke abnormalities of

continues

continued

the ECG which are recognised to be associated with sudden death in other conditions and this observation offers a possible mechanism to explain the phenomenon.

- Hypoglycaemia also produces changes in plasma viscosity and capillary perfusion which may increase the risk of myocardial ischaemia, although the clinical evidence that this is responsible for myocardial infarction in people with diabetes is limited.
- The intense sympathoadrenal response provoked by severe hypoglycaemia may also provoke changes that could also worsen established microvascular complications although to date this is primarily hypothetical, with little supportive evidence.

REFERENCES

Arky RA, Veverbrants E and Abramson EA (1968). Irreversible hypoglycemia. A complication of alcohol and insulin. *Journal of the American Medical Association* **206**: 575–8.

Avogaro A, Crepaldi C, Miola M et al (1994). Sequelae of acute hypoglycaemia on 24 hour blood pressure and metabolic parameters in normal and type 1 (insulin-dependent) diabetic individuals. *Diabetic Medicine* **11**: 573–7.

Baxter MA, Garewal C, Jordan R, Wright AD and Nattrass M (1990). Hypoglycaemia and atrial fibrillation. *Postgraduate Medical Journal* **66**: 981.

Borch-Johnsen K and Helweg-Larsen K (1993). Sudden death and human insulin: is there a link? *Diabetic Medicine* **10**: 255–9.

Botstein P (1993). Is QT prolongation harmful? A regulatory perspective. *American Journal of Cardiology* **72**: 50–2B.

Brown SW, Mawer GE, Lawler W et al (1990). Sudden death and epilepsy. *Lancet* **335**: 606–7.

Campbell I (1991). Dead in bed syndrome: a new manifestation of nocturnal hypoglycaemia? *Diabetic Medicine* **8**: 3–4.

Collier A, Matthews DM, Young RJ and Clarke BF (1987). Transient atrial fibrillation precipitated by hypoglycaemia: two case reports. *Postgraduate Medical Journal* **63**: 895–7.

Critchley JAJH, Proudfoot AT, Boyd SG, Campbell IW, Brown NS and Gordon A (1984). Deaths and paradoxes after intentional insulin overdosage. *British Medical Journal* **289**: 225.

Ewing DJ, Campbell IW and Clarke BF (1980). The natural history of diabetic autonomic neuropathy. *Quarterly Journal of Medicine* **49**: 95–108.

Ewing DJ and Neilson JMM (1990). QT interval length and diabetic autonomic neuropathy. *Diabetic Medicine* **7**: 23–6.

Ewing DJ, Boland O, Neilson JMM, Cho CG and Clarke BF (1991). Autonomic neuropathy, QT interval lengthening, and unexpected deaths in male diabetic patients. *Diabetologia* **34**: 182–5.

Fisher BM, Gillen G, Dargie HJ, Inglis GC and Frier BM (1987). The effects of insulin-induced hypoglycaemia on cardiovascular function in normal man: studies using radionuclide ventriculography. *Diabetologia* **30**: 841–5.

Fisher BM and Frier BM (1993). Effect on vascular disease. In: *Hypoglycaemia and Diabetes: Clinical and Physiological Aspects*. Frier BM and Fisher BM, eds. Edward Arnold, London: 355–61.

Frier BM and Hilsted J (1985). Does hypoglycaemia aggravate the complications of diabetes? *Lancet* **326**: 1175–7.

Jackman WM, Friday KJ, Anderson JL, Aliot EM, Clark M, Lazzara R (1988). The long QT syndromes: a critical review, new clinical observations and a unifying hypothesis. *Progress in Cardiovascular Diseases* **31**: 115–72.

Kalimo H and Olsson Y (1980). Effects of severe hypoglycemia on the human brain. Neuropathological case reports. *Acta Neurologica Scandinavica* **62**: 345–56.

Laing SP, Swerdlow AJ, Slater SD et al (1999). The British Diabetic Association Cohort Study, II: cause-specific mortality in patients with insulin-treated diabetes mellitus. *Diabetic Medicine* **16**: 466–71.

MacCuish AC (1993). Treatment of hypoglycaemia. In: *Hypoglycaemia and Diabetes: Clinical and Physiological Aspects*. Frier BM and Fisher BM, eds. Edward Arnold, London: 212–21.

Malins J (1968). Hypoglycaemia. In: *Clinical Diabetes Mellitus*. Eyre and Spottiswoode, London: 425–46.

Marques JLB, George E, Peacey SR, Harris ND, Macdonald IA, Cochrane T and Heller SR (1997). Altered ventricular repolarization during hypoglycaemia in patients with diabetes. *Diabetic Medicine* **14**: 648–54.

Nabarro JDN, Mustaffa BE, Morris DV, Walport MJ and Kurtz AB (1979). Insulin deficient diabetes. Contrasts with other endocrine deficiencies. *Diabetologia* **16**: 5–12.

Nashef L and Brown S (1996). Epilepsy and sudden death. *Lancet* **348**: 1324–5.

Odeh M, Oliven A and Bassan H (1990). Transient atrial fibrillation precipitated by hypoglycemia. *Annals of Emergency Medicine* **19**: 565–7.

Pladziewicz DS and Nesto RW (1989). Hypoglycemia-induced silent myocardial ischemia. *American Journal of Cardiology* **63**: 1531–2.

Pramming S, Thorsteinsson B, Bendtson I and Binder C (1991). Symptomatic hypoglycaemia in 411 type 1 diabetic patients. *Diabetic Medicine* **8**: 217–22.

Sartor G and Dahlquist G (1995). Short-term mortality in childhood onset insulin-dependent diabetes mellitus: a high frequency of unexpected deaths in bed. *Diabetic Medicine* **12**: 607–11.

Shenfield GM, Bhalla IP, Elton RA and Duncan LJP (1980). Fatal coma in diabetes. *Diabete & Metabolisme (Paris)* **6**: 151–5.

Tattersall RB and Gale EAM (1993). Mortality. In: *Hypoglycaemia and Diabetes: Clinical and Physiological Aspects*. Frier BM and Fisher BM, eds. Edward Arnold, London: 191–8.

Tattersall RB and Gill GV (1991). Unexplained deaths of type 1 diabetic patients. *Diabetic Medicine* **8**: 49–58.

The DCCT Research Group (1991). Epidemiology of severe hypoglycemia in the Diabetes Control and Complications Trial. *American Journal of Medicine* **90**: 450–9.

The Diabetes Control and Complications Trial Research Group (1993). The effect of intensive treatment of diabetes on the development and progression of long-term complications in insulin-dependent diabetes mellitus. *New England Journal of Medicine* **329**: 977–86.

Thordarson H and Sovik O (1995). Dead in bed syndrome in young diabetic patients in Norway. *Diabetic Medicine* **12**: 782–7.

Tunbridge WMG (1981). Factors contributing to deaths of diabetics under fifty years of age. *Lancet* **318**: 569–72.

Vaughan NJA, Home PD for the Diabetes Audit Working Group of the Research Unit of the Royal College of Physicians and the British Diabetic Association (1995). The UK Diabetes Dataset: a standard for information exchange. *Diabetic Medicine* **12**: 717–22.

Weston PJ, Panerai RB, McCullough A, McNally PG, James MA, Potter JF, Thurston H and Swales JD (1996). Assessment of baroceptor-cardiac reflex sensitivity using time domain analysis in patients with IDDM and the relation to left ventricular mass index. *Diabetologia* **39**: 1385–91.

8

Long-term Effects of Hypoglycaemia on Cognitive Function and the Brain in Diabetes

PETROS PERROS and IAN J. DEARY*
Freeman Hospital, Newcastle upon Tyne and *Department of Psychology, The University of Edinburgh

INTRODUCTION

Almost one-third of all diabetic patients treated with insulin experience one or more episodes of severe hypoglycaemia every year (MacLeod et al, 1993), this being defined as an episode which requires the help of another person to effect a recovery. Strict glycaemic control, and intensified insulin treatment are associated with a three-fold increase in the probability of developing severe hypoglycaemia (see Chapter 6). In this chapter the effects of diabetes on the brain are reviewed, with an emphasis on the chronic complications of hypoglycaemia.

"Hypos" are usually perceived as a temporary and reversible complication of insulin therapy by people with diabetes and their relatives. However, severe and prolonged hypoglycaemia lasting for several hours can cause serious and permanent brain damage and, rarely, can be fatal (Malouf and Brust, 1985). Fortunately, such devastating complications

Hypoglycaemia in Clinical Diabetes. Edited by B. M. Frier and B. M. Fisher.

are rare. The vast majority of people who experience an episode of severe hypoglycaemia appear to make a full recovery. However, it is possible that repeated exposure to severe hypoglycaemia may have subtle progressive long-term effects on brain function and mental functions of people with type 1 (insulin dependent) diabetes. Currently, there is evidence for and against the possibility that recurrent episodes of severe, and apparently reversible, hypoglycaemia in adult patients with type 1 diabetes may have a small detrimental effect on mental capacities. Thus, the brain may not be immune from diabetic complications. The concept of "diabetic encephalopathy", i.e. a disorder of the brain associated with some aspects of diabetes, is gaining acceptance. Its causes are complex, and may be related to several factors, only one of which is hypoglycaemia (Dejgaard et al, 1991; McCall, 1992; Biessels et al, 1994).

COGNITIVE FUNCTION AND HYPOGLYCAEMIA

Hypoglycaemia and Mental Functions in Children and Adolescents

In addition to the severity of hypoglycaemia, the age of the individual is important in determining the potential impact of hypoglycaemia on the brain (Ack et al, 1961). The human brain develops rapidly until the age of five years, and during this critical period any insult can have long-lasting effects. In diabetic children important risk factors for the development of later cognitive impairment are (Ryan, 1988):

- early onset of diabetes
- long duration of diabetes
- poor metabolic control
- severe hypoglycaemia.

Children with type 1 diabetes who suffer repeated and severe hypoglycaemia while younger than five years old have lower mental abilities later on in life, and may show more difficult behaviour (Ryan et al, 1984; Rovet et al, 1987; Golden et al, 1989). The combination of an early onset of diabetes (before five years of age) and recurrent severe hypoglycaemia appears to be associated with reduced attention and psychomotor efficiency in adolescence (Rovet and Alvarez, 1997; Bjorgaas et al, 1998). Adolescents who had developed type 1 diabetes after the age of five years have been shown to have lower verbal IQ than their peers, but this may be related in part to learning-related problems at school and loss of formal education rather than with hypoglycaemia (Fallstrom, 1974).

Most of the studies mentioned above are cross-sectional, i.e. they have tested groups of children, with and without diabetes, and have tried to review the children's clinical records to estimate the amount of previous hypoglycaemia experienced by each child with diabetes. A more robust type of study is one in which groups of children are followed prospectively. One such study is ongoing in Melbourne, Australia (Northam et al, 1995). Over 100 children with newly diagnosed type 1 diabetes have been compared with a matched control group of non-diabetic children. No differences in mental abilities or in educational attainments were discernible between the two groups. Therefore, when children develop type 1 diabetes they do not begin with any mental decrements when they are compared with their non-diabetic peers. An initial report from this invaluable study has indicated that within two years of the development of diabetes the mental abilities of the diabetic children may begin to lag behind their non-diabetic peers (Northam et al, 1998). However, the roles of hyper- and hypoglycaemia and other possible effects of having diabetes in promoting these changes, remain to be elucidated.

Examination of electroencephalograms (EEGs), the electrical signals that can be detected from living brains (Haumont et al, 1979), and of visual evoked potentials, (signals generated in the brain in response to a stimulus (Seidl et al, 1996), has found that abnormalities are commoner in children with early-onset diabetes who have had recurrent severe hypoglycaemia. The brain's electrical responses to stimuli are significantly slowed in almost three-quarters of adolescents with type 1 diabetes (Uberall et al, 1996). However, this same study found no differences in the mental ability of children with diabetes when they were compared to non-diabetic controls, and the neurophysiological changes in the diabetic children were not related to age at onset of diabetes, duration of diabetes, quality of metabolic control or the presence of peripheral neuropathy. In children, repeated exposure to severe hypoglycaemia has its most deleterious effects on the front and central regions of the brain's cerebral hemispheres (Bjorgaas et al, 1996). During controlled, modest hypoglycaemia induced in the laboratory, the EEGs of children with diabetes were more disturbed than those of non-diabetic children (Bjorgaas et al, 1998).

In summary, there is convincing evidence to suggest that children with type 1 diabetes who have repeated exposure to severe hypoglycaemia, especially when this occurs below the age of five years, will subsequently have lower mental ability levels with evidence of detrimental effects on the physiological activity of their brains.

Evidence for Neuropsychological Deterioration Following Repeated Hypoglycaemia in Adults

Adults with type 1 diabetes perform less well on mental ability tests than do non-diabetic subjects (Ryan, 1988), but the differences are subtle and the underlying causes unclear. This is a complex and difficult area of clinical research with a number of possible causative factors that are hard to tease apart; these include the metabolic disturbances of diabetes and its treatment, and the social and educational impact of chronic illness on intelligence. Recently a few carefully controlled studies have focused on adult subjects with insulin-treated diabetes who have a history of severe recurrent hypoglycaemia. These patients seem to recover mentally and physically after each episode of hypoglycaemia, but when they are tested in the laboratory with standardised mental tests they display subtle chronic impairment of some mental functions. Abnormal neurological symptoms and signs are usually absent. The evidence from the small number of retrospective studies that are available indicates an association between a history of recurrent severe hypoglycaemia and a modest reduction in IQ (Deary, 1993). The main findings from some of the more influential studies can be summarised as follows.

1. Wredling et al (1990) performed a carefully controlled study in two small groups of patients with type 1 diabetes, with and without histories of recurrent severe hypoglycaemia. They demonstrated impaired performance on a number of mental function tests in the group with a history of severe hypoglycaemia. The study design could not exclude the possibility that the patients with a history of hypoglycaemia had a lower pre-morbid IQ.
2. Langan et al (1991) conducted a study in 100 patients with type 1 diabetes, using more detailed tests of cognitive functions. Within this sample of people with diabetes, the group of patients with more than five episodes of severe hypoglycaemia displayed a small, but significant, decline in IQ (averaging about six IQ points) compared to the diabetic patients who had experienced no episodes of severe hypoglycaemia (Figure 8.1). Pre-morbid IQ was similar in patients with and without severe hypoglycaemia, thus strengthening the hypothesis that repeated, severe hypoglycaemia was responsible for the lower IQ (Langan et al, 1991; Deary et al, 1993). Taking the 100 diabetic patients as a whole, they had lower IQs than healthy, non-diabetic subjects with similar ages and social and educational backgrounds (Deary et al, 1993). Impaired performance IQ was closely associated with repeated, severe hypoglycaemia. Making decisions and initiating

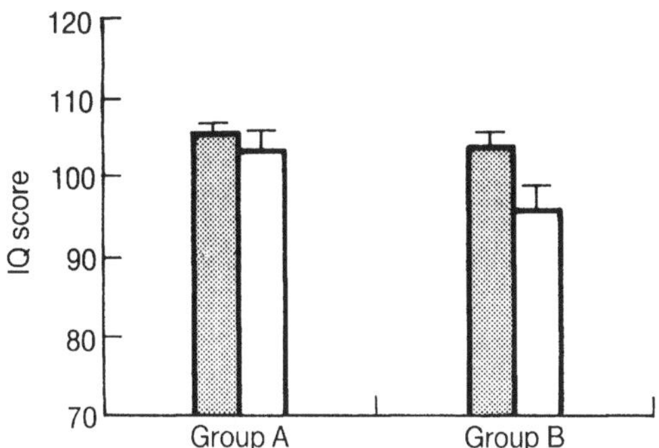

Figure 8.1 Pre-morbid (solid bars) and present (open bars) IQ levels for Group A (subjects with type 1 with no history of severe hypoglycaemia) and Group B (subjects with type 1 with at least five episodes of severe hypoglycaemia). Premorbid versus present IQ comparison for Group A is non-significant, comparison for Group B is significant at $p < 0.001$. Reproduced from Langan et al (1991) by permission of Springer-Verlag

responses appeared to be affected specifically by recurrent severe hypoglycaemia (Deary et al, 1992). Verbal IQ was lower in people with type 1 diabetes compared to healthy control subjects, regardless of their history of hypoglycaemia. This may result from the social impact of the disorder (Deary et al, 1993).

3. The results of Langan et al (1991) have been confirmed by another team of researchers (Lincoln et al, 1996) using an identical study design.
4. A small group of patients with type 1 diabetes has been described (Gold et al, 1994), in which the individuals have suffered many episodes of severe hypoglycaemia over several years of treatment with insulin, and have subsequently developed severe mental and memory problems and devastating social and psychological deficits, causing premature retirement from employment and disrupting social and family life.

Retrospective studies suggest that recurrent severe hypoglycaemia has a detrimental effect on cognitive functions. By contrast, the limited evidence from prospective studies of intensified insulin therapy, namely the Diabetes Control and Complications Trial (DCCT) (The Diabetes Control and Complications Trial Research Group, 1996) and the Stockholm Diabetes Intervention Study (Reichard and Pihl, 1994) appears to indicate that cognitive function does not deteriorate in patients who suffer recurrent hypoglycaemia, at least in the timescale (less than 10 years) of these studies.

At present, it cannot be concluded for certain that recurrent severe hypoglycaemia causes significant long-term effects on cognitive function (Deary, 1997). The benefits of strict glycaemic control in reducing the microvascular complications of diabetes are undoubted, but there is a price to pay: a substantial increase in the risk of severe hypoglycaemia. Within the timescale of the study, the DCCT cohort seem not to have suffered a detrimental effect in cognitive function, but the participants were young, highly motivated, of above average intelligence, free of advanced complications with no history of severe hypoglycaemia before entering the study, and they received a very high level of support from health professionals. In most diabetes outpatient clinics where resources are limited, such model patients are not the norm. It seems entirely justifiable to aim for strict glycaemic control for patients who fit the entry criteria used in the DCCT. It is probably also appropriate to extrapolate the lessons of the DCCT to older patients with more advanced diabetic complications and reasonable life expectancy, who have not previously experienced recurrent severe hypoglycaemia. There still remains a sizeable group of patients with type 1 diabetes whose glycaemic control is sub-optimal by the standards of the DCCT, yet they have suffered recurrent severe hypoglycaemia in the past. The targets of glycaemic control should be set less rigidly for these patients, who are entitled to be informed of the potential risks of further hypoglycaemia on cognitive function.

FUNCTIONAL EFFECTS OF HYPOGLYCAEMIA

Hypoglycaemia-induced Neurological Syndromes

Hypoglycaemia can cause a wide range of neurological symptoms and clinical signs, which can be subtle or severe, reversible or permanent. The effects of hypoglycaemia on the brain depend on several factors:

- the blood glucose nadir reached during hypoglycaemia
- the duration of hypoglycaemia
- the frequency of hypoglycaemia
- the presence of previous brain insults (e.g. head injury, chronic alcohol abuse).

Reversible Effects of Hypoglycaemia on the Brain

An acute fall in blood glucose causes mental slowness which, if untreated, can proceed to loss of consciousness. Recovery is usually rapid (within 30 to 45 minutes) after the blood glucose concentration returns to normal but patients often complain of headache, malaise and memory problems for several hours, and although most aspects of intellectual performance recover within a day of the event, altered mood may take much longer to recover (Strachan et al, 1998). In some patients hypoglycaemia triggers stereotypical responses (Box 8.1).

Diagnostic confusion may arise because of an atypical presentation, a post-ictal state, and if it is measured, blood glucose concentration either may be in the normal range, or even elevated, by the time of arrival at hospital, because of the compensatory counterregulatory response (Chapter 1).

Convulsions and Associated Morbidity

Focal or generalised convulsions can be precipitated by hypoglycaemia and have been estimated to occur with a frequency of two convulsions per 100 diabetic patients per year in up to 10% of all patients treated with insulin (MacLeod et al, 1993). There is an obvious risk of injury during convulsions (Hepburn et al, 1989), including:

- fracture-dislocation of joints
- vertebral compression fractures (Figure 8.2)
- soft tissue injury
- head injury.

Idiopathic epilepsy (which occurs in insulin-treated diabetic patients with the same frequency as in the non-diabetic population) may be misdiagnosed and patients may be treated unnecessarily with anticonvulsant drugs, which are thought to be ineffective in preventing hypoglycaemia-induced convulsions. The distinction between idiopathic epilepsy and hypoglycaemia-induced convulsions can be difficult. The EEG is

Box 8.1 Transient neuropsychological manifestations of severe hypoglycaemia

Neurological
- Focal or generalised convulsions
- Hemiparesis
- Focal neurological syndromes

Psychosocial
- Mental slowness
- Inappropriate behaviour
- Automatic behaviour
- Aggressive behaviour

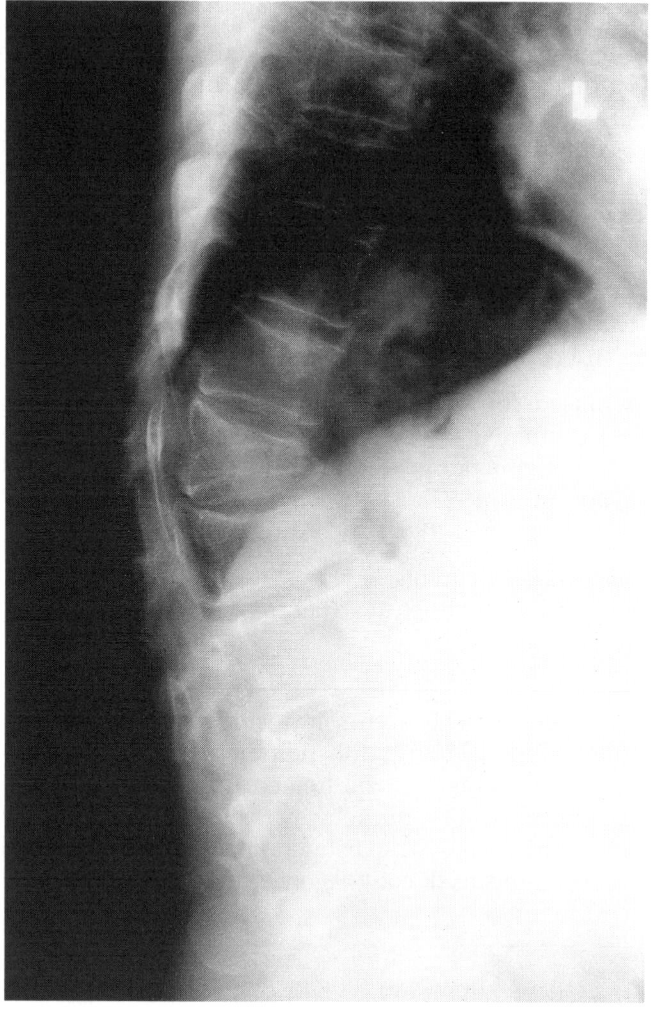

Figure 8.2 Lateral X-ray of thoracic spine demonstrating a vertebral compression fracture sustained during a hypoglycaemia-induced convulsion (courtesy of Dr B. M. Frier)

often unhelpful as changes occur with acute hypoglycaemia (Figure 8.3), and abnormalities can persist for several days following an episode of hypoglycaemia. EEG examination should therefore be deferred for at least a week and blood glucose should be estimated at the time of examination. Permanent EEG abnormalities have been identified in 30–80% of diabetic patients (Haumont et al, 1979; Pramming et al, 1988).

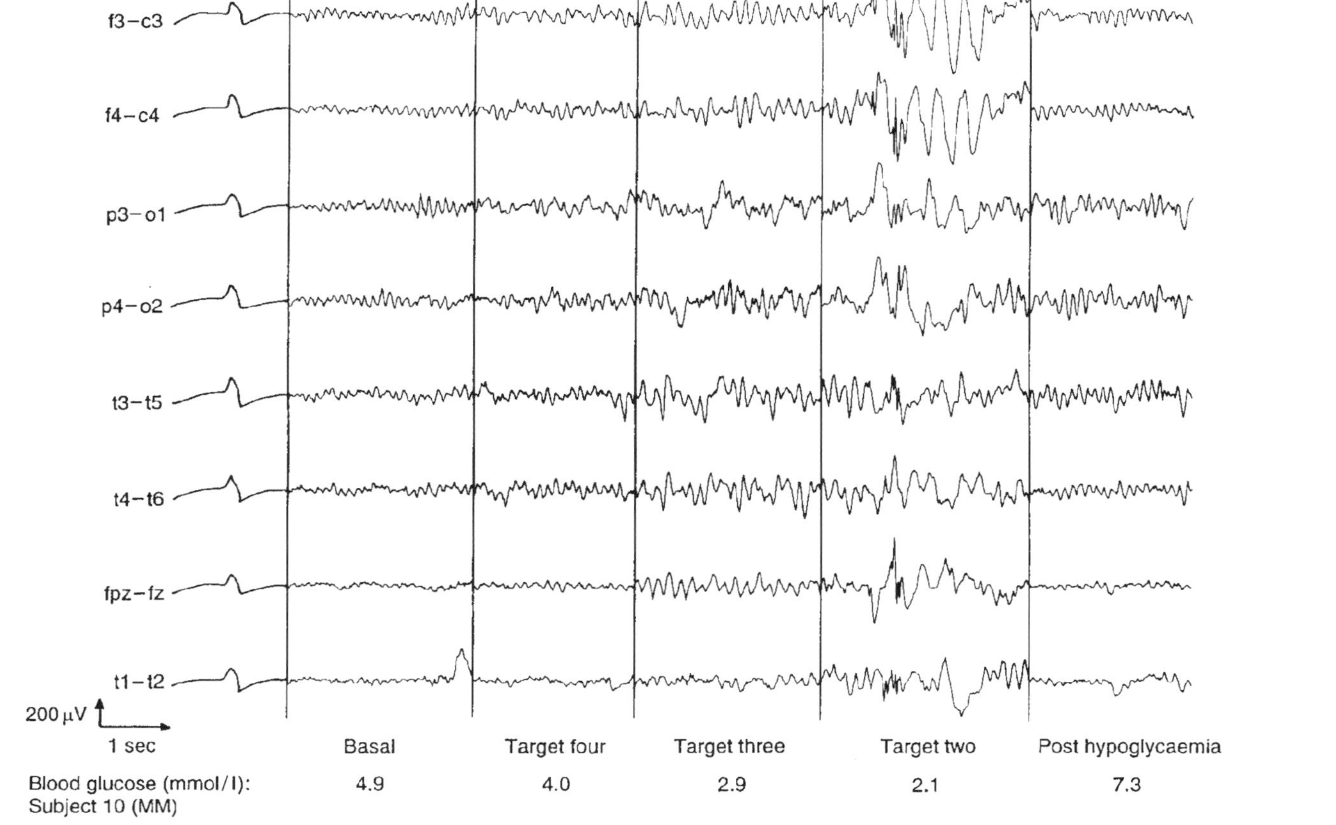

Figure 8.3 EEG changes during hypoglycaemia in a child with type 1 diabetes who experienced hypoglycaemia-induced convulsions. There is progressive slow activity leading to epileptiform spikes at blood glucose of 2.1 mmol/l. Reproduced from Bjorgaas et al, 1998, by permission of John Wiley & Sons

Cerebral oedema is a dreaded complication of severe insulin-induced hypoglycaemia and should be suspected if further deterioration or false localising signs ensue (MacCuish, 1993). Hypoglycaemia-associated cerebral oedema is often very resistant to treatment and is usually fatal. Urgent imaging of the brain is imperative to exclude other potentially remediable causes of neurological abnormalities or coma.

Permanent Neurological Effects of Hypoglycaemia on the Brain

Rarely, severe and protracted hypoglycaemia can cause permanent brain damage, but this has often been associated with excessive consumption of alcohol, (see Chapter 3) and is occasionally the sequel of attempted suicide or unintentional insulin overdose. Some patients survive but remain in a persistent vegetative state (Agardh et al, 1983). Some recover partially with focal neurological deficits such as hemiparesis, ataxia or severe memory loss (Malouf and Brust, 1985; Lins and Adamson, 1993) (Box 8.2). Patients with neurological complications of severe hypoglycaemia are usually admitted to hospital. Patients who require hospital admission for treatment of severe hypoglycaemia have been observed to have a high incidence of psychiatric disturbance and increased mortality within a few months of discharge (Hart and Frier, 1998).

Box 8.2 Long-term neuropsychological manifestations of severe insulin-induced hypoglycaemia

Neurological

- Persistent vegetative state
- Hemiparesis
- Focal abnormalities (motor, sensory)
- Brainstem syndrome
- Ataxia; choreoathetosis
- Epilepsy

Psychological

- Cognitive impairment
- Behavioural abnormalities
- Automatism; psychosis
- Psychosocial problems

STRUCTURAL AND FUNCTIONAL CHANGES IN THE CENTRAL NERVOUS SYSTEM

Structural Changes of the Brain in Diabetes

Hypertension and hyperlipidaemia are common in diabetes and cerebrovascular disease is a recognised macrovascular complication. Atheromatous cerebral artery occlusion involving major vessels, embolism from cervical arteries, and lacunar strokes are more extensive and occur at an earlier age in diabetic patients compared with the non-diabetic population (McCall, 1992). Whether microvascular disease affects the brain is uncertain. Following the death of a group of young patients with long-standing type 1 diabetes, meningeal fibrosis, pseudocalcinosis and diffuse degeneration of grey and white matter were observed in their brains (Reske-Nielsen et al, 1965). However, these patients had uraemia and hypertension secondary to renal failure with diabetic nephropathy, and the neuropathological changes could not be attributed to diabetes *per se*. Despite the vulnerability of retinal vessels to microvascular disease, the cerebral microcirculation appears to be protected from diabetic microangiopathy. However, subtle changes in cerebral capillaries have been described (increased endothelial basal membrane thickness and, infrequently, microaneurysms) using sensitive techniques in specimens from the brains of diabetic subjects (Johnson et al, 1982). The premise that the brain is not susceptible to microvascular diabetic complications is as yet unproven. This is an important consideration because of the hypothesis that the haemodynamic and haemorrheological changes induced by hypoglycaemia may precipitate ischaemia in tissues with established disease of the macro- and microvasculature (Fisher and Frier, 1993) (see Chapter 7).

Effect of Hypoglycaemia on Cerebral Blood Flow and Structure

Hypoglycaemia promotes a redistribution of regional cerebral blood flow (Tallroth et al, 1992; MacLeod et al, 1994) which may encourage localised neuronal ischaemia, particularly if the cerebral macro- or microcirculation is already compromised in subjects with type 1 diabetes. Using techniques such as Single Photon Emission Tomography, the blood flow to the frontal lobes has been shown to be increased during acute hypoglycaemia in non-diabetic subjects (Tallroth et al, 1992). In patients with a history of previous severe hypoglycaemia (MacLeod et al, 1994) and in patients with impaired hypoglycaemia awareness (MacLeod et al, 1996) this altered pattern in regional cerebral blood flow appears to be a

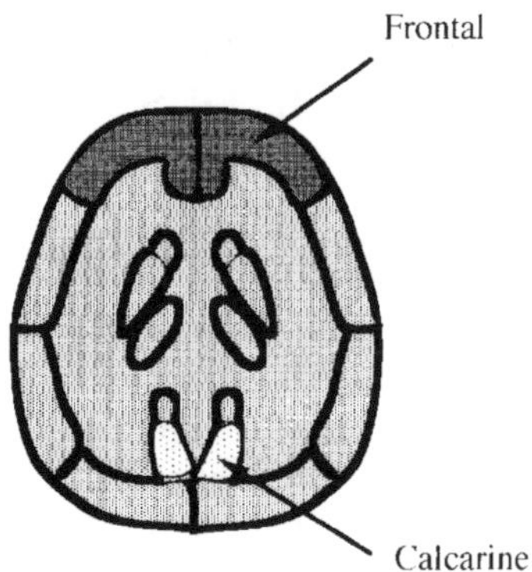

Figure 8.4 Schematic representation of regions of interest in the brain in a neuroanatomical template used for transaxial (horizontal) slices at the level of the basal ganglia, examining cerebral blood flow. By using single photon emission tomography (SPET) during acute hypoglycaemia, increased uptake of isotope in the frontal area indicated increased blood flow while in the calcarine area it was reduced compared to euglycaemia, thus demonstrating redistribution of regional blood flow (MacLeod et al, 1994)

permanent sequel (Figure 8.4). This permanent increase in regional cerebral blood flow to the frontal lobes may be an adaptive response to protect an area of the brain that is most vulnerable to the effects of hypoglycaemia. This susceptibility of the frontal areas has been shown by other techniques, including EEG (Pramming et al, 1988), and tests of cognitive function (see Chapter 2). Neuropathological observations have indicated that the brain is susceptible to neuroglycopenia in a rostrocaudal direction with the cerebral cortex and hippocampus being most sensitive and the brainstem and spinal cord being most resistant (Auer et al, 1984) (Figure 8.5).

Other imaging techniques of the brain have yielded complementary information about abnormal brain structure in diabetes (Figure 8.6). Studies using CT and MRI scanning have shown a high prevalence of cerebral atrophy in people with diabetes (36–53% compared to 12% in age-matched non-diabetic controls), that occurs earlier in life than in non-diabetic control subjects and tends to be more extensive (Figure 8.7) (Araki et al, 1994). Ventricular enlargement also occurs more frequently in patients with diabetes than in healthy controls (Lunetta et al, 1994).

Studies of the brains of people with diabetes using magnetic resonance imaging (MRI) demonstrated a high prevalence (69% in type 1 diabetes versus 12% in healthy non-diabetic subjects) of small periventricular high-intensity lesions known as "leukoaraiosis" (Dejgaard et al, 1991). Leukoaraiosis is an age-related radiological finding that is also associated with hypertension, vascular disease, dementia and demyelination (Pan-

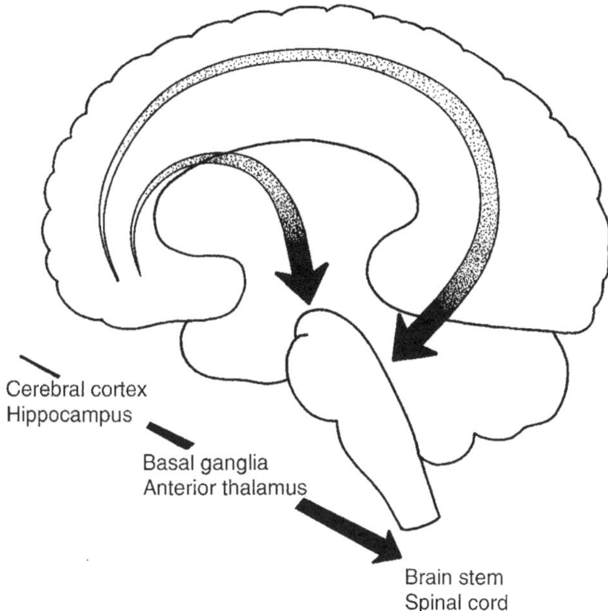

Figure 8.5 Diagram indicating the sensitivity of regions of the brain to acute neuroglycopenia. The cortex and hippocampus are most vulnerable and the brainstem and spinal cord are most resistant

toni and Garcia, 1996). Pathologically, leukoaraiosis has non-specific features consisting of areas of gliosis, loss of myelin sheaths and increased water content (Awad et al, 1986). The significance of leukoaraiosis in diabetes is unknown, but may represent localised ischaemia. In one study it was associated with advanced microvascular diabetic complications (Dejgaard et al, 1991) (Box 8.3, see page 202). Recently, a high incidence of cerebral atrophy (33%), cerebellar atrophy (11%) and leukoaraiosis (56%) was observed in diabetic patients with the 3243 mitochondrial tRNA mutation (Suzuki et al, 1996). Some abnormal patterns of the appearance of MRI scans of the brain are shown schematically in Figure 8.8.

Structural Changes Associated with Hypoglycaemia (Box 8.4)

Human subjects who have succumbed to severe hypoglycaemia have been studied at post-mortem, and are shown to have areas of cortical necrosis, particularly in the frontal lobes and hippocampus, with relative sparing of the hindbrain (Auer et al, 1984). Cortical and hippocampal atrophy and ventricular enlargement have been described in long-term

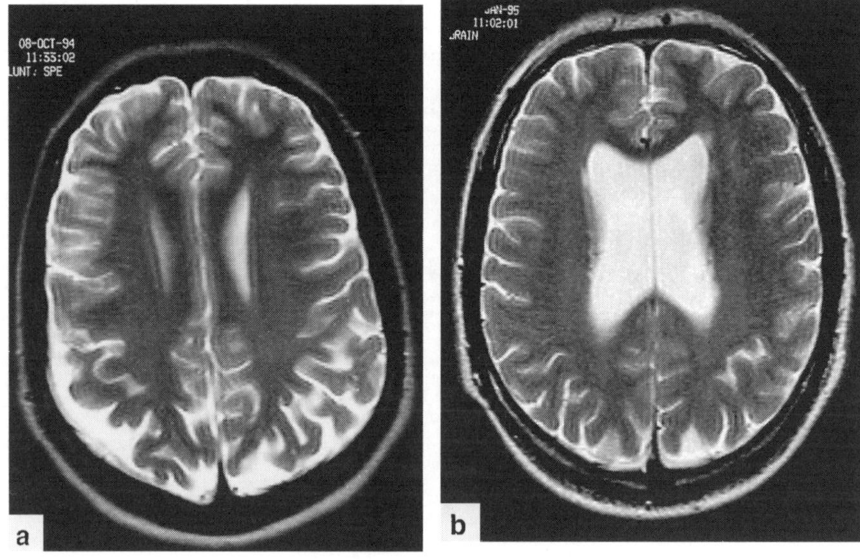

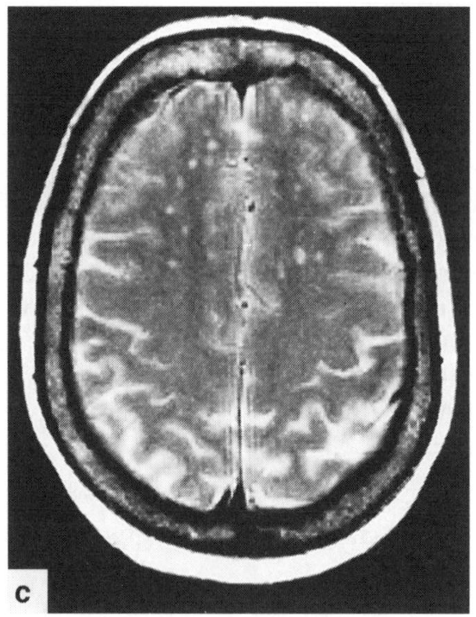

Figure 8.6 Common asymptomatic neurological abnormalities observed with MRI in patients with type 1 diabetes. (a) Cortical atrophy; (b) ventricular dilatation; (c) leukoaraiosis

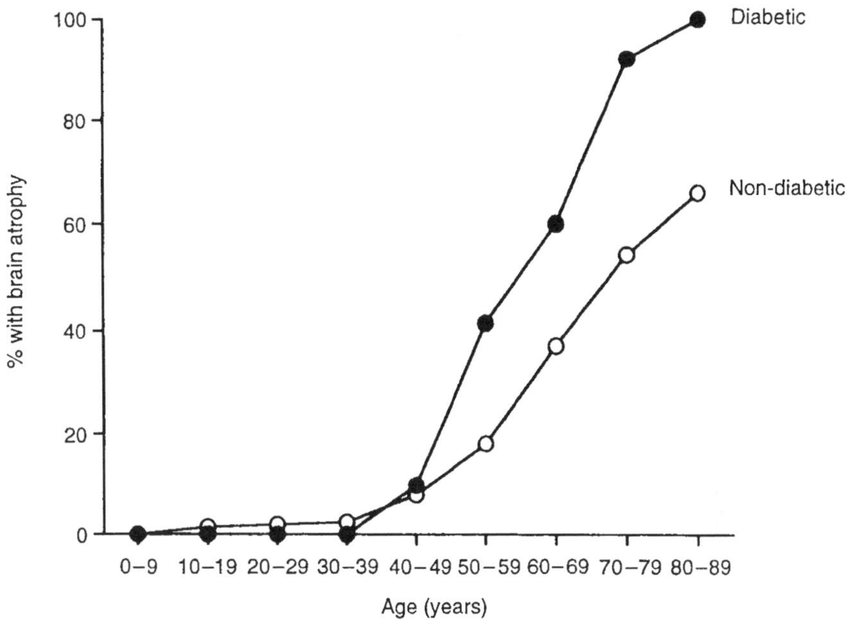

Figure 8.7 The prevalence of brain atrophy with increasing age as demonstrated by MRI. This is more common in diabetic subjects (type 1 and type 2) at an earlier age. Reproduced from Araki et al (1994) by permission of Springer-Verlag

survivors of severe hypoglycaemia (McCall, 1992). The neurohistological features, however, are non-specific and are similar to those of anoxic brain damage. Human studies are further confounded by the fact that many subjects have suffered secondary brain damage as a result of cardiorespiratory collapse (Patrick and Campbell, 1990). In hypoglycaemic brain damage there is selective neuronal acidophilia with shrinkage of the cells which have a bright red cytoplasm (Figure 8.9). These cannot be differentiated from ischaemic neurones, but the *pattern* of neuronal injury characterises hypoglycaemic damage with cells in specific layers of the cortex being destroyed.

A few case reports have described abnormalities of brain structure detected by CT scanning or MRI, associated with focal neurological deficit following one or more episodes of severe hypoglycaemia. Marked global cerebral atrophy has been described in a young patient with type 1 diabetes within a few months of a severe episode of hypoglycaemia which was associated with severe neurological deficit and cortical blindness (Gold and Marshall, 1996). Following severe hypoglycaemia, lesions have been located in the hippocampus in diabetic patients with severe

Box 8.3 Structural abnormalities of the brain associated with diabetes

Gross pathology
Severe cerebral atheroma
Cerebral infarction
Lacunar strokes

*Histological abnormalities**
Meningeal fibrosis
Pseudocalcinosis
Diffuse degeneration of grey and white matter
Increased endothelial basement membrane thickness
Microaneurysms

Abnormal imaging (Figure 8.6)
Cortical atrophy
Ventricular dilatation
Leukoaraiosis

* Some changes were observed in patients who died with coexisting uraemia and hypertension—changes may not be specific to diabetes.

amnesia (Chalmers et al, 1991; Boeve et al, 1995). A lesion with similar appearance on MRI (Figure 8.10) was found in the pons of a patient with persistent ataxia and hemiparesis after an episode of severe hypoglycaemia (Perros et al, 1994).

The neuropathology of mild cognitive impairment (in the absence of abnormal neurological signs) associated with recurrent severe hypoglycaemia is unknown, but may either be a milder form of structural neuronal damage similar to that described in lethal cases, or a functional (metabolic) defect. In support of the former hypothesis is a recent study using brain MRI, in which a group of 11 diabetic patients with a history of severe recurrent hypoglycaemia had a high prevalence of cortical atrophy (45%) compared to none in a matched diabetic control group (Perros et al, 1997).

Mechanisms of Hypoglycaemia-induced Brain Injury

The principal mechanism by which hypoglycaemia leads to its acute neuropsychological manifestations is thought to be the direct effect of lack of glucose on neurones, causing energy failure. Additional alterations in the cerebral circulation induced by hypoglycaemia may cause transient and localised ischaemia, provoking focal neurological abnorm-

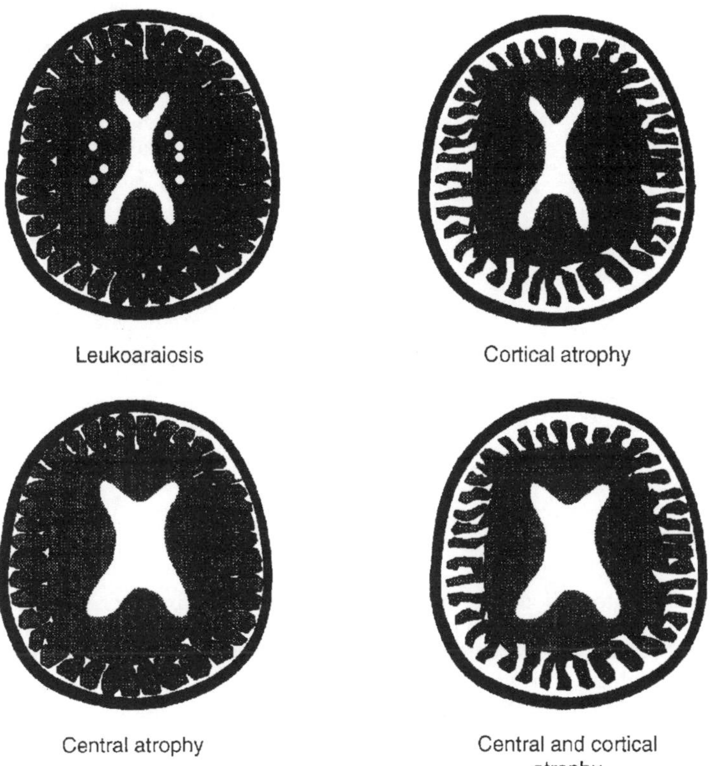

Figure 8.8 Diagrammatic representations of the patterns of abnormal appearance observed in MRI scans of brains in subjects with type 1 diabetes

Box 8.4 Structural abnormalities of the brain associated with profound hypoglycaemia

Lethal hypoglycaemia
Cortical necrosis
Hippocampal necrosis

Survivors of severe hypoglycaemia with gross neurological deficit
Cortical atrophy
Hippocampal atrophy
Ventricular dilatation

Patients with severe recurrent hypoglycaemia and no neurological signs
Cortical atrophy

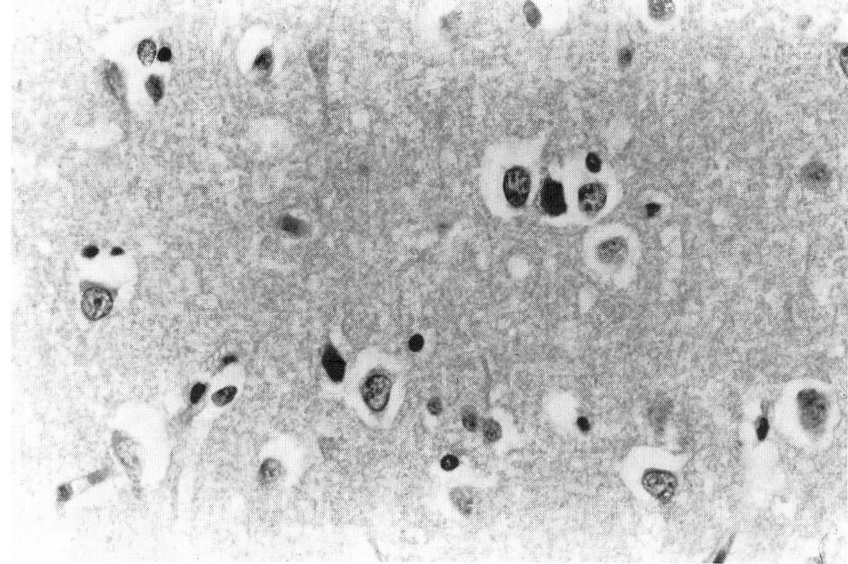

Figure 8.9 Histopathological appearance of neurones in layer 2 of the parietal cortex destroyed by exposure to severe hypoglycaemia in a fatal case of a patient with type 1 diabetes, showing pronounced shrinkage of neurones which appeared acidophilic and were stained bright red (not demonstrable in black and white print). Photograph by courtesy of Dr G. A. Lammie, Department of Neuropathology, Western General Hospital, Edinburgh

alities such as hemiparesis. Less is known about the pathogenesis of permanent neurological damage following severe prolonged hypoglycaemia. In animal models, activation of postsynaptic neurocytotoxin receptors by neurotransmitters (glutamate and N-acetyl aspartate) released from presynaptic neurones as a result of hypoglycaemia, appear to be an important cause of neuronal death (Choi, 1990; Cotman and Iversen, 1987). Increased influx of calcium, which may be linked to stimulation of neurocytotoxin receptors, is also toxic and can cause cell death (Siesjo and Bengsston, 1989). These mechanisms may explain the selective nature of hypoglycaemia-induced neuronal damage which spares glial and vascular tissue in the brain.

Evidence for Diabetic Encephalopathy

Considerable evidence indicates an association between neuropsychological dysfunction and diabetes. The nature of this association is unclear but four main contributing factors have been identified:

- poor glycaemic control

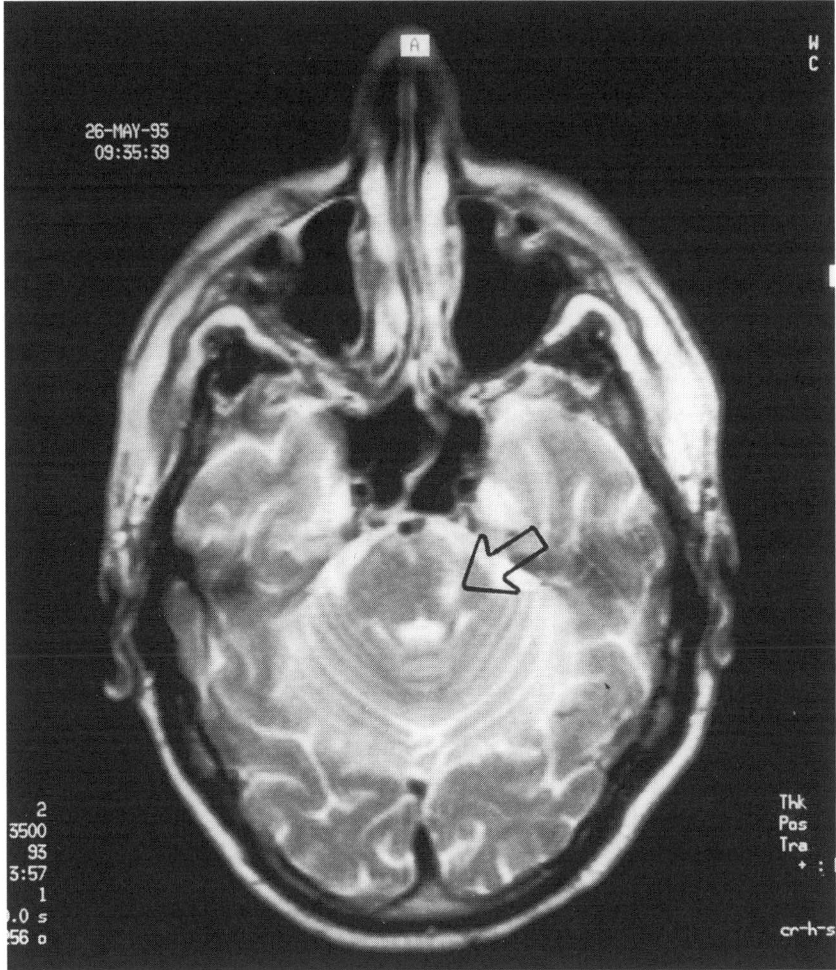

Figure 8.10 MRI scan showing an irregular area of high signal intensity in the left pons in a patient with type 1 diabetes who suffered permanent ataxia and hemiparesis following a single episode of severe hypoglycaemia. From Perros et al (1994) by permission of the American Diabetes Association

- cerebrovascular disease
- hypoglycaemia
- the psychosocial impact of diabetes *per se*.

Hypoglycaemia is of particular importance because it is potentially avoidable, and the subtle cumulative effects on cognitive function may not be noticed until its severity compromises the social and psychological functioning of the affected individual. The misplaced enthusiasm by which some health professionals (and patients) pursue and implement strict glycaemic control when this may not be prudent or appropriate (such as in people with impaired awareness of hypoglycaemia), may place some people at risk of developing diabetic encephalopathy. In a clinical context, severe hypoglycaemia is encountered in three broad categories of patients:

- patients with type 1 diabetes who have strict glycaemic control with no or minimal microvascular complications
- patients with long duration of type 1 diabetes, moderate or poor glycaemic control (often due to inadequate diabetes self-management, erratic lifestyle, inappropriate insulin dose or regimen, coexistent social and psychological problems), associated with advanced microvascular complications
- patients who have suffered a single devastating episode of hypoglycaemia as a result of deliberate or accidental overdose of insulin or sulphonylurea.

Whereas the evidence so far suggests that younger patients in the first category (resembling the highly selected population of patients with type 1 diabetes studied in the DCCT) may not be susceptible to cumulative cognitive deterioration (The Diabetes Control and Complications Trial Research Group, 1996; Reichard and Pihl, 1994), in clinical practice a sizeable proportion of patients belongs to the second category. They have elevated glycated haemoglobin concentrations and established microvascular complications. It has been suggested that hypoglycaemia can aggravate established micro- and macrovascular disease (Fisher and Frier, 1993) and potentiate the risk of hypoglycaemia-induced damage to the brain. The evidence from retrospective studies suggests that chronic deterioration in cognitive function may be a real risk should the conclusions of the DCCT be applied indiscriminately to these patients (Deary and Frier, 1996).

CONCLUSIONS

- It is vital that every effort is made to avoid exposure to severe hypoglycaemia in very young children with type 1 diabetes.
- The targets for glycaemic control should be set flexibly and individually for patients with a history of recurrent severe hypoglycaemia.

continues

continued

- The brain, like the retina, kidney and peripheral nervous system, can be regarded as a target organ in diabetes.
- Hypoglycaemia should be considered as a possible diagnosis in all diabetic patients presenting with any neurological syndrome.
- Hypoglycaemia should be considered in insulin-treated diabetic patients who present with a convulsion. Cerebral oedema should be sought if a patient does not quickly recover consciousness after treatment.
- A wide range of relatively minor and non-specific abnormalities on brain imaging that resemble the changes of normal ageing, are common in diabetic patients. In otherwise asymptomatic patients these abnormalities do not necessarily warrant further investigation.
- The pathogenesis of diabetic encephalopathy is as yet unknown, but hypoglycaemia probably plays a significant contributory role.
- Research in this area and the application of new imaging techniques of the brain are likely to shed further light on this important complication of diabetes.

REFERENCES

Ack M, Miller I, Weil WB (1961). Intelligence of children with diabetes mellitus. *Pediatrics* **28**: 764–70.

Agardh C-D, Rosen I, Ryding E (1983). Persistent vegetative state with high cerebral blood flow following profound hypoglycemia. *Ann Neurol* **14**: 482–6.

Araki Y, Nomura M, Tanaka H, Yamamoto T, Tsukaguchi I, Nakamura H (1994). MRI of the brain in diabetes mellitus. *Neuroradiology* **36**: 101–3.

Arky RA, Veverbrants E, Abramson EA (1968). Irreversible hypoglycemia. A complication of alcohol and insulin. *J Am Med Assoc* **206**: 575–8.

Auer RN, Wieloch T, Olsson Y, Siesjo BK (1984). The distribution of hypoglycemic brain damage. *Acta Neuropathol (Berl)* **64**: 177–91.

Awad IA, Johnson PC, Spetzler RF, Hodak JA (1986). Incidental subcortical lesions identified on magnetic resonance imaging in the elderly, II: postmortem pathological correlations. *Stroke* **17**: 1090–7.

Biessels GJ, Kappelle AC, Bravenboer B, Erkelens DW, Gispen WH (1994). Cerebral function in diabetes mellitus. *Diabetologia* **37**: 643–50.

Bjorgaas M, Sand T, Gimse R (1996). Quantitative EEG in type 1 diabetic children with and without episodes of severe hypoglycemia: a controlled, blind study. *Acta Neurol Scand* **93**: 398–402.

Bjorgaas M, Gimse R, Vik T, Sand T (1997) Cognitive function in type 1 diabetic children with and without episodes of severe hypoglycaemia. *Acta Paediatr* **86**: 148–53.

Bjorgaas M, Sand T, Vik T, Jorde R (1998). Quantitative EEG during controlled hypoglycaemia in diabetic and non-diabetic children. *Diabet Med* **15**: 30–7.

Boeve BF, Bell DG, Noseworthy JH (1995). Bilateral temporal lobe MRI changes in uncomplicated hypoglycemic coma. *Can J Neurol Sci* **22**: 56–8.

Chalmers JC, Risk MTA, Kean DM, Grant R, Ashworth B, Campbell IW (1991). Severe amnesia after hypoglycemia. Clinical, psychometric, and magnetic resonance imaging correlations. *Diabetes Care* **14**: 922–5.

Choi DW (1990). Methods for antagonizing glutamate neurotoxicity. *Cerebrovasc Brain Metab Rev* **2**: 105–47.

Cotman CW, Iversen LL (1987). Excitatory amino acids in the brain-focus on NMDA receptors. *Trends Neurosci* **10**: 263–5.

Deary IJ (1993). Neuropsychological manifestations. In: *Hypoglycaemia and Diabetes: Clinical and Physiological Aspects*. BM Frier and BM Fisher, eds. Edward Arnold, London: 337–46.

Deary IJ (1997). Hypoglycemia-induced cognitive decrements in adults with type 1 diabetes: a case to answer? *Diabetes Spectrum* **10**: 42–7.

Deary IJ, Frier BM (1996). Severe hypoglycaemia and cognitive impairment in diabetes. *BMJ* **313**: 767–9.

Deary IJ, Langan SJ, Graham KS, Hepburn D, Frier BM (1992). Recurrent severe hypoglycemia, intelligence, and speed of information processing. *Intelligence* **16**: 337–59.

Deary IJ, Crawford JR, Hepburn DA, Langan SJ, Blackmore LM, Frier BM (1993). Severe hypoglycemia and intelligence in adult patients with insulin-treated diabetes. *Diabetes* **42:** 341–4.

Dejgaard A, Gade A, Larsson H, Balle V, Parving A, Parving H-H (1991). Evidence for diabetic encephalopathy. *Diabetic Med* **8**: 162–7.

Fallstrom K (1974). On the personality structure in diabetic school children aged 7–15 years. *Acta Paediatr Scand* **251** (suppl 1): 1–70.

Fisher BM, Frier BM (1993). Effect on vascular disease. In: *Hypoglycaemia and Diabetes: Clinical and Physiological Aspects*. BM Frier and BM Fisher, eds. Edward Arnold, London, 355–61.

Gold AE, Marshall SM (1996). Cortical blindness and cerebral infarction associated with severe hypoglycemia. *Diabetes Care* **19**: 1001–3.

Gold AE, Deary IJ, Jones RW, O'Hare JP, Reckless JPD, Frier BM (1994). Severe deterioration in cognitive function and personality in five patients with long-standing diabetes: a complication of diabetes or a consequence of treatment? *Diabetic Med* **11**: 499–505.

Golden MP, Ingersol GM, Brack CJ, Russell BA, Wright JC, Huberty TJ (1989). Longitudinal relationship of asymptomatic hypoglycemia to cognitive function in IDDM. *Diabetes Care* **12**: 89–93.

Hart SP, Frier BM (1998). Causes, management and morbidity of acute hypoglycaemia in adults requiring hospital admission. *Q J Med* **91**: 505–10.

Haumont D, Dorcy H, Pelc S (1979). EEG abnormalities in diabetic children. Influence of hypoglycemia in children and adolescents with IDDM. *Clin Pediatr* **18**: 750–3.

Hepburn DA, Steel JM, Frier BM (1989). Hypoglycemic convulsions cause serious musculoskeletal injuries in patients with IDDM. *Diabetes Care* **12**: 32–4.

Johnson PC, Brendel K, Meezan E (1982). Thickened cerebral cortical capillary basement membranes in diabetics. *Arch Pathol Lab Med* **106**: 214–7.

Langan SJ, Deary IJ, Hepburn DA, Frier BM (1991). Cumulative cognitive impairment following recurrent severe hypoglycaemia in adult patients with insulin-treated diabetes mellitus. *Diabetologia* **34**: 337–44.

Lincoln NB, Faleiro RM, Kelly C, Kirk BA, Jeffcoate WJ (1996). Effect of long-term glycemic control on cognitive function. *Diabetes Care* **19**: 656–8.

Lins PE, Adamson U. Neurological manifestations of hypoglycaemia. In: *Hypoglycaemia and Diabetes: Clinical and Physiological Aspects*. BM Fisher and BM Frier, eds. Edward Arnold, London, 347–54.

Lunetta M, Damanti AR, Fabbri G, Lombardo M, Di Mauro M, Mughini L (1994). Evidence by magnetic resonance imaging of cerebral alterations of atrophy type in young insulin-dependent diabetic patients. *J Endocrinol Invest* **17**: 241–5.

MacCuish AC (1993). Treatment of hypoglycaemia. In: *Hypoglycaemia and Diabetes: Clinical and Physiological Aspects*. BM Frier and BM Fisher, eds. Edward Arnold, London, 212–21.

MacLeod KM, Hepburn DA, Frier BM (1993). Frequency and morbidity of severe hypoglycaemia in insulin-treated diabetic patients. *Diabet Med* **10**: 238–45.

MacLeod KM, Hepburn DA, Deary IJ, Goodwin GM, Ebmeier KP, Frier BM (1994). Regional cerebral blood flow in IDDM patients: effects of diabetes and of recurrent severe hypoglycaemia. *Diabetologia* **37**: 257–63.

MacLeod KM, Gold AE, Ebmeier KP, Hepburn DA, Deary IJ, Goodwin GM, Frier BM (1996). The effects of hypoglycemia on relative cerebral blood flow distribution in patients with type 1 (insulin-dependent) diabetes and impaired hypoglycemia awareness. *Metabolism* **45**: 974–80.

Malouf R, Brust JC (1985). Hypoglycemia: causes, neurological manifestations, and outcome. *Ann Neurol* **17**: 421–30.

McCall AL (1992). The impact of diabetes on the CNS. *Diabetes* **41**: 557–70.

Northam E, Anderson P, Werther G, Adler R, Andrewes D (1995). Neuropsychological complications of insulin-dependent diabetes in children. *Child Neuropsychol* **1**: 74–87.

Northam EA, Anderson PJ, Werther GA, Warne GL, Adler RG, Andrewes D (1998). Neuropsychological complications of IDDM in children 2 years after disease onset. *Diabetes Care* **21**: 379–84.

Pantoni L, Garcia JH (1996). The significance of cerebral white matter abnormalities 100 years after Binswanger's report. *Stroke* **26**: 1293–301.

Patrick AW, Campbell IW (1990). Fatal hypoglycaemia in insulin-treated diabetes mellitus: clinical features and neuropathological changes. *Diabet Med* **7**: 349–54.

Perros P, Sellar RJ, Frier BM (1994). Chronic pontine dysfunction following insulin-induced hypoglycemia in an IDDM patient. *Diabetes Care* **17**: 725–7.

Perros P, Deary IJ, Sellar RJ, Best JJK, Frier BM (1997). Brain abnormalities demonstrated by magnetic resonance imaging in adult IDDM patients with and without a history of recurrent severe hypoglycemia. *Diabetes Care* **20**: 1013–8.

Pramming S, Thorsteinsson B, Stigsby B, Binder C (1988). Glycaemic threshold for changes in electroencephalograms during hypoglycaemia in patients with insulin dependent diabetes. *BMJ* **296**: 665–7.

Reichard P, Pihl M (1994). Mortality and treatment side-effects during long-term intensified conventional insulin treatment in the Stockholm Diabetes Intervention Study. *Diabetes* **43**: 313–7.

Reske-Nielsen E, Lundbaek K, Rafaelson OJ (1965). Pathological changes in the central and peripheral nervous system of young long-term diabetics. *Diabetologia* **1**: 233–41.

Rovet J, Alvarez M (1997). Attentional functioning in children and adolescents with IDDM. *Diabetes Care* **20**: 803–10.

Rovet JF, Ehrlich RM, Hoppe M (1987). Intellectual deficits associated with early onset of insulin-dependent diabetes mellitus in children. *Diabetes Care* **10**: 510–5.

Ryan CM (1988). Neuropsychological complications of type 1 diabetes. *Diabetes Care* **11**: 86–93.

Ryan C, Vega A, Longstreet C, Drash A (1984). Neuropsychological changes in adolescents with insulin-dependent diabetes. *J Consult Clin Psychol* **52**: 335–42.

Seidl R, Birnbacher R, Hauser E, Bernert G, Freilinger M, Schober E (1996). Brainstem auditory evoked potentials and visually evoked potentials in young patients with IDDM. *Diabetes Care* **19**: 1220–4.

Siesjo BK, Bengsston F (1989). Calcium fluxes, calcium antagonists, and calcium related pathology in brain ischemia, hypoglycemia and spreading depression: a unifying hypothesis. *J Cereb Blood Flow Metab* **9**: 127–40.

Strachan MWJ, Deary IJ, Ewing FME, Frier BM (1998). Recovery of cognitive function and mood following a single episode of spontaneously occurring severe hypoglycaemia in insulin-treated diabetic patients. *Diabet Med* **15** (suppl 1): S4 (abstract).

Suzuki Y, Hata, T, Miyaoka H, Atsumi Y, Kadowaki H, Taniyama M, Kadowaki T, Odawara M, Tanaka Y, Asahina T, Matsuoka K (1996). Diabetes with the 3243 mitochondrial tRNA Leu(UUR) mutation. *Diabetes Care* **19**: 739–84.

Tallroth G, Ryding E, Agardh C-D (1992). Regional cerebral blood flow in normal man during insulin-induced hypoglycemia and in the recovery period following glucose infusion. *Metabolism* **41**: 717–21.

The Diabetes Control and Complications Trial Research Group (1996). Effects of intensive diabetes therapy on neuropsychological function in adults in the Diabetes Control and Complications Trial. *Ann Int Med* **124**: 379–88.

Uberall MA, Renner C, Edl S, Parzinger E, Wenzel D (1996). VEP and ERP abnormalities in children and adolescents with prepubertal onset of insulin-dependent diabetes mellitus. *Neuropediatrics* **27**: 88–93.

Wredling R, Levander S, Adamson U, Lins P-E (1990). Permanent neuropsychological impairment after recurrent episodes of severe hypoglycaemia in man. *Diabetologia* **33**: 152–7.

9

Hypoglycaemia in Children with Diabetes

PETER G. F. SWIFT
Children's Hospital, Leicester Royal Infirmary, Leicester

INTRODUCTION

"Hypos are hell. It is difficult to overestimate their significance."
(Quote: a doctor with diabetes.)

The uniquely intrusive demands which diabetes imposes upon children and their families is highlighted by the impact of hypoglycaemia. All children with diabetes will expect to experience hypoglycaemia at some time because the essential treatment (insulin) causes hyperinsulinaemia (see Chapter 6) and childhood itself is inherently labile and unpredictable. A child's development, growth, nutritional demands, activity levels and metabolism are constantly changing, every day and every night. The signs, symptoms, frequency and biopsychosocial consequences of hypoglycaemia are distinctly different in children than in adults and they change during the course of childhood and adolescence. Childhood diabetes is a constantly moving target.

If the threat of even mild hypoglycaemia resulting in difficult or regressive behaviour is sufficient to induce chronic parental anxiety, then the terrifying experience of a severe nocturnal hypoglycaemic seizure will destroy self-confidence. Both experiences may undermine attempts to achieve near normoglycaemia. Parents are faced with the cruel dilemma of negotiating a perilous course for their child between tighter control

---

Hypoglycaemia in Clinical Diabetes. Edited by B. M. Frier and B. M. Fisher.

with the greater risk of hypoglycaemia, and more lenient control with the prospect of developing long-term vascular complications. Nevertheless, a significant proportion of children are able to achieve excellent metabolic control without frequent severe hypoglycaemia, and this outcome should be the aim in all children's diabetic clinics.

PHYSIOLOGICAL IDIOSYNCRASIES OF CHILDHOOD

There are some fundamental metabolic characteristics of young children, especially in the fasted state, which allow them to tolerate starvation much less well than adults (Aynsley-Green et al, 1993) and make them vulnerable to hypoglycaemia.

- The young child has a large brain relative to total body weight. The brain is growing and utilises large amounts of glucose as its major fuel independent of insulin action.
- The liver is also a relatively large organ with a glucose production rate that is two to four times greater than in adults. Glycogen stores are therefore more rapidly exhausted in the fasting state.
- The muscle mass of children is low compared with adults, muscle glycogen is more readily depleted and mobilisation of gluconeogenic precursors is less effective (Haymond et al, 1982).
- Ketogenesis is two to three times more rapid in children than in adults (Haymond et al, 1982). Ketone bodies can be utilised as an alternative fuel for the brain.

Thus in the normal fasting state, despite suppression of endogenous insulin, there is a threat of rapid glycogen depletion and inadequate gluconeogenesis. In the diabetic child, unphysiological hyperinsulinaemia exacerbates the tendency to hypoglycaemia because not only are glycogenolysis and proteolysis inhibited, but the alternative fuel of ketones is readily turned off. These risks may become greater with increasing duration of diabetes and intensive insulin treatment as a result of progressive failure of catecholamine and glucagon counterregulatory mechanisms (see Chapter 4).

Younger children with diabetes are particularly likely to experience hypoglycaemia, not only because of the above metabolic characteristics, but also because parents (or the children themselves) adhere responsibly to regular administration of insulin, although food intake is variable. In addition, the child goes to bed earlier and has a longer period of nocturnal starvation. By adolescence the metabolic and practical idiosyncrasies of early childhood may have changed, to be replaced by the equally challenging problems of erratic frequency of insulin injections and risk-taking behaviour, making ketoacidosis a greater threat than hypoglycaemia.

CAN HYPOGLYCAEMIA BE USEFULLY DEFINED IN CHILDREN?

"What is a 'high-pow'?—We should call it a 'low-po'!"
(Quote: A seven-year-old child with diabetes.)

Studies have shown that a low blood glucose is usually, but not always, associated with neurophysiological changes or with recognisable signs and symptoms. Therefore the definition of "low" remains debatable because of considerable individual variation in response to a particular level of blood glucose. When some *non-diabetic* children have been fasted they may occasionally exhibit concentrations of blood glucose which could be considered to be in a hypoglycaemic range, and may even experience autonomic responses to a reduction in blood glucose following the ingestion of sugar drinks (Jones et al, 1995). Haymond et al (1982) showed that during 18 hours of fasting the blood glucose concentration was usually maintained above 4.0 mmol/l but decreased thereafter and studies on young non-diabetic children during the night have revealed a decline in blood glucose to 3.4 mmol/l but rarely to lower levels (Matyka et al, 1996). However, after fasting for surgery, non-diabetic children have been shown to develop hypoglycaemia (Kelnar, 1976), and when blood glucose was measured during overnight endocrine tests Stirling et al (1991) found that 5% of children had a blood glucose below 3.0 mmol/l.

In any individual a *physiological and functional* definition of hypoglycaemia may be the blood glucose threshold below which there are cognitive or physiological changes sufficient to interfere with normal activities and so require intervention. However, neurophysiological changes may be unrecognised or asymptomatic and the longer-term significance of such hypoglycaemia is not known. In children with diabetes asymptomatic biochemical hypoglycaemia is certainly common, particularly at night, in young children and in those with strict glycaemic control (Porter et al, 1997), but should not be tolerated as a frequent event as it may affect the responses to subsequent hypoglycaemia (see Chapter 5).

Several prevalence studies have used *clinical definitions* of hypoglycaemia in children (Box 9.1). These descriptions of severity may be applicable to schoolchildren and teenagers but not to children who are too young to self-treat or to recognise symptoms of hypoglycaemia. In adults, no distinction is made between "moderate" and "severe" categories. If

Box 9.1 Clinical definitions of hypoglycaemia

- *Mild hypoglycaemia* – episodes not requiring external assistance (self-treated)
  – episodes easily reversed by glucose or food
- *Moderate hypoglycaemia* – episodes requiring external assistance (with additional carbohydrate)
- *Severe hypoglycaemia* – episodes causing coma/convulsions or requiring parenteral therapy

external assistance is required, significant neuroglycopenia is present and this is classified as "severe". Davis et al (1997) have suggested that moderate hypoglycaemia in pre-school children should include episodes with obvious neuroglycopenia manifesting as confusion or drowsiness and requiring immediate oral carbohydrate. It has been emphasised that any episode which causes an increase in risk to the patient is important (The Diabetes Control and Complications Trial Research Group, 1994). Thus, an academic biochemical definition of hypoglycaemia is unhelpful, and it is unwise to accept blood glucose values of less than 3.5 mmol/l either during the day or night. The safest advice is to suggest that blood glucose should be maintained above 4.0 mmol/l (i.e. "make four the floor").

FREQUENCY

"When is it going to happen, this hypo . . . ?"
(Quote: Anxious parent.)

All children with diabetes can expect to experience some degree of hypoglycaemia, whatever their quality of metabolic control. The time of occurrence of the first episode of severe hypoglycaemia is unpredictable and the reported prevalence of severe events varies because of different definitions, variations in severity and whether studies are retrospective or prospective.

A large prospective study (Davis et al, 1997) of 657 children on conventional twice-daily insulin regimens showed:

- an incidence of *severe* (coma/convulsions) episodes of 5 per 100 patient years
- an incidence of *moderate* (requiring assistance) episodes of 30 per 100 patient years

- an incidence of *severe/moderate* episodes of 40 per 100 patient years in children less than 7 years
- 75% of severe episodes occurred at night
- during one year, 15% of children experience a *moderate/severe* episode
- if one episode of severe hypoglycaemia occurred there was a 32% risk of recurrence within three years
- the incidence per 100 patient years was inversely related to glycaemic control (HbA1c) (Table 9.1).

Other major studies have documented *severe* hypoglycaemic events. In the subgroup of adolescent subjects (aged 13–17 years) in the Diabetes Control and Complications Trial (DCCT) (The Diabetes Control and Complications Trial (DCCT) Research Group, 1994):

- an incidence was recorded of 27 per 100 patient years on intensive therapy (HbA1c 8.1%) using multiple insulin injection or pump regimens
- an incidence was recorded of 10 per 100 patient years on conventional therapy (HbA1c 9.8%), usually with twice-daily insulin regimens
- 82% of the intensively treated group experienced a severe event during the seven years of the DCCT.

An international study of diabetic control in children (Mortensen and Hougaard, 1997) showed:

- an incidence of 58 per 100 patient years in children aged <5 years
- an incidence of 30 per 100 patient years in children aged 5–8 years
- an incidence of 14 per 100 patient years in children aged 9–18 years
- the incidence increased with lower HbA1c although some centres achieving excellent glycaemic control did not report an increased frequency of hypoglycaemia.

Table 9.1 Percentage of children experiencing hypoglycaemia of different severity in one year

HbA1c (%)	Severe	Moderate	Combined
<7	15	32	47
7–8	7	28	35
>8	4	12	16

Derived from Davis et al (1997)

A single-centre survey of 146 children maintaining a near-physiological mean HbA1c of 6.9%, using predominantly multiple injection treatment reported an incidence of 19 per 100 patient years. (Nordfeldt and Ludvigsson, 1997) The authors maintain that this rate, which was lower than that recorded in the DCCT, can be achieved by an educational programme which teaches active problem-solving and self-management, but this requires intensive psychosocial support.

A prospective survey over eight years by Egger et al (1991) of 155 children with type 1 diabetes reported a rising incidence of hypoglycaemic coma from 4.4 per 100 patient years in the first four years of the study to 7.4 per 100 patient years in the second four years (Figure 9.1). This was associated with intensification of insulin treatment and a reduction in mean glycated haemoglobin. A prospective study of 133 children and adolescents with type 1 diabetes in Hungary (Barkai et al, 1998) demonstrated an overall incidence of hypoglycaemia of 38.5 episodes per 100 patient years and of coma or seizure of 6.2 per 100 patient years, although another prospective study of 287 children and adolescents with type 1 diabetes, all of whom were on multiple injection therapy, recorded a much lower rate of 3.1 episodes per 100 patient years (Tupola et al, 1998b).

Incidence of Nocturnal Hypoglycaemia

"I sleep very lightly at night . . . to hear if she's hypo."
(Quote: Anxious mother.)

Overnight blood glucose profiles confirm that nocturnal hypoglycaemia is very common (Table 9.2). Matyka et al (1996), in studies of young

Table 9.2 Frequency of nocturnal hypoglycaemia in children with diabetes

Blood glucose during the night (mmol/l)	Incidence (%)	Reference
Hospital studies		
<3.6	18	Winter, 1981
<3.0	19	Baumer et al, 1982
<3.0	34	Whincup and Milner, 1987
<3.3	14	Shalwitz et al, 1990
<3.0	25	Simell et al, 1993
<3.3	47	Beregszaszi et al, 1997
Studies at home		
<3.5	18	Porter et al, 1997
<3.5	60–70	Matyka et al, 1996

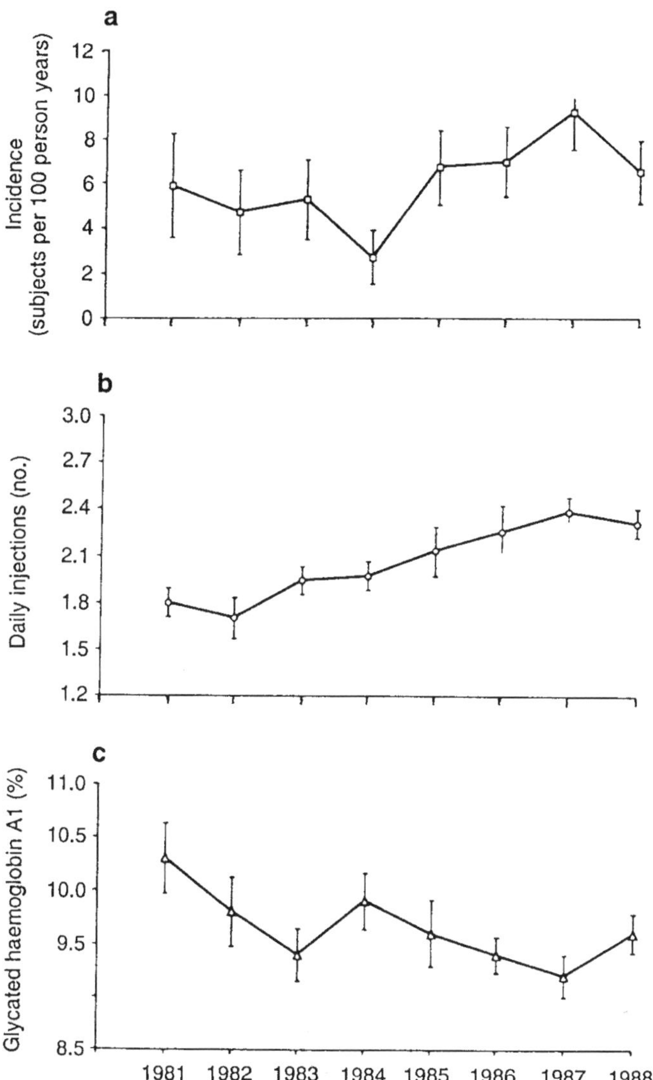

Figure 9.1 Incidence of hypoglycaemic coma (a), number of daily insulin injections (b) and mean HbA1c levels (c) in 155 children with type 1 diabetes, from 1981 to 1988 (mean ± SE). From Egger et al (1991) with permission of the American Diabetes Association

children in their homes, have reported that 65% on conventional insulin therapy have a blood glucose below 3.5 mmol/l during the night, some remaining profoundly hypoglycaemic for hours, with concentrations as low as 1.6 mmol/l. These episodes are almost entirely asymptomatic but might be expected to affect symptomatic awareness of hypoglycaemia the following day. However, simultaneous EEG recordings and cognitive tests performed the following morning have not revealed significant abnormalities (K. Matyka, personal communication).

Practice Points

- Any child with a falling blood glucose may experience autonomic symptoms
- From 6 to 27% of children have one severe hypoglycaemic episode per year (a significant proportion being at night)
- The risk of hypoglycaemia is doubled if HbA1c $<8\%$
- The risk is increased five times if age <6 years
- The risk of recurrence is increased following an episode of severe hypoglycaemia
- Blood glucose <3.5 mmol/l occurs during the night in at least 15% of children on conventional insulin regimens

CAUSES OF HYPOGLYCAEMIA

Hypoglycaemia in the diabetic child is caused by:

- excessive insulin action
- inadequate carbohydrate absorption
- excessive glucose utilisation (often exercise-induced)
- a combination of the above.

In various cohort studies, identifiable precipitants of hypoglycaemia often could not be identified—from 15% (Daneman et al, 1989) to 38% (Davis et al, 1997).

Excessive Insulin Action

1. There is a risk that newly diagnosed children experience confidence-shattering hypoglycaemia soon after going home because inadequate guidance has been given about insulin therapy. With improved education from organised diabetes teams severe hypoglycaemia in the first year after diagnosis may now be less common (Davis et al, 1997), and retention of residual endogenous insulin secretion during this period diminishes the degree of fluctuation of blood glucose.
2. Insulin absorption is unpredictably variable, so causing sudden

surges of hyperinsulinaemia and resulting hypoglycaemia. A number of children with sudden unexpected hypoglycaemia, on careful questioning, describe bleeding and pain from the injection site, probably because insulin had been injected intramuscularly promoting more rapid absorption. Lipohypertrophy at injection sites also increases the variability of absorption.

3. Current insulin regimens make nocturnal hyperinsulinaemia almost inevitable.
4. Particular insulin regimens in children may increase the risk of hypoglycaemia. The excessive use of short-acting (soluble) insulin in the morning may cause hypoglycaemia before lunch, particularly in young children who sometimes appear to be exquisitely "sensitive" to soluble (unmodified) insulin. By contrast, the new rapid-acting insulin analogue, insulin lispro, may reduce hypoglycaemic events in adolescents (Garg et al, 1996). Although some studies have suggested that twice-daily regimens are associated with more hypoglycaemia than multiple injection therapy, the DCCT has refuted this, and other studies show variable rates of hypoglycaemia on multiple injection therapy (Aman et al, 1989; Nordfeldt and Ludvigsson, 1997). Dorchy (1994) and Dorchy et al (1997) have provided "recipes" for good glycaemic control on twice-daily insulin which include advice on increasing the intake of carbohydrate at mid-morning to match the plasma insulin profile.

   Although the plasma insulin profile needs careful consideration, particularly in children with recurrent hypoglycaemia, the frequency of episodes often depends on factors other than the insulin regimen *per se*.
5. Errors in insulin administration:
   - Mistakes are common human errors. They are unpredictable, inevitable and unpreventable, accounting for less than 10% of episodes (Davis et al, 1997).
   - Factitious injections of insulin are associated with psychological disturbance. Clinic staff occasionally recognise a child who injects excessive insulin to provoke recurrent episodes of hypoglycaemia. Although these children present with recurrent hypoglycaemia they may report that their insulin dose is decreasing: "Doctor, do you think the diabetes is going away?" A high index of suspicion is needed to recognise this problem and astute detective work may be required to uncover the precipitants—often a distressed family, or a child experiencing school or peer group problems.
6. Failure to reduce insulin during strenuous exercise (see below).

Inadequate Carbohydrate Absorption

Several reports have sounded a note of surprise that no close correlation exists between total insulin dose and rate of hypoglycaemia, or that sometimes there is no direct relationship between the frequency of hypoglycaemia and mean glycated haemoglobin. Almost certainly this is because the importance of providing a regular intake of high-fibre carbohydrate to balance the unphysiological hyperinsulinaemia is underestimated. It is not difficult for children to establish eating patterns with regular snacks and main meals but it is impossible for these meals to be always taken on time, to contain similar quality and quantity of carbohydrate or to be absorbed homogeneously.

Delayed or Missed Food

About one-third of episodes of hypoglycaemia have been attributed to delayed or inadequate ingestion of food (Bhatia and Wolfsdorf, 1991; Daneman et al, 1989). This is probably an underestimate, especially when children become less dependent upon parental organisation. Adolescents experiment with alternative or missed meals just as they experiment with insulin doses. Children and parents sometimes forget a bedtime snack or reduce the intake of carbohydrate if blood glucose is high.

Inappropriate Carbohydrate Intake

In young children a common cause of recurrent hypoglycaemia is an inappropriately regulated diet. There is little doubt that when children can be guided to take regular quantities of high fibre, starchy carbohydrate, the frequency of hypoglycaemia declines.

In certain circumstances, such as prolonged or vigorous exercise, particularly if associated with hazardous activities such as water-sports or rock-climbing, the carbohydrate intake should be significantly increased (Akerblom et al, 1980; Thompson et al, 1995). Many children continue to be constrained in their carbohydrate intake by outdated concepts of a calculated intake of carbohydrate, counting grams or exchanges of carbohydrate that are infrequently revised despite growth and changing activities (Frost, 1995). These have little proven scientific credibility (Price et al, 1993; Waldron, 1996) and during heavy exercise may well inhibit adequate food intake rather than increase it. This has been highlighted by studies of hypoglycaemia at summer camps for children with diabetes (Braatvedt et al, 1997; Swift, 1997).

Gastro-intestinal Upsets

A common childhood infection which causes hypoglycaemia, rather than the opposite, is gastroenteritis with diarrhoea and vomiting. Carbohydrate absorption may be severely compromised. The hypoglycaemia sometimes precedes the diarrhoea and may be profound and prolonged.

Excessive Glucose Utilisation

Muscular activity with vigorous exercise can cause acute and sometimes prolonged falls in blood glucose because:

- insulin is mobilised from injection sites
- glucose uptake is enhanced
- insulin sensitivity is improved
- insulin inhibits hepatic glucose production.

If the exercise is particularly prolonged, muscle and hepatic glycogen stores are depleted and during later repletion hypoglycaemia may occur again (MacDonald, 1987). Exercise always features as an important factor in studies of childhood hypoglycaemia (Daneman et al, 1989; Bhatia and Wolfsdorf, 1991; Davis et al, 1997) and is well known to clinicians who take children on adventure holidays (Akerblom et al, 1980; Hillson, 1987). Children most at risk may not be those who frequently perform strenuous exercise with games and sporting activities, but those who are not accustomed to it (Chadwick and Brown, 1992).

Miscellaneous Causes

1. A combination of inappropriately adjusted insulin and too little carbohydrate during physical exercise is one of the commonest preventable causes of hypoglycaemia in children.
2. Alcohol inhibits gluconeogenesis, and in combination with the inhibition of glycogenolysis by insulin may cause profound nocturnal hypoglycaemia after an evening binge. The metabolic effects of alcohol are more pronounced in young people and can cause problems other than intoxication in teenagers with type 1 diabetes who are experimenting with alcohol.
3. It has been speculated that deficient secretion of endogenous glucagon in response to hypoglycaemia might exacerbate severity. This does not seem to be an important factor because it is usually compensated for by vigorous secretion of adrenaline. However, when antecedent hypoglycaemia has occurred, counterregulatory hormonal deficiency may be significant (see Chapter 5).

4. Unexplained recurrent episodes of hypoglycaemia must be rigorously investigated, including tests to exclude the conditions of coeliac disease and adrenocortical insufficiency (Addison's disease), that are associated with type 1 diabetes.

Changes in Routine

Most of the precipitants of hypoglycaemia described above are associated in one way or another with changes in daily routine, habit or activity. Insulin doses are relatively stable but increase greatly through childhood; food intake cannot be tightly regulated and the absorption varies markedly; exercise and its effects are unpredictable. Tupola et al (1998b) observed that severe hypoglycaemia was most common in summer (Figure 9.2), attributing this to accelerated absorption of insulin in warm weather, increased physical activity and changes in daily routine at school. Hypoglycaemia is more common on holidays, especially in the first few days when the usual routines are altered and parental vigilance may be relaxed. At weekends, on holiday or at special events, meal planning is different, insulin timing goes awry, activity levels vary and

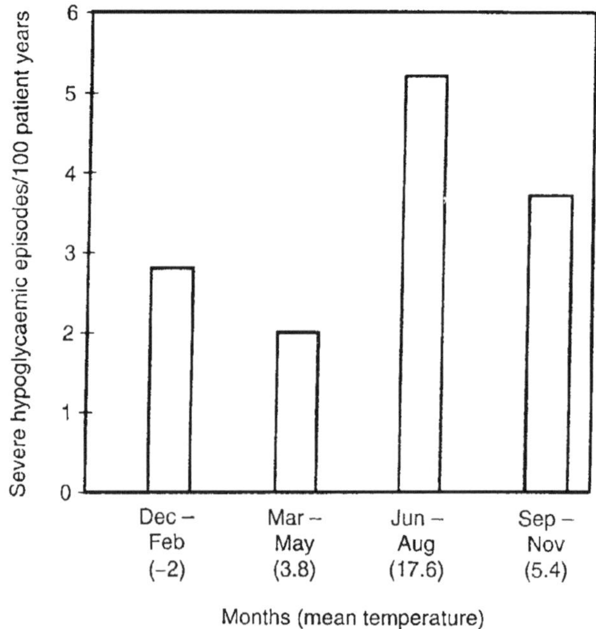

Figure 9.2 Seasonal variation in rate of severe hypoglycaemia with mean temperatures (°C) in Helsinki in a study of children with diabetes from 1990 to 1995. Reproduced from Tupola et al (1998b) with permission of *Diabetic Medicine*

surveillance may slip—all recipes for destructive hypoglycaemia to ruin the fun (Swift and Waldron, 1990). Unfortunately diabetes also goes on holiday but does not relax its grip!

PHYSIOLOGICAL RESPONSES TO HYPOGLYCAEMIA

Autonomic Nervous System Responses

Certain signs (early pallor; later sweating) and symptoms (hunger, trembling, feeling hot, pounding heart) are generated by activation of the autonomic nervous system. The blood glucose concentration at which activation occurs varies between and within individuals in different circumstances and is associated with the release of adrenaline (see Figure 9.3).

Hypoglycaemia studies using the glucose clamp technique have demonstrated:

- secretion of adrenaline in adults with type 1 diabetes at variable blood glucose concentrations from 4.1 to 2.7 mmol/l (Amiel et al, 1987)
- exaggerated catecholamine responses in non-diabetic children (aged 13 ± 2 years) occurring at a higher mean blood glucose (3.9 mmol/l) than adults (3.2 mmol/l) (Jones et al, 1991)
- autonomic activation and symptoms occurring at a higher blood glucose concentration (4.9 mmol/l) in poorly controlled children with diabetes than in those with better glycaemic control (2.6 mmol/l) (Amiel et al, 1988; Jones et al, 1991)
- adrenaline release occurs at a wide range of blood glucose thresholds (4.7–2.7 mmol/l) in adolescents with diabetes who have average glycaemic control (Bjorgaas et al, 1997)
- that the level of blood glucose *per se* is more important than the rate of fall of blood glucose for the activation of autonomic symptoms (Amiel et al, 1987).

Clinical studies in adults have shown major discrepancies between the development of symptoms of hypoglycaemia and the level of blood glucose. In one study only 11% of episodes showed concurrence between symptoms and biochemical hypoglycaemia (Pramming et al, 1990). Discrepancies between symptoms, measured blood glucose (of questionable precision) and variable blood glucose thresholds for autonomic activation make advice and management difficult. Parents often say "my child feels better when blood glucose levels are high," or "hypos occur when blood glucose is above 4 or 6 mmol/l or even higher". This phenomenon (a feature of poor glycaemic control) may sabotage attempts to improve control. If there is doubt about the blood glucose threshold for hypoglycaemic symptoms, the level should be estimated by careful monitoring and if the blood glucose is in the higher "non-hypoglycaemic" range, the quantity of carbohydrate given to treat symptoms should be much less than that required for a genuinely low blood glucose (below 3.5 mmol/l) or for severe disabling hypoglycaemia. Overtreatment of very mild hypoglycaemia often provokes prolonged hyperglycaemia for the following 24 hours.

Central Nervous System (Neuroglycopenic) Responses

The signs (glazed, 'spaced-out', altered behaviour) and symptoms (dizziness, tingling of lips, agitation, confusion, tiredness) differ from the autonomic features described above, and are provoked by the direct effect of hypoglycaemia causing dysfunction of the central nervous system (neuroglycopenia).

Studies by Koh et al (1988) showed that:

- alterations (i.e. delayed conduction) occur in brainstem and auditory evoked potentials in children and babies when blood glucose falls below 2.6 mmol/l
- neural function may still be normal (in children aged more than one year) at a blood glucose as low as 1.9 mmol/l
- neurological dysfunction persists for several hours after blood glucose has returned to normal
- abnormal neurophysiology may not necessarily be associated with any recognisable symptoms.

Ryan et al (1990) showed that subtle tests of cognitive function (e.g. decision-making, attention, speed responses) in children with diabetes revealed disturbances at a mean blood glucose of 3.7 mmol/l and these became more abnormal below 3.3 mmol/l, but with significant individual variation in response. Considerable delays in recovery were observed. When the blood glucose is as low as 2.2 mmol/l, electroencephalogram (EEG) abnormalities may also be generated (Hawarth and Coodin, 1960). Ketones may offer a degree of protection to electrophysiological abnormalities, but the importance of this in recovery from hypoglycaemia is uncertain (Koh et al, 1988). In a similar manner to the autonomic responses to hypoglycaemia, the blood glucose threshold for neurological dysfunction varies considerably between and within individuals in different circumstances (see Figure 9.3).

Recognisable autonomic signs or symptoms are essential to the individual child or carer if prevention and treatment of hypoglycaemia are to

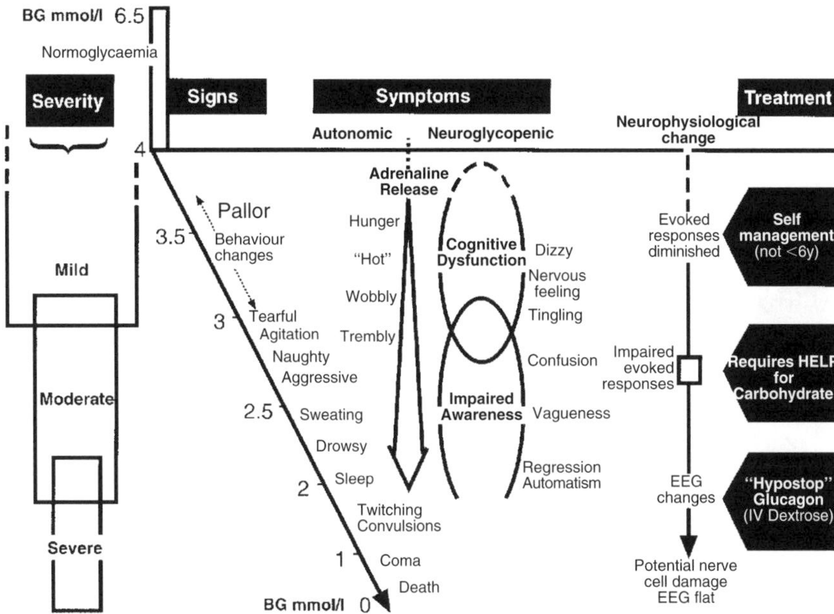

Figure 9.3 Relationship between clinical and physiological changes at different levels of glycaemia

be successful. These clinical changes must trigger *awareness of hypoglycaemia* or *recognition* which in turn should promote a corrective response (see Figure 9.4). In children less than six years of age the full pathway of recognition and responsiveness is virtually impossible, because at this age symptoms cannot be linked in abstract thought to action. In older children neuroglycopenia may precede or override autonomic responses, and the risk of this may be greater in children who are treated more intensively. The claim that impaired awareness of hypoglycaemia occurs in children below the age of six years (Barkai et al, 1998) is unfounded, although older children and teenagers may develop this problem.

There are therefore several circumstances which may sabotage appropriate responsiveness:

- when neuroglycopenia precedes autonomic activation
- very young children who cannot respond
- older children who are distracted by other activities
- true impaired awareness of hypoglycaemia
- personal behavioural limitations of self-care.

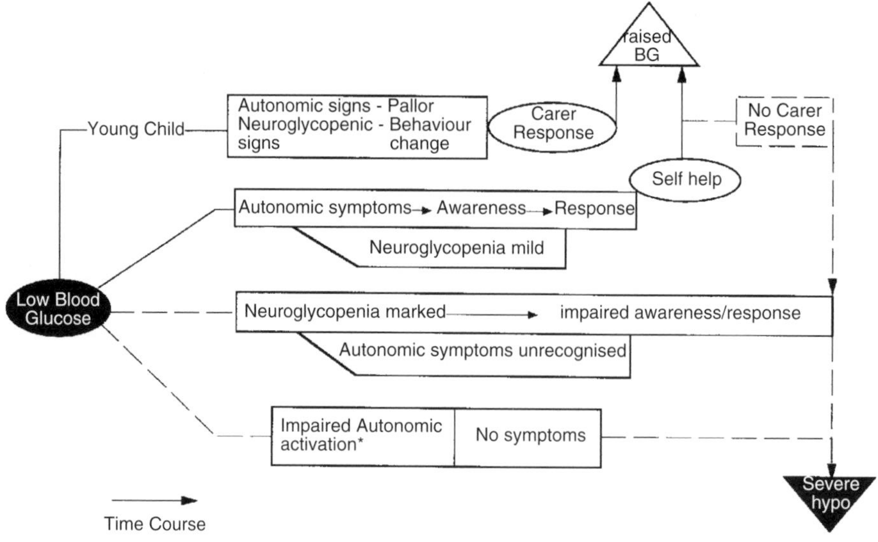

Figure 9.4 Response pathways to hypoglycaemia

SIGNS AND SYMPTOMS

"It feels like my batteries have dropped out."
(Quote: 10-year-old boy with diabetes.)

"He woke me up screaming and terrified. I gave him some holy water and he seemed more relaxed. He screamed again and I thought to give him some food. What do you think this was, doctor?" (Quote: a frightened parent.)

Although many signs and symptoms of hypoglycaemia in children are non-specific, individual children exhibit changes which usually alert parents or carers to the possibility of an impending crisis (see Figures 9.4 and 9.5).

The characteristic symptomatology in children has been described in several reports (Aman et al, 1989; Macfarlane et al, 1989) and confirmed recently by similar studies in which parents and children rated the

How I feel when I'm healthy.

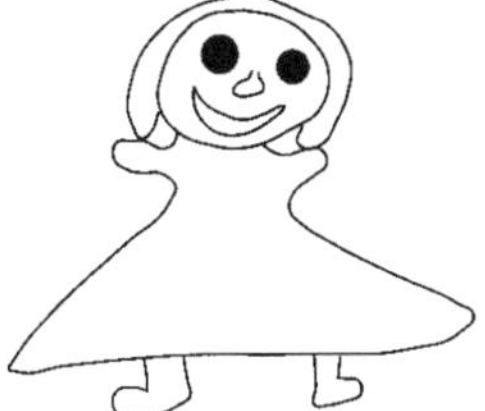

How I feel when I feel all....

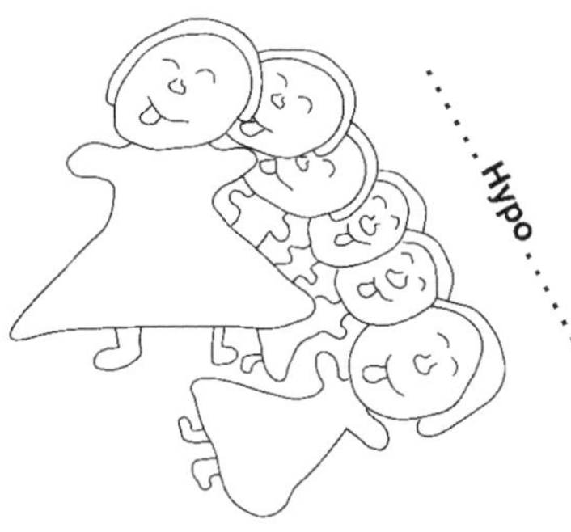

K.W. (8 1/2y)

Figure 9.5 A child's impression of hypoglycaemia

frequency and intensity of a large number of hypoglycaemic symptoms (McCrimmon et al, 1995; Ross et al, 1998). Both studies emphasised the coalescence of autonomic, neuroglycopenic and behavioural symptoms making interpretation, prevention and management difficult. Neuroglycopenic and non-specific symptoms are usual in very young children (aged less than six years) in whom autonomic symptoms are not recognised (Tupola and Rajantie, 1998). The changes most commonly reported by more than two-thirds of parents and children are shown in Box 9.2.

Parents and carers often blame themselves (quite wrongly) for not recognising the subtle shift from mild behavioural changes to significant cognitive impairment. Such changes are impossible to recognise on all occasions. Equally subtle are symptoms such as night sweats (clammy skin), nightmares, morning headache, refusal to eat, poor school performance or stubborn non-cooperation (Goldstein et al, 1981). Children sometimes exhibit much more overt and distressing symptoms such as regression towards infantile behaviour (dribbling, thumb sucking, inconsolable crying) which is alarming to the parents who fear that brain damage has been induced. Occasionally, distinctive focal neurological

Box 9.2 Features of hypoglycaemia in children

Signs	*Behavioural changes*	*Symptoms*
Pallor	Tearful	Weakness
Hunger (young children)	Confused	Hunger
Sweating	Tired	Trembling
	Irritable	Dizziness
	Aggressive	Poor concentration
		Drowsiness

signs occur transiently, such as squints and hemiparesis (Spallino et al, 1998). The ultimate shock for unwary parents and carers is the occasional, completely unpredictable, episode of severe hypoglycaemia associated with myoclonic jerking in a stuporose, clammy, sweating, deathly white, screaming child.

> *"She just collapsed before breakfast. There was no warning."*
> (Quote: mother of child with diabetes.)

Unrecognised nocturnal hypoglycaemia may have another important effect on the following day, namely the subsequent inhibition of sympatho-adrenal and other counterregulatory responses with an associated impairment of awareness (see Chapter 5). It is not known how often this occurs in children, but experience suggests that the possibility of antecedent nocturnal hypoglycaemia should be explored when other unexplained neurological symptoms occur or there is impaired awareness of hypoglycaemia in a child. In one study, young children with type 1 diabetes experienced no warning symptoms when hypoglycaemia occurred before breakfast, almost certainly an indication of preceding nocturnal hypoglycaemia (Porter et al, 1997).

RISKS OF COGNITIVE IMPAIRMENT

The risk of recurrent, severe or prolonged hypoglycaemia provoking cognitive impairment are difficult to dispute in young children.

- Numerous follow-up studies of children with diabetes of preschool onset who have experienced severe hypoglycaemia (usually with convulsions) have shown significant but small intellectual deficits sometimes associated with schooling problems (Ack et al, 1961; Ryan et al, 1985; Rovet et al, 1987).

- Persistent EEG abnormalities have been reported in children with diabetes of early onset who had a history of convulsion caused by severe hypoglycaemia (Soltesz and Acsadi, 1989) or severe hypoglycaemia alone (Bjorgaas et al, 1996).
- Some paediatric clinics have an occasional unfortunate child in whom severe prolonged hypoglycaemia with secondary cerebral oedema has resulted in cerebral damage and secondary epilepsy, although epilepsy *per se* is not considered to be more common in children with diabetes.

A more recent prospective study has indicated that recurrent mild hypoglycaemia does not impair the child's intellectual development (Rovet et al, 1991) and confirms that mild attention deficits are most likely the result of hypoglycaemia-induced seizures in very young children with diabetes (Rovet and Alvarez, 1997).

Following the publication of the DCCT, statements were made that intensification of insulin therapy in pre-pubertal children should be approached with caution (Drash, 1993) because of the dangers of hypoglycaemia. However, this should not be a licence for accepting sub-optimal metabolic control. So long as severe hypoglycaemia is avoided in pre-school children, there should be no significant impairment in cognitive function associated with good glycaemic control. Chronic recurrent hypoglycaemia, however, may have a detrimental effect (Northam et al, 1998).

OTHER HYPOGLYCAEMIC THREATS

The short-term morbidity of acute hypoglycaemia should not be under-estimated. During and after episodes of hypoglycaemia:

- Children may function poorly at school both mentally and physically, affecting their academic or sporting performance
- Behavioural changes may lead uninformed observers and peers to accuse young people with diabetes of being stupid, childish, uncooperative, anti-social or even drunk
- Accidents may occur if the blood glucose is low during potentially dangerous activities such as cycling, driving, swimming, climbing, riding ski-lifts and the like
- At night there are dangers of falling out of bed (or down stairs), convulsions, aspiration of vomit and perhaps the unquantified threat of sudden death (Thordarson and Sovik, 1995) (see Chapter 7).

Panic Attacks

The fear of hypoglycaemia in adolescents may cause considerable anxiety and sometimes even panic. Severe panic attacks with autonomic symptoms such as tremor, pounding heart and anxiety may occur and it is difficult to distinguish these from the symptoms of hypoglycaemia. Both may coexist and require careful investigation and counselling.

MANAGEMENT

Prevention of severe hypoglycaemia is the ideal management (see later) but inevitably unexpected episodes occur. Remember the 5 'R' s (Box 9.3).

Box 9.3 The five 'R's

Recognition
Response
Recovery
Review
Reminder

Recognition

Individual daytime and night-time signs and symptoms are quickly learned by parents. They need to be described to other carers, particularly babysitters, relatives, friends, school teachers and leaders of group activities for children (e.g. Brownies, swimming clubs, etc.), most of whom have little or no knowledge of diabetes and its management.

Response

An urgent and clear treatment programme (Figure 9.6) is required, but without inducing panic. Parents or carers are often alarmed by the onset of hypoglycaemia and overtreatment is common. It is very difficult to assess how much carbohydrate should be given to treat an individual hypoglycaemic episode. Post-hypoglycaemic hyperglycaemia is almost inevitable because:

- too much immediate (fast-acting) glucose is given
- too much slower onset carbohydrate is given (to prevent another episode)

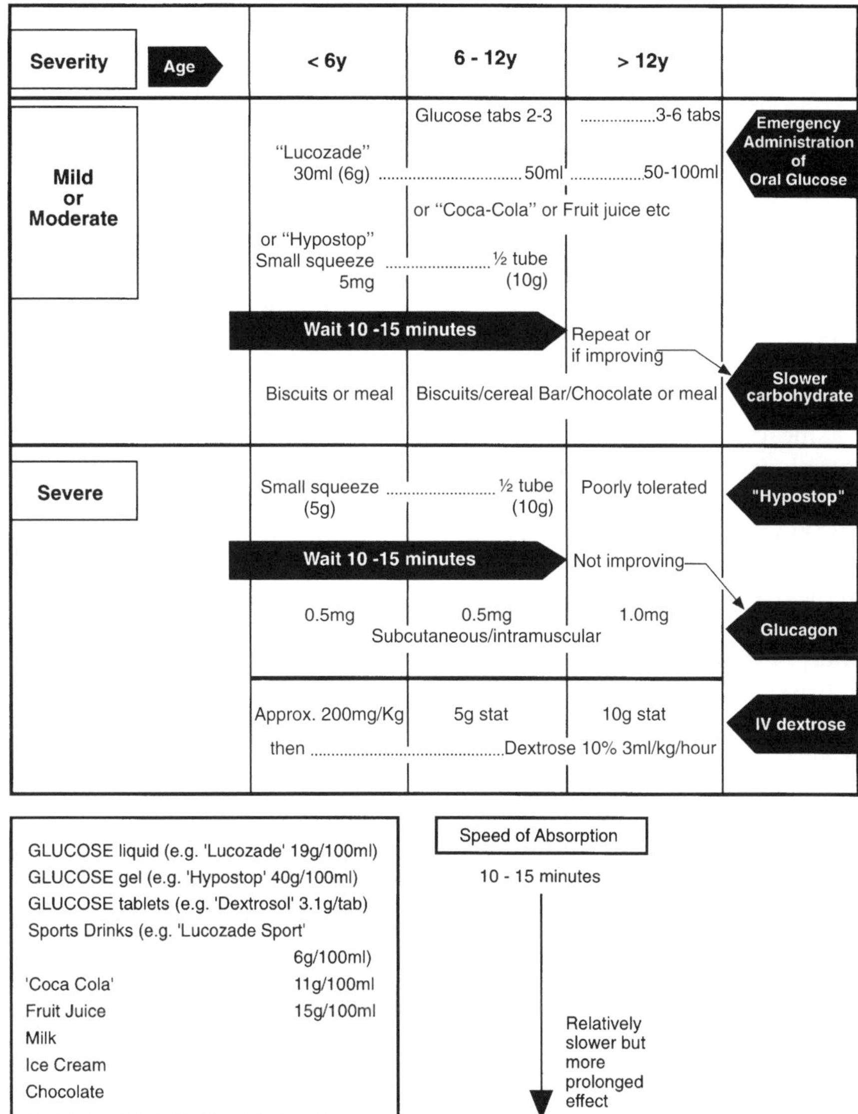

Figure 9.6 Treatment of hypoglycaemia in different age groups

- counterregulatory hormones are activated by hypoglycaemia
- the plasma insulin concentration may be falling during recovery.

Monitoring of the blood glucose response is helpful and when the blood glucose is 4.0 mmol/l or more, the child is safe and the amount of ingested carbohydrate can be more restrained. In severe hypoglycaemia if spitting, swallowing or gag reflexes are still present, sips of a glucose drink can be tried or glucose gel squeezed into the buccal cavity against the cheek. Even honey or jam smeared on the inside of the mouth may be effective. Hypostop (Bio-Diagnostics Ltd, Worcester, UK) is a glucose gel (40 g/100 ml) applied to the gums or cheek inside the mouth and with gentle massaging glucose will be absorbed through the buccal mucosa. It has been claimed that Hypostop is not absorbed from the mouth in adults, but this is successful in children and widespread paediatric experience has shown Hypostop to be effective in treating hypoglycaemia (Chaussain et al, 1984). If unsuccessful, or the child is deeply unconscious, convulsing or vomiting, parenteral administration of glucagon or dextrose will be the safest and most rapidly effective treatment.

Glucagon, given subcutaneously or intramuscularly, effectively raises the blood glucose within 5–15 minutes in profoundly hypoglycaemic children (Aman and Wranne, 1988) and will maintain the blood glucose for one to two hours. The dose is 0.5 mg in small children and 1 mg for older children (see Figure 9.6). The technique for administering glucagon in a crisis may appear formidable to parents, who should receive repeated instructions, reassurance that glucagon (even in excess) is safe, and prescriptions should be renewed regularly to ensure that the glucagon is "in date". Unfortunately many parents, despite instructions, do not use glucagon and prefer to contact the emergency services (Daneman et al, 1989; Davis et al, 1997) so it is equally important that paramedical ambulance crews and staff in the hospital emergency department are confident in the use of glucagon. Glucagon has been blamed too readily for causing nausea and vomiting. Hypoglycaemia *per se* is more likely to induce vomiting than subcutaneous glucagon. In hospital 50% dextrose has traditionally been used and is readily available in emergency departments. However, it is hyperosmolar, may damage precious veins and if given in excessive amounts can precipitate cerebral oedema. It is best diluted with water for injection and given in specified limited amounts (Figure 9.6), followed if necessary by intravenous dextrose as a 10% infusion.

Recovery

Even after severe hypoglycaemia, recovery is usually rapid and apparently complete, and children often return to their activities remarkably quickly. However, subtle cognitive changes can be present for 24–48 hours (Ryan et al, 1990). More worryingly, after a severe prolonged convulsive episode (often occurring overnight or in the early morning), abnormal behaviour, neurological deficits, mood change and obtunded concentration may persist for several hours. Parents need reassurance that if the blood glucose is maintained above 4–6 mmol/l during this anxious time, full recovery will occur.

Review

The likely causes of each episode of severe hypoglycaemia should be sought and may reveal evidence of:

- a change of routine
- more strenuous exercise
- a meal or snack that has been forgotten, delayed or only partly consumed
- preceding (nocturnal) hypoglycaemia.

All of these may be potentially avoidable. There is a tendency for physicians (especially those dealing with emergency treatment of hypoglycaemia and not the routine diabetic care) and also parents, to decrease the insulin dose, even when a preventable cause of the hypoglycaemia can be identified (Tupola et al, 1998a). Thus the adverse experience of hypoglycaemia leads to poorer glycaemic control.

Reminder

Analysis of severe hypoglycaemia should prompt a review of the insulin regimen, food intake, exercise advice, preventive measures and whether the episode can be used positively as a learning experience to improve future management.

PREDISPOSITION, PREDICTION AND PREVENTION

> *"I'm depressed about good control and having these sudden hypos—I'm going to ease up and start living . . . "* (Quote: young student with type 1 diabetes.)

If up to 27% of young people experience severe hypoglycaemia each year, why do the other 73% escape such an experience? Many young people without hypoglycaemia are older and "ease up" on their control, and indeed some young people never achieve blood glucose levels that approach normality. In addition, the activation of autonomic symptoms in children with poorly controlled diabetes occurs at a higher blood glucose concentration which may prevent the risk of developing severe hypoglycaemia during waking hours. Recurrent hypoglycaemia appears to be more common in boys, particularly during adolescence, than in girls, and is unrelated to quality of glycaemic control (Herskowitz Dumont et al, 1995).

Predisposition towards hypoglycaemia may be associated with:

- young pre-school age
- longer duration of diabetes with deficient hormonal counterregulation
- high total insulin dose
- low glycated haemoglobin (within or near non-diabetic range)
- change of routine/unstable lifestyle
- unaccustomed or strenuous exercise
- failure to eat snacks, particularly at bedtime
- spring/early summer (altered physical activity)
- preceding low bedtime blood glucose or asymptomatic nocturnal hypoglycaemia
- alcohol ingestion.

Predicting and Preventing Nocturnal Hypoglycaemia

Measurement of a bedtime blood glucose is often advised as a safeguard for children but is not a consistently reliable predictor of nocturnal hypoglycaemia, particularly as young children go to bed much earlier than adults. A more useful time for measuring blood glucose in the child is around 23.00–24.00 hours but this may present practical difficulties and waken the child. Although a routine high fibre carbohydrate snack at bedtime is also recommended, the effects of extra carbohydrate eaten at bedtime will not counteract prolonged nocturnal hyperinsulinaemia. Pre-breakfast (asymptomatic) hypoglycaemia may indicate antecedent and protracted hypoglycaemia during the night. Parents whose child has experienced previous nocturnal hypoglycaemia should be advised to measure their child's blood glucose around 23.00–24.00 hours, and if the level is below 7.0 mmol/l, to waken them and give additional slowly digested carbohydrate. It may also be useful to perform a physical check to see if the child's nose or forehead is cold and clammy or if the child shows no movement when lightly disturbed. Occasional blood tests at 02.00–03.00 hours are also informative when asymptomatic nocturnal hypoglycaemia is suspected. Staff at diabetic camps may perform a night round for similar reassurance. Nevertheless, practical experience at many local camps and skiing holidays has shown that when children eat an adequate supper late in the evening, symptomatic nocturnal hypoglycaemia is unusual. Therefore, at many such camps, blood glucose measurements are not performed routinely after bedtime on sleeping children, especially as studies have not shown convincing evidence of predictability (Table 9.3).

Pre-breakfast hyperglycaemia and ketonuria have also been the subject of much debate because of the long-standing belief that they reflect preceding nocturnal hypoglycaemia. It is still quite commonly stated that nocturnal hypoglycaemia elicits the release of counterregulatory hormones (Winter, 1981), resulting in a rise in blood glucose that manifests as fasting hyperglycaemia (the "Somogyi effect"). In the USA this concept has encouraged the examination of the urine each morning for glucose and ketones. Although it is well established that the secretion of adrenaline is more marked in children with diabetes than in non-diabetic children or in adults (Jones et al, 1991), cumulative evidence suggests that the early morning hyperglycaemia (after nocturnal hypoglycaemia) is most likely caused by a lack of biologically active insulin in the hours before awakening (Gale et al, 1980). This is particularly important in the adolescent and the effect is exacerbated by the effects of high levels of nocturnal growth hormone and insulin-like growth factor 1 (IGF-1) in this age group (Dunger, 1992). Thus pre-breakfast hyperglycaemia (with ketonuria) is not a good indicator of antecedent nocturnal hypoglycaemia.

When the young adult with diabetes leaves home, new friends and partners and those supervising residential accommodation at University or college should be forewarned of the possibilities of nocturnal hypoglycaemia. Students should be advised to eat a large bedtime snack, particularly after parties and the ingestion of alcohol.

Table 9.3 Predictability of nocturnal hypoglycaemia in children with diabetes

Reference	BG measurements at 2200–2300 hours (mmol/l)	Frequency of blood glucose <3 mmol/l at 2am (%)
Studies in hospital:		
Whincup and Milner, 1987*	<7	80
	>7	17
Shalwitz et al, 1990**	<5.6	24
Study at home:		
Porter et al, 1997***	<7	35
	<4	60

*Nocturnal hypoglycaemia prevented by 10 g carbohydrate; no association between hypoglycaemia at 0200 hours and blood glucose at 0800 hours
**No significant rebound hyperglycaemia
***Nocturnal hypoglycaemia not prevented by additional carbohydrate

Predicting and Preventing Daytime Hypoglycaemia

Pre-school Children

Hypoglycaemia in this age group can only be recognised by careful surveillance and a high level of suspicion by the child's carers. Symptoms may be non-specific, with changes of behaviour, particularly irritability or quietness, gently drifting into hypoglycaemia and stupor. Prevention in this age group is important to avoid progression to severe convulsive hypoglycaemia. The morning dose of short-acting (soluble) insulin may have to be small, particularly if breakfast is likely to be inadequate. Even the very young child should be encouraged to eat regular high fibre starchy snacks and main meals. The use of the rapid-acting insulin analogue, insulin lispro, may be valuable in this situation, as it can be given *after* meals, the dose being determined by how much food the child has eaten. This avoids the problem of a young child refusing to eat after insulin has been injected.

Primary School Children

Close liaison between the parents, the diabetes team and school teachers is the best prevention of hypoglycaemia at primary school. Booklets providing guidance for school teachers and nurses and provision of a description of the child's idiosyncratic symptoms of hypoglycaemia are useful. Rapidly absorbed carbohydrate must be readily available close to the child in the classroom or at the games hall or playing field, and not in a distant office.

Secondary School

The teenager must be instructed:

- to respond to symptoms of hypoglycaemia immediately, and not to resist them
- to ensure that glucose tablets are always immediately available (especially in the sporting arena)
- that friends are made aware of the features of hypoglycaemia.

School Trips

Some schools still avoid taking children with diabetes on outside activities because of the added responsibilities. Teachers need help and guidance from parents and the diabetes team.

Weekends, Holidays and Travel

Parents and young people must be educated and re-educated in symptom awareness and in particular the times when hypoglycaemia is most likely, particularly during exercise and when routine is altered. The following holiday advice may be useful to parents:

- obsessional planning is necessary
- make reminder lists of things to take
- be prepared for hazards, e.g. travel delays, mishaps, tiredness, tummy upsets
- take extra supplies of food, equipment and "hypo kits"
- regular blood glucose monitoring, more food, less insulin may be required
- beware changes in nature and quality of food (and standards of hygiene) in foreign countries
- anticipate the effects of high activity holidays
- be alert to the potential dangers of the first day and night away when the development of severe hypoglycaemia can destroy a holiday (Swift and Waldron, 1990).

"How many Mars Bars does it take to swim the Clyde?"
(A questioning parent quoted by Oman Craig, in his book *Childhood Diabetes and Its Management* (1977).)

Guidelines are available to help the management of diabetes during high levels of activity and hazardous holidays such as hill and rock climbing, walking in mountains, water-sports and skiing (Hillson, 1987; Chadwick and Brown, 1992; Thompson et al, 1995). During winter skiing holidays, insulin may have to be reduced by 20% or more on the first day, although some youngsters who regularly partake in active sports may not need this reduction (see Chapter 11).
More importantly, great emphasis should be given to:

- increasing overall carbohydrate intake by 30–50% especially at breakfast and bedtime snack
- taking two or three dextrosol tablets before commencing dangerous activities, e.g. riding on ski lifts, skiing down difficult slopes
- not going to sleep after exercise without first having a snack.

Most of the children graze on snack bars and some have frequent small sips of sports drinks which they carry with them. Carbohydrate constraint on holidays can be calamitous (Swift, 1997).

Education

"Let me down easy ... Tell me on a Sunday please."
(Quote: Andrew Lloyd-Webber.)

"You didn't tell me he could have a fit."
(Quote: parent of child with diabetes.)

Some sensitivity has to be given to the timing and level of education about hypoglycaemia for parents and young people. It is obvious that all parents and children need considerable information about how hypoglycaemia occurs, the symptomatology and its management. However, there is always concern about how and when parents should be told about the possibility of severe hypoglycaemia causing a convulsion, particularly as a night-time event. A basic understanding of hypoglycaemia is important for parents and even young children from the first day or two after diagnosis and commencing insulin therapy, concentrating mainly on the symptoms that we all experience when we are extremely hungry and how insulin can cause a fall in blood glucose. In practice most children will begin to experience mild hypoglycaemic symptoms in the first week or so after diagnosis as the blood glucose approaches normality, and the management of these episodes may prove the most effective learning experience. Progressing from there in a graduated approach to education, parents should then be informed about the risks of developing more severe hypoglycaemia and its emergency treatment.

In some diabetes centres attempts to provoke hypoglycaemia are still made immediately after diagnosis while the child is in hospital. Supervision of the procedure is often left to inexperienced junior medical staff and nurses and such an experience can be frustrating, frightening, risky and often unsuccessful. It may also represent yet another unhappy hospital experience for the child. Some parents may be made more anxious about hypoglycaemia because healthcare professionals have introduced the threat of severe hypoglycaemia at too early a stage in the educational process. Some parents suppress concerns of the potential risks of severe hypoglycaemia. When a hypoglycaemia-induced convulsion occurs some months or years after education has been imparted, they deny having received any information about this problem and often do not respond appropriately. This underlines the need for continuing, repetitive and timely education.

CONCLUSIONS

- Optimal metabolic control of diabetes is important in children of all ages to prevent long-term vascular complications.
- Near-normal blood glucose and glycated haemoglobin concentrations are achieved with insulin regimens that cause unphysiological hyperinsulinaemia, and this induces hypoglycaemia.
- Recurrent hypoglycaemia may cause impaired hypoglycaemia awareness.
- Mild hypoglycaemia may not be harmful and may be associated with attempts to achieve near normoglycaemia
- Severe episodes or repeated nocturnal hypoglycaemia should be rigorously avoided, particularly in pre-school children.
- Prevention of severe hypoglycaemia may be helped by:
  - paying individual attention to balancing each child's insulin and food regimens
  - encouragement of regular ingestion of high-carbohydrate, high-fibre foods
  - advising flexible and increased carbohydrate intake with and after strenuous/unusual exercise to prevent immediate and delayed hypoglycaemia.
  - making parents aware that any change of routine (particularly excitement, late nights, travelling, holidays) may predispose a child to hypoglycaemia.
- Repeated education is important in helping parents and young people to manage hypoglycaemia successfully, especially ensuring availability and appropriate use of quick-acting glucose and glucagon.

REFERENCES

Ack M, Miller I, Weil WB (1961). Intelligence of children with diabetes mellitus. *Pediatrics* **28**: 764–0.

Akerblom HK, Koivukangas T, Ilkka J (1980). Experience from a winter camp for teenage diabetics. *Acta Paed Scand*, **283** (Suppl.): 50–2.

Aman J, Karlsson I, Wranne L (1989). Symptomatic hypoglycaemia in childhood diabetes: a population-based questionnaire study. *Diabetic Med* **6**: 257–61.

Aman J, Wranne L (1988). Hypoglycaemia in childhood diabetes II Effect of subcutaneous or intramuscular injection of different doses of glucagon. *Acta Paed Scand* **77**: 548–53.

Amiel S, Simonson DC, Sherwin RS, Lauritano AA, Tamborlane WV (1987).

Exaggerated epinephrine responses to hypoglycemia in normal and insulin-dependent diabetic children. *J Pediatr* **110**: 832–7.

Amiel SA, Sherwin RS, Simonson DC, Tamborlane WV (1988). Effect of intensive insulin therapy on glycemic thresholds for counterregulatory hormone release. *Diabetes* **37**: 901–7.

Aynsley-Green AS, Eyre JA, Soltesz G (1993). Hypoglycaemia in diabetic children. In *Hypoglycaemia and Diabetes. Clinical and Physiological Aspects* (eds BM Frier and BM Fisher). Edward Arnold, London, pp 228–40.

Barkai L, Vámosi I, Lukács K (1998). Prospective assessment of severe hypoglycaemia in diabetic children and adolescents with impaired and normal awareness of hypoglycaemia. *Diabetologia*, **41**: 898–903.

Baumer JH, Edelstein AD, Howlett BC et al (1982). Impact of home blood glucose monitoring on childhood diabetes. *Arch Dis Child* **57**: 195–9.

Beregszaszi M, Tubiana-Rufi N, Benali K, Noel M, Bloch J, Czernichow P (1997). Nocturnal hypoglycemia in children and adolescents with insulin-dependent diabetes mellitus: prevalence and risk factors. *J Pediatr* **131**: 27–33.

Bhatia V, Wolfsdorf JI (1991). Severe hypoglycemia in youth with insulin-dependent diabetes mellitus: frequency and causative factors. *Pediatrics* **88**: 1187–93.

Bjorgaas M, Sand T, Gimse R (1996). Quantitative EEG in type 1 diabetic children with and without episodes of severe hypoglycemia: a controlled, blind study. *Acta Neurol Scand*, **93**: 398–402.

Bjorgaas M, Vik T, Sand T et al (1997). Counterregulatory hormone and symptom responses to hypoglycaemia in diabetic children. *Diabetic Med* **14**: 433–41.

Braatvedt GD, Mildenhall L, Patten C, Harris G (1997). Insulin requirements and metabolic control in children with diabetes mellitus attending a summer camp. *Diabetic Med* **14**: 258–61.

Chadwick J, Brown KGE (1992). A party of 43 young people with diabetes go skiing. *Diabetic Med* **9**: 671–3.

Chaussain JL, Bernard MM, Artavia E (1984). Study of the hyperglycaemic effect of a glucose gel in paediatric hypoglycaemia after injection of insulin. *Theor Pract Thér* 43–50.

Daneman D, Frank M, Perlman K, Tamm J, Ehrlich R (1989). Severe hypoglycemia in children with insulin-dependent diabetes mellitus: frequency and predisposing factors. *J Pediatr* **115**: 681–5.

Davis EA, Keating B, Byrne GC, Russell M, Jones TW (1997). Hypoglycemia: incidence and clinical predictors in a large population-based sample of children and adolescents with IDDM. *Diabetes Care* **20**: 22–5.

Dorchy H (1994). Dorchy's recipes explaining the "intriguing efficacity of Belgian conventional therapy". *Diabetes Care* **17**: 458–60 (letter).

Dorchy H, Roggemans M-P, Willems D (1997). Glycated hemoglobin and related factors in diabetic children and adolescents under 18 years of age: a Belgian experience. *Diabetes Care*, **20**: 2–6.

Drash AL (1993). The child, the adolescent and the Diabetes Control and Complications Trial. *Diabetes Care* **16**: 1515–6.

Dunger DB (1992). Diabetes in puberty. *Arch Dis Child* **67**: 569–70.

Egger M, Gschwend S, Davey Smith G, Zuppinger K (1991). Increasing incidence of hypoglycemic coma in children with IDDM. *Diabetes Care* **14**: 1001–5.

Frost G (1995). Is carbohydrate a complex problem? *Practical Diabetes* **12**: 160–3.

Gale EAM, Kurtz AB, Tattersall RB (1980). In search of the Somogyi effect. *Lancet* **ii**: 279–82.

Garg SK, Carmain JA, Braddy KC et al (1996). Pre-meal insulin analogue insulin lispro vs. Humulin R insulin treatment in young subjects with type 1 diabetes. *Diabetic Med* **13**: 47–52.

Goldstein DE, England JD, Hess R, Rawlings SS, Walker B (1981). A prospective study of symptomatic hypoglycemia in young diabetic patients. *Diabetes Care* **4**: 601–5.

Haymond MW, Karl IE, Clarke WL et al (1982). Differences in circulating gluconeogenic substrates during short-term fasting in men, women and children. *Metabolism* **31**: 33–42.

Hawarth J, Coodin FJ (1960). Idiopathic spontaneous hypoglycemia in children. Report of seven cases and review of the literature. *Pediatrics* **25**: 748–65.

Herskowitz Dumont R, Jacobson AM, Cole C, Hauser ST, Wolfsdorf JI, Willett JB, Milley JE, Wertlieb D (1995). Psychosocial predictors of acute complications of diabetes in youth. *Diabetic Med* **12**: 612–8.

Hillson R (1987). British Diabetic Association activities for young people—safety while adventuring. *Practical Diabetes* **4**: 233–4.

Jones TW, Boulware SD, Kraemer DT, Caprio S, Sherwin RS, Tamborlane WV (1991). Independent effects of youth and poor diabetes control on responses to hypoglycemia in children. *Diabetes* **40**: 358–63.

Jones TW, Borg WP, Boulware SD et al (1995). Enhanced adrenomedullary response and increased susceptibility to neuroglycopenia: mechanisms underlying the adverse effects of sugar ingestion in healthy children. *J Pediatr* **126**: 171–7.

Kelnar CJH (1976). Hypoglycaemia in children undergoing adenotonsillectomy. *BMJ* **1**: 751–2.

Koh THHG, Aynsley-Green A, Tarbit M, Eyre JA (1988). Neural dysfunction during hypoglycaemia. *Arch Dis Child* **63**: 1353–8.

MacDonald MJ (1987). Postexercise late-onset hypoglycemia in insulin-dependent diabetic patients. *Diabetes Care* **10**: 584–8.

Macfarlane PI, Walters M, Stutchfield P, Smith CS (1989). A prospective study of symptomatic hypoglycaemia in childhood diabetes. *Diabetic Med* **6**: 627–30.

McCrimmon RJ, Gold AE, Deary IJ, Kelnar CJH, Frier BM (1995). Symptoms of hypoglycemia in children with IDDM. *Diabetes Care* **18**: 858–61.

Matyka KA, Watts AP, Stores G, Dunger DB (1996). High prevalence of nocturnal hypoglycaemia in young children with insulin dependent diabetes mellitus studied overnight at home. *Diabetic Med* **13** (Suppl. 3): S13 (abstract).

Mortensen HB, Hougaard P (1997). Comparison of metabolic control in a cross-sectional study of 2,873 children and adolescents with IDDM from 18 countries. *Diabetes Care* **20**: 714–20.

Nordfeldt S, Ludvigsson J (1997). Severe hypoglycemia in children with IDDM. *Diabetes Care* **20**: 497–503.

Northam EA, Anderson PJ, Werther GA, Warne GL, Adler RG, Andrews D (1998). Neuropsychological complications of IDDM in children 2 years after disease onset. *Diabetes Care* **21**: 379–84.

Porter PA, Keating B, Byrne G, Jones TW (1997). Incidence and predictive criteria of nocturnal hypoglycemia in young children with insulin-dependent diabetes mellitus. *J Pediatr* **130**: 366–72.

Pramming S, Thorsteinsson B, Bendtson I, Binder C (1990). The relationship between symptomatic and biochemical hypoglycaemia in insulin-dependent diabetic patients. *J Intern Med* **228**: 641–6.

Price KJ, Lang JD, Eiser C, Tripp JH (1993). Prescribed versus unrestricted carbohydrate diets in children with type 1 diabetes. *Diabetic Med* **10**: 962–7.

Ross LA, McCrimmon RJ, Frier BM, Kelnar CJH, Deary IJ (1998). Hypoglycaemic symptoms reported by children with type 1 diabetes and by their parents. *Diabetic Med* **15**: 836–43.

Rovet JF, Ehrlich RM, Hoppe M (1987). Intellectual deficits associated with early onset of insulin-dependent diabetes mellitus in children. *Diabetes Care* **10**: 510–5.

Rovet J, Czuchta D, Ehrlich RM (1991). Neuropsychological sequelae of diabetes in childhood. A three year prospective study. *Diabetes* **40** (Suppl.1): 430A (abstract).

Rovet J, Alvarez M (1997). Attentional functioning in children and adolescents with IDDM. *Diabetes Care* **20**: 803–10.

Ryan C, Vega A, Drash A (1985). Cognitive deficits in adolescents who developed diabetes early in life. *Pediatrics* **75**: 921–7.

Ryan CM, Atchison J, Puczynski SS et al (1990). Mild hypoglycemia associated with deterioration of mental efficiency in children with insulin-dependent diabetes mellitus. *J Pediatr* **117**: 32–8.

Shalwitz RA, Farkas-Hirsch R, White NH, Santiago JV (1990). Prevalence and consequences of nocturnal hypoglycemia among conventionally treated children with diabetes mellitus. *J Pediatr* **116**: 685–9.

Simell T, Simell O, Lammi E-M et al (1993). Glucose profiles in children two years after the onset of type 1 diabetes. *Diabetic Med* **10**: 524–9.

Soltesz G, Acsadi G (1989). Association between diabetes, severe hypoglycaemia, and electroencephalographic abnormalities. *Arch Dis Child* **64**: 992–6.

Spallino L, Stirling HF, O'Regan M, Ross L, Zampolli M, Kelnar CJH (1998). Transient hypoglycemic hemiparesis in children with IDDM. *Diabetes Care* **21**: 1567–8 (letter).

Stirling HF, Darling JAB, Kelnar CJH (1991). Nocturnal glucose homeostasis in normal children. *Hormone Res* **35** (Suppl. 2): 54 (abstract).

Swift PGF (1997). Flexible carbohydrate. *Diabetic Med* **14**: 187–8.

Swift PGF, Waldron S (1990). Have diabetes — will travel. *Practical Diabetes* **7**: 101–4.

The Diabetes Control and Complications Trial Research Group (1994). Effect of intensive diabetes treatment on the development and progression of long-term complications in adolescents with insulin-dependent diabetes mellitus: Diabetes Control and Complications Trial. *J Pediatr* **125**: 177–88.

Thordarson H, Sovik O (1995). Dead in bed syndrome in young diabetic patients in Norway. *Diabetic Med* **12**: 782–7.

Thompson C, Greene SA, Newton RW (1995). Camps for diabetic children and teenagers. In: *Childhood and Adolescent Diabetes* (ed. CJH Kelnar). Chapman and Hall Medical, London, pp 483–92.

Tupola S, Rajantie J (1998). Documented symptomatic hypoglycaemia in children and adolescents using multiple daily insulin injection therapy. *Diabetic Med* **15**: 492–6.

Tupola S, Rajantie J, Akerblom HK (1998a). Experience of severe hypoglycaemia may influence both patient's and physician's subsequent treatment policy of insulin-dependent diabetes mellitus. *Eur J Pediatr* **157**: 625–7.

Tupola S, Rajantie J, Mäenpää J (1998b). Severe hypoglycaemia in children and adolescents during multiple-dose insulin therapy. *Diabetic Medicine* **15**: 695–9.

Waldron S (1996). Current controversies in the dietary management of diabetes in childhood and adolescents. *B J Hosp Med* **56**: 450–5.

Whincup G, Milner RDG (1987). Prediction and management of nocturnal hypoglycaemia in diabetes. *Arch Dis Child* **62**: 333–7.

Winter RJ (1981). Profiles of metabolic control in diabetic children—frequency of asymptomatic nocturnal hypoglycemia. *Metabolism* **30**: 666–72.

10

Hypoglycaemia and Pregnancy

SIMON R. HELLER
Northern General Hospital, Sheffield

INTRODUCTION

Long before the results of the Diabetes Control and Complications Trial (DCCT) confirmed that near normoglycaemia could prevent microvascular complications, those caring for patients with diabetes had recognised that intensive insulin therapy dramatically improved the outcome of pregnancy. Home blood glucose monitoring and multiple injection regimens for the administration of insulin had helped women to achieve average blood glucose values that were close to normal. This approach has been rewarded with a perinatal mortality rate which now approaches that of non-diabetic women. However, just as in the DCCT, where the reduction in the risk of complications was accompanied by a marked increase in frequency of severe hypoglycaemia (see Chapter 6), the benefits of strict glycaemic control during pregnancy are generally bought at a similar price.

It is now standard practice to aim for near normoglycaemia in any antenatal clinic where women with insulin-treated diabetes receive care. In practice, this clinical model is more representative of intensive insulin therapy than the experimental approach pursued in the DCCT. Clinical observations derived from the management of diabetic pregnancy could be used to guide attempts to achieve strict glycaemic control in the non-pregnant state. However, the usefulness of this model may be limited if

Hypoglycaemia in Clinical Diabetes. Edited by B. M. Frier and B. M. Fisher.

pregnancy itself modifies the physiological response to hypoglycaemia. None the less, if this is the case then it may shed light on factors which can impair physiological responses to hypoglycaemia and cause hypoglycaemia unawareness. This section examines the epidemiology, physiology and risks to both mother and baby of hypoglycaemia in women with type 1 diabetes during pregnancy and considers some practical approaches which may reduce the risks of severe hypoglycaemia.

CARBOHYDRATE METABOLISM DURING PREGNANCY

Carbohydrate metabolism alters in pregnancy, presumably to ensure that fuel delivery to the fetus is maintained. Under the influence of placental hormones, glucose output from the liver is increased. Higher rates of lipolysis enhance gluconeogenesis and this is accompanied by the increased production of ketones. However, fasting blood glucose is lower in pregnancy despite the increased hepatic glucose output, because of glucose uptake by the placenta. The fasting blood glucose in non-diabetic women is around 4.8 mmol/l, compared to 4.1 mmol/l when pregnant. (Johnston et al, 1995). Plasma insulin concentrations are raised throughout pregnancy in non-diabetic women, yet the postprandial increment in blood glucose is higher than in the non-pregnant state. This is associated with insulin resistance which presumably is mediated by the placental hormones, human placental lactogen and progestagens, as well as higher plasma cortisol levels.

In women with type 1 diabetes the change in carbohydrate metabolism during pregnancy increases their insulin requirement. This starts to rise during the first trimester, although the greatest increase usually occurs between 26 and 30 weeks of gestation. The exact amount of insulin that will eventually be required is impossible to predict. By the end of their pregnancy some women have had to increase their insulin dose by about 50% while others will be using two or three times their original total daily dose.

Despite increased insulin resistance, many women are prone to repeated episodes of severe hypoglycaemia early in pregnancy. Several studies have shown that severe hypoglycaemia is more common during the first 20 weeks of gestation. The causes are not entirely clear. The rate of gastric emptying is unpredictable and hyperemesis may affect the absorption of carbohydrate in women with type 1 diabetes. However, it is possible that physiological defences to hypoglycaemia become impaired in early pregnancy, either as a direct result of the pregnancy itself, or as women succeed in improving their glycaemic control. As described in Chapters 5 and 6, there is experimental evidence that patients may develop a vicious circle of deficient counterregulation, impaired hypoglycaemia awareness and recurrent severe hypoglycaemia.

EPIDEMIOLOGY OF HYPOGLYCAEMIA

Various studies have reported the frequency of hypoglycaemia during pregnancy, but comparison of data is often difficult. Different investigators have not defined mild and severe episodes of hypoglycaemia in the same way and the reported frequency of biochemical hypoglycaemia clearly depends upon how often patients have recorded their blood glucose. Table 1 summarises some of the studies that have examined this problem. Rates of severe hypoglycaemia vary widely but most studies have reported a high frequency. Lankford and Bartholomew (1992) recorded six episodes of coma and one road traffic accident caused by hypoglycaemia in five of 15 women with type 1 diabetes.

Rosenn et al (1995) reported the results of a retrospective study of 84 women who were pregnant between 1989 and 1993. Glycaemic targets were similar to those of the DCCT: preprandial values of less than 5.5 mmol/l and postprandial values up to 8.0 mmol/l, with patients testing blood glucose six or more times every day. Moderate hypoglycaemia was defined as those needing help for recovery, and severe hypoglycaemia as those episodes producing coma or seizure. Thirty-four per cent of women suffered severe episodes, which occurred on an average of 1.5

Table 10.1 Frequency of severe hypoglycaemia during pregnancy in type 1 diabetes

Reference	*n*	Proportion of pregnancies where women experience coma or seizures (%)	Proportion of pregnancies where women needed assistance for recovery (%)
Rayburn et al (1986)	72	(one death)	33
Steel et al (1989)	143		44
Persson and Hanson (1993)	113		4.4
Kimmerle et al (1992)	85	41	
Rosenn et al (1995)	84	17	6.7 ± 1.2
DCCT (originally intensive therapy) (1996)	135	17	
DCCT (originally conventional therapy) (1996)	135	20	

times during each pregnancy. Moderate episodes occurred in 71% of women at an average of seven times during each pregnancy. Severe hypoglycaemia was four times as common before 20 weeks of gestation compared to the second 20 weeks while moderate episodes occurred three times more frequently during the first half of the pregnancy compared to the second. The rate of severe episodes reached a peak at 10–15 weeks and then declined. Surprisingly, there was no difference in HbA1c between those experiencing either a high or low rate of severe hypoglycaemia.

The experience of the 180 women who became pregnant during the DCCT has also been reported (The Diabetes Control and Complications Trial Research Group, 1996). Those randomised to conventional therapy were treated intensively throughout their pregnancy and encouraged to improve their glycaemic control as soon as they were contemplating becoming pregnant. Despite this approach at the start of their pregnancies, their glycaemic control was generally poorer than those in the intensively treated group. Congenital abnormalities were more common in the conventionally treated group compared to those who were on intensive insulin therapy from the outset, emphasising the importance of strict glycaemic control during the first trimester. In addition, hypoglycaemia was more common in women who were transferred to intensive insulin therapy; there were 35 episodes of severe hypoglycaemia in 17 women compared to 23 episodes in 16 women who were on intensive insulin therapy throughout. There were fewer hypoglycaemic episodes during the third trimester. These data suggest that tightening glycaemic control in those where it was poor initially, may impose an additional risk of severe hypoglycaemia, perhaps as a result of acquired defects in the physiological defences to hypoglycaemia.

Kimmerle et al (1992) have reported the frequency of severe hypoglycaemia in 85 pregnancies of women with type 1 diabetes. They studied 77 women who experienced 94 episodes of severe hypoglycaemia. They also concluded that these rates were high compared to intensive insulin therapy in the non-pregnant state and that hypoglycaemia was more common during the first trimester (Figure 10.1).

In summary, rates of severe hypoglycaemia during pregnancy in patients with insulin-treated diabetes vary between 19% and 44%, and several groups of investigators have concluded that the risk of severe hypoglycaemia is greater than in the non-pregnant state. In a pattern similar to that observed during intensive insulin therapy in the DCCT, hypoglycaemia is generally more common at night, frequently accompanied by impaired awareness of hypoglycaemia, and those with a previous history of severe hypoglycaemia have a significantly greater risk. However, episodes of severe hypoglycaemia are not inevitable.

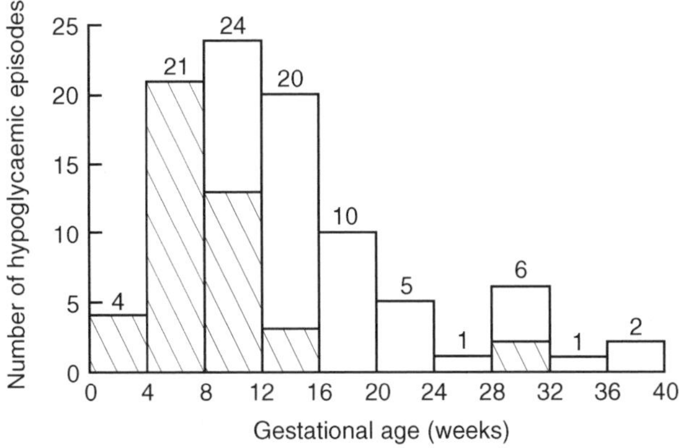

Figure 10.1 Frequency of episodes of severe hypoglycaemia during 35 pregnancies according to four week periods of gestational age. Shaded bars: severe hypoglycaemia that occurred before the first visit to the pregnancy clinic. Open bars: severe hypoglycaemia that occurred after the first visit. Reproduced from Kimmerle et al (1992) with permission of the American Diabetes Association

Persson and Hansson (1993) have reported a much lower incidence of 4.4% in 113 pregnant women.

These data suggest that the same pathogenetic mechanisms which are responsible for severe hypoglycaemia in the non-pregnant state operate in pregnancy. It is difficult to know why women in some centres seldom experience hypoglycaemia. During the DCCT a wide variation was noted in the rates of hypoglycaemia reported from different participating centres. It remains unclear whether these differences were a consequence of varied approaches in diabetes management or were associated with different characteristics in the patients.

RISKS OF HYPOGLYCAEMIA IN THE MOTHER

Severe hypoglycaemia brings with it the potential risk of morbidity and even mortality from the effect of neuroglycopenia on the brain, or cardiac arrhythmias, and indirectly if patients become severely hypoglycaemic while engaged in activities such as driving. There have been reports of death as a result of hypoglycaemia during pregnancy (Rayburn et al, 1986). However, there is no evidence that the risk to the pregnant mother with diabetes is greater than her risk when not pregnant.

Impaired hypoglycaemia awareness is common during pregnancy. It is presumably related to improved glycaemic control and acquired defects in the physiological responses to hypoglycaemia. To what extent these impairments are related to the direct effect of the pregnancy remains unclear. No studies have examined the degree of reversibility of impaired hypoglycaemia awareness when this develops during pregnancy. If impaired hypoglycaemia awareness was a consequence of pregnancy then those affected should recover their symptoms immediately after delivery. If impaired hypoglycaemia awareness has resulted from repeated episodes of antecedent hypoglycaemia, it is likely that it would take weeks to months to resolve as the rise in average blood glucose concentrations reduced the frequency of hypoglycaemia.

As described in Chapters 1 and 4, those with diabetes rely on physiological defences to hypoglycaemia to mitigate the effects of high plasma insulin concentrations. Acquired defects in the hormonal and symptomatic responses to hypoglycaemia increase the risk of severe hypoglycaemia. Different groups of investigators have tried to answer the question of whether these defects are present during pregnancy, by examining physiological responses to experimentally induced hypoglycaemia during pregnancy in animals, and in humans with and without diabetes.

Diamond et al (1992) examined the physiological response to hypoglycaemia during pregnancy in nine women with type 1 diabetes using a hyperinsulinaemic glucose clamp. They showed that the adrenaline response was markedly suppressed compared to a non-pregnant control group of seven non-diabetic women (Figure 10.2), and the glycaemic threshold for the secretion of adrenaline was set at a lower level of 2.5 mmol/l compared to 3.0 mmol/l in the control subjects. Increments in growth hormone were also diminished in the pregnant diabetic women, although cortisol failed to rise significantly in either group. As expected in those with longstanding type 1 diabetes, no rise in glucagon occurred during hypoglycaemia. The difficulty of interpreting this study is to determine whether changes were related to diabetes, the effect of strict glycaemic control during pregnancy or pregnancy *per se*. The same investigators used an animal model to test the hypothesis that these lower responses might have been a consequence of pregnancy itself (Rossi et al, 1993). They measured the responses of glucagon and adrenaline to hypoglycaemia in non-diabetic pregnant rats. The glucagon response was absent and the adrenaline response was diminished in contrast to a brisk response of both hormones in non-pregnant animals.

However, other studies have reported an unchanged response of adrenaline to hypoglycaemia in pregnant women with diabetes. In nine women with diabetes, Nisell et al (1994) induced hypoglycaemia with insulin administered as an intravenous bolus on two separate occasions, during the third trimester of pregnancy and 8–12 weeks post-partum. The subjects reached similar blood glucose nadirs on both occasions although the insulin doses required were different. Peak plasma adrena-

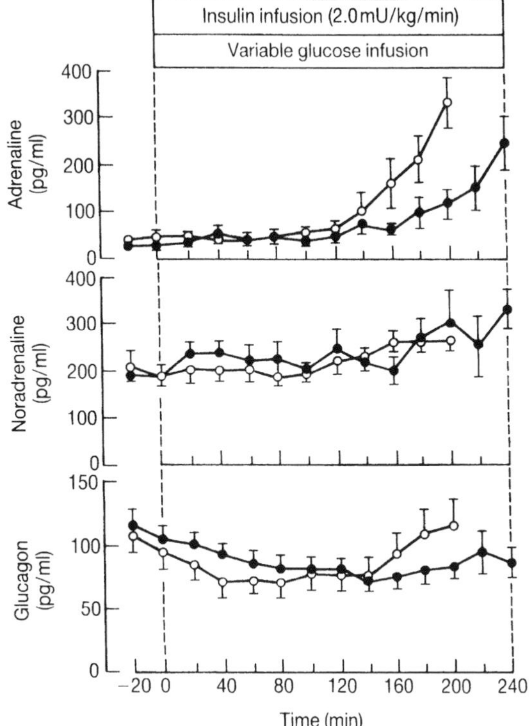

Figure 10.2 Plasma adrenaline, noradrenaline and glucagon responses to hypoglycaemia in pregnant insulin-treated diabetic women (on intensive insulin treatment) (●) and non-pregnant, non-diabetic control women (○). Reproduced from Diamond et al (1992) with permission of the *American Journal of Obstetrics and Gynecology*

line concentrations did not differ significantly, although the rise on both occasions was under 1.0 nmol/l, reflecting the relatively mild hypoglycaemic stimulus at a blood glucose nadir of 3.2 mmol/l. The contradictory conclusions of this study may in part reflect the alternative study design and the inclusion of a patient with gestational diabetes. Furthermore, women were studied within eight weeks of delivery. If the impaired counterregulatory responses have resulted from repeated hypoglycaemia during pregnancy, they may take several weeks to months to recover, although this would depend upon how frequently hypoglycaemia was being experienced.

Björklund et al (1998a) studied 10 women with type 1 diabetes during the third trimester of pregnancy and 5–13 months post-partum, using a hyperinsulinaemic glucose clamp to induce hypoglycaemia (blood glucose 2.2 mmol/l). No significant differences were observed in the adrenaline and noradrenaline responses between the pregnant and non-pregnant state but the increase in pituitary growth hormone was attenuated during pregnancy. By contrast, placental growth hormone was significantly increased during pregnancy (Björklund et al, 1998b), although the biological role of the rise in this hormone is unclear. Other placental hormones were not significantly elevated. These studies suggest that the counterregulatory responses to hypoglycaemia are not impaired during pregnancy in diabetic patients.

The question of whether pregnancy *per se* impairs the physiological responses to hypoglycaemia would best be answered by measuring responses during hypoglycaemia induced in pregnant non-diabetic women. Although many would feel that such a study presents serious ethical problems, Rosenn et al (1996) included a pregnant non-diabetic control group when comparing the counterregulatory hormonal responses at a blood glucose of 3.3 mmol/l in women with type 1 diabetes during the second and third trimesters, and post-partum. The peak plasma adrenaline responses were reduced in pregnant women with diabetes compared to controls in the pregnant and non-pregnant state (Figure 10.3). The diabetic patients had a slight but significantly attenuated rise in adrenaline during pregnancy compared to the post-partum period, particularly when the responses were tested in the third trimester. In the non-diabetic group, the glucagon and growth hormone responses were markedly reduced by the end of the third trimester compared to those measured after the pregnancy was over. The data in the women with diabetes suggested that counterregulation is impaired during pregnancy. However, those obtained from the non-diabetic women indicated that the altered hormonal milieu may modify the physiological responses to hypoglycaemia by preventing normal counterregulation. This hypothesis is supported by Davis et al (1996), who demonstrated that the infusion of cortisol causes lower episodes of responses of growth hormone, adrenaline and glucagon during a subsequent episode of experimental hypoglycaemia. Furthermore, Björklund et al (1998a) have reported increased cortisol responses during hypoglycaemia in women with type 1 diabetes during pregnancy. Further research is needed to test these concepts which have implications for patients with diabetes beyond pregnancy.

RISKS OF HYPOGLYCAEMIA TO THE FETUS

The potential effects of hypoglycaemia on the fetus can be divided into:

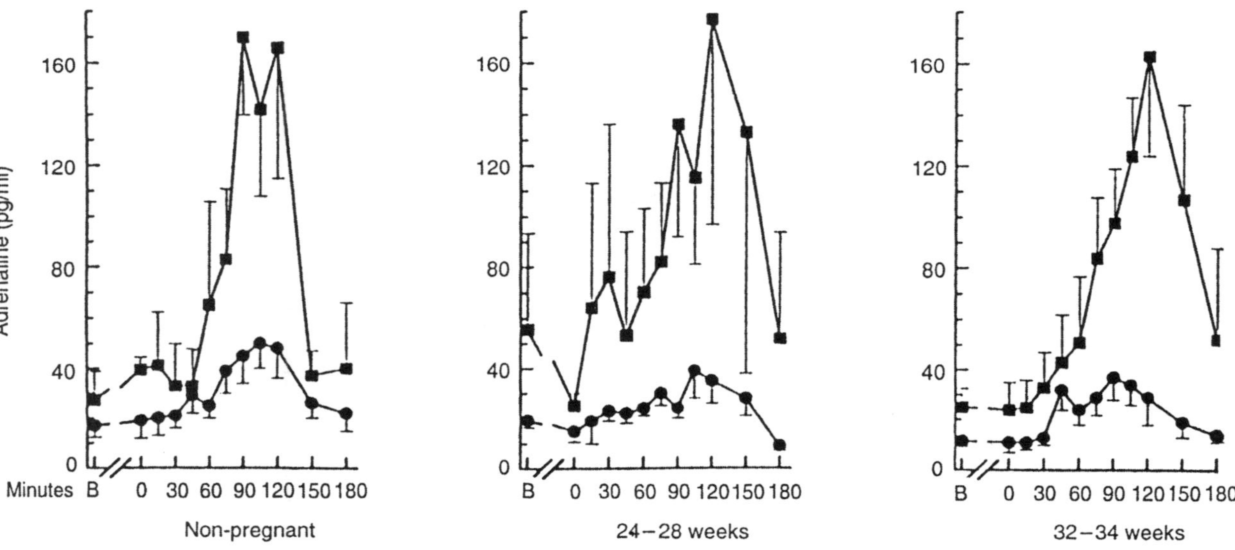

Figure 10.3 Adrenaline (epinephrine) responses to hypoglycaemia (mean ± standard error) in diabetic and non-diabetic women during pregnancy and in the non-pregnant state. ●: insulin-treated diabetic patients; ■: non-diabetic controls. Reproduced from Rosenn et al (1996), with permission of *Obstetrics and Gynecology*

- teratogenic effects
- immediate effects on the fetus *in utero*
- developmental effects post-partum.

Teratogenic Effects

The possibility that hypoglycaemia may contribute to the risks of congenital abnormalities was initially raised by *in vivo* studies in which pregnant rats exposed to profound and prolonged hypoglycaemia produced increased numbers of offspring with congenital malformations compared to animals whose blood glucose was maintained at a normal level (Buchanan et al, 1986). These experiments encouraged others to examine this question in the laboratory. Rat embryos were exposed to low concentrations of glucose (<2.0 mmol/l) at critical times of neurological development and developed malformations such as neural tube defects (Ellington, 1987). Importantly, there was a direct relationship between the depth and duration of hypoglycaemia and the rate of congenital malformations, suggesting that hypoglycaemia was causing these effects. This is powerful evidence to suggest that, at least in rodents, hypoglycaemia occurring early in gestation can cause congenital defects. The studies which have incorporated periods of hypoglycaemia lasting for many hours may have limited clinical significance since this is probably equivalent to a period of hypoglycaemia lasting a day or more in human pregnancy. However, one study in the mouse fetus has indicated that exposure to just two hours of mild hypoglycaemia at a critical period of gestation results in an increased rate of congenital malformation (Smoak and Sadler, 1990).

In psychiatric conditions, insulin shock treatment has been used during pregnancy, in non-diabetic women, in whom hypoglycaemic coma was induced for five hours (Impastato et al, 1964). The fetus was affected in six of the 19 pregnancies, the authors reporting two spontaneous abortions, two late stillbirths and two congenital abnormalities. In only two of the 13 unaffected pregnancies was the hypoglycaemia induced before 11 weeks, compared to five of the six pregnancies reported above. The clinical situation in patients with diabetic pregnancy is different. Blood glucose fluctuates between high and low levels even in women whose glycaemic control is fairly strict. However, most studies of strict glycaemic control generally indicate that the better the control of blood glucose, the greater the frequency of severe hypoglycaemia. If severe hypoglycaemia does contribute to the risk of congenital malformations one would expect to find either no difference or a higher malformation rate in clinical studies where blood glucose was strictly controlled. In fact, most of the evidence suggests that the opposite is the case and that during the first trimester, elevated blood glucose values increase the rate of congenital malformations. Fuhrmann et al (1983) have described much lower malformation rates in those women who undertook intensive insulin therapy before conception, compared to those who did not attend for antenatal care until later in the pregnancy and in whom glycaemic control was poor. Similar results have been published by others (Steel et al, 1990; Kitzmiller et al, 1991). Clearly these data do not exclude the possibility that episodes of severe hypoglycaemia may contribute to causing congenital malformations. In clinical practice, periods of hyperglycaemia are tolerated for much longer than episodes of hypoglycaemia since the latter are corrected far more rapidly. Nevertheless, the potential teratogenic effect of prolonged episodes of hypoglycaemia provide yet another reason to devise approaches to intensive insulin therapy during pregnancy which minimise the frequency of severe hypoglycaemia, particularly during the night.

In summary the data suggest that women with diabetes benefit most by keeping their glucose as strictly controlled as possible and that the potential teratogenic effects of hypoglycaemia are far outweighed by the effects of a chronically raised blood glucose. However, the question is by no means answered and additional research is needed.

Immediate Effects on the Fetus *in Utero*

Maternal hypoglycaemia can potentially affect the fetus in other ways. Physiological responses such as a sudden rise in plasma catecholamines may reduce uterine blood flow, depriving the fetus of oxygen and other fuels. This could be detected either by measuring uterine blood flow, or alternatively by examining the alteration in fetal physiology directly. The stress caused by a fall in fetal fuel delivery may stimulate the release of stress hormones and alter fetal cardiovascular responses. A number of studies have examined these responses during experimentally induced hypoglycaemia.

Reece et al (1995) lowered maternal blood glucose to 2.5 mmol/l and found that fetal limb and body movements tended to rise initially as the glucose fell before returning to baseline. There were no changes in fetal blood flow or respiratory rate despite increases in maternal plasma catecholamines and other counterregulatory hormones. They concluded that fetal well-being was unaltered by mild maternal hypoglycaemia in pregnancy. In contrast, Björklund et al (1996), at a maternal blood glucose of 2.2 mmol/l, demonstrated increased fetal heart accelerations (Figure 10.4), a reduction in the pulsatility index of the umbilical artery (Figure 10.5) and a rise in maternal catecholamines. Other studies have reported increased fetal activity during maternal hypoglycaemia (Patrick et al,

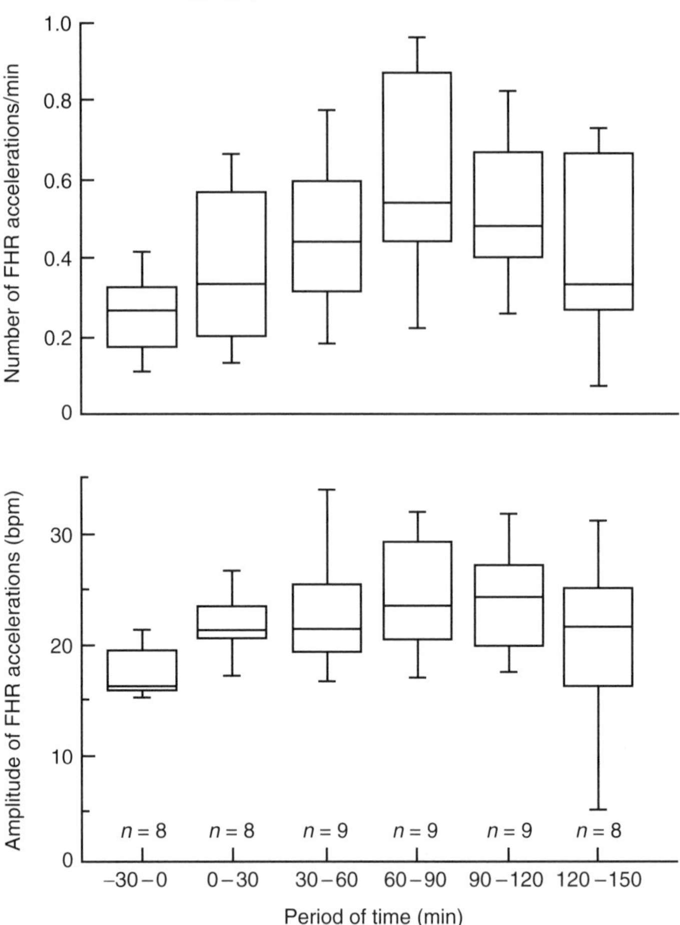

Figure 10.4 Fetal heart rate (FHR) acceleration shown as number per minute (upper graph) and amplitude (lower graph), during each 30-minute period from 30 minutes before start of induction of hypoglycaemia (zero time) until the end of the glucose clamp procedure at 150 minutes. (n = number of FHR tracings accepted for analysis each period; bpm = beats per minute. Reproduced from Björklund et al (1996) with permission of the *British Journal of Obstetrics and Gynaecology*

1982; Holden et al, 1984). More severe maternal hypoglycaemia induced by an intravenous bolus of insulin produces a decrease in fetal heart rate variability (Stangenberg et al, 1983). Nevertheless, none of the data suggest that moderate experimental hypoglycaemia in the mother has a profound and harmful effect upon the fetus. Whether this is because the fetus can maintain its blood glucose when the maternal blood glucose

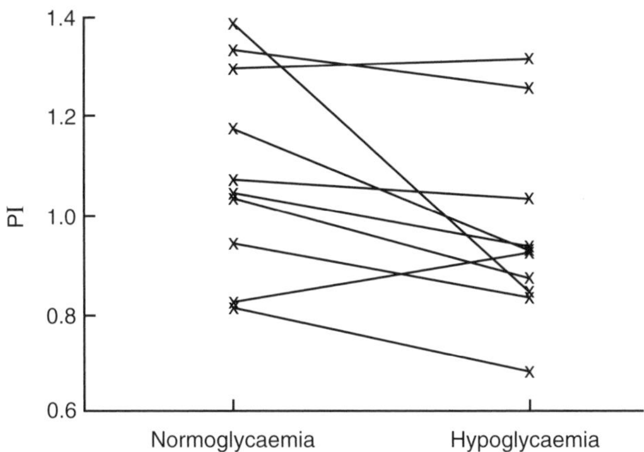

Figure 10.5 Individual changes of pulsatility index (PI) in the umbilical artery, from the examination at induction of normoglycaemia to the examination during established hypoglycaemia. Reproduced from Björklund et al (1996) with permission of the *British Journal of Obstetrics and Gynaecology*

falls or is resistant to the effects of fetal hypoglycaemia, possibly by utilising alternative fuels, is not clear.

Developmental Effects Post-partum

The adverse effects of maternal hypoglycaemia upon the fetus, particularly those upon the brain, may not be apparent at birth or in early infancy, but become apparent as developmental delay or impaired intellectual attainment later on in childhood. However, although it may be possible to demonstrate impairment using neuropsychological testing, attempting to relate these measurements retrospectively to episodes of severe hypoglycaemia in the mother is fraught with difficulty. Both high and low concentrations of blood glucose have potentially adverse effects, and trying to separate these in the same individual is almost impossible, particularly when recording events which may have occurred many years before. In an early study, Farquhar (1969) suggested that diabetic pregnancy had considerable long-term implications for the children. When reviewed during adolescence, of 210 children born to insulin-treated diabetic women, 10% were less than the third percentile for height and 20% were obese. Yssing (1974) reported evidence of cerebral dysfunction and difficulties with reading and speech in a significant proportion of children born to mothers with diabetes. A tentative association was noted with poor maternal glycaemic control but the influence of maternal hypoglycaemia was not examined in either study.

More recent studies have looked at the effect of severe hypoglycaemia on subsequent child development. Churchill et al (1969) reported lower mental test scores at the age of four years in children whose mothers had developed ketonuria during the last trimester. Rizzo et al (1991) also found a correlation between concentrations of maternal plasma ketones during pregnancy and impaired IQ in children of women with diabetes when measured at four years of age. In both studies, maternal hypoglycaemia was reported to have no demonstrable effect on subsequent cognitive function of the children. Therefore, as in other outcomes of diabetic pregnancy, the limited evidence suggests that poor glycaemic control can lead to mild but measurable neurological impairment in the children of women with diabetes. Subsequent neurological attainment does not appear to be affected by rates of maternal hypoglycaemia, although long-term prospective studies are required to answer this question definitively.

PRINCIPLES OF MANAGEMENT

The principles of achieving strict glycaemic control with the minimum risk of hypoglycaemia are, of course, those which are applied to diabetic patients who are not pregnant. Most specialist centres devote a large proportion of their clinical resources to a relatively small number of pregnant women. Each centre has their own approach and that followed by my own unit is described below (Box 10.1). However, the detailed principles of management during pregnancy are probably less important

Box 10.1 Principles of management in diabetic pregnancy to minimise the risk of hypoglycaemia

- Frequent contact (at least weekly) between patient and diabetes nurse specialist
- Frequent blood glucose monitoring
- Education of patient and partner to encourage insulin self-adjustment
- Basal/bolus insulin regimens for those with nocturnal hypoglycaemia
- Regular snacks (two-hourly)
- Supply of Hypostop and glucagon
- Increased energy intake or reduced insulin dose when breastfeeding

in ensuring successful outcomes than the strength of the relationship that develops between the patient and the diabetes nurse specialist.

The diabetes nurses on my unit maintain contact with all women by telephone each week during their pregnancy, giving patients their home telephone number and always seeing them personally when they attend the antenatal clinic. A joint obstetric/diabetic clinic attended by the physician, nurse and dietitian is not essential in ensuring strict glycaemic control but improves the likelihood that patients will receive consistent messages from all the team and helps the obstetric staff to understand the burden of hypoglycaemia during pregnancy. Considerable re-education is usually undertaken when patients become pregnant, usually on a one-to-one basis. Although the reported success of pre-pregnancy clinics in some centres is impressive (Steel et al, 1989), despite our best efforts only about half the women with type 1 diabetes who become pregnant achieve strict glycaemic control before conception.

Patients are given a glucose meter to use throughout their pregnancy and they are encouraged to monitor their blood glucose pre-prandially and post-prandially, on alternate days. In my clinic, our glycaemic targets are 5.0–6.0 mmol/l before, and 6.0–9.0 mmol/l after meals. A few women achieve these blood glucose levels on twice-daily insulin but most split their evening dose early in pregnancy, taking the isophane insulin at bedtime to reduce their risk of nocturnal hypoglycaemia. The majority of those attending the antenatal clinic eventually find that a basal-bolus regimen, with pre-meal soluble insulin and bedtime isophane insulin, suits them best. Fast-acting insulin analogues offer the prospect of strict glycaemic control with lower rates of hypoglycaemia. However, more evidence of their safety in pregnancy is required before they can be recommended routinely.

Partners should be involved as soon as a couple start to plan a pregnancy, as they need to learn when hypoglycaemia is most likely to occur and how to treat it. Couples are always issued with a supply of glucagon and Hypostop. They are also told that one episode of hypoglycaemia increases the risk of further hypoglycaemia and are encouraged to measure their blood glucose occasionally during the night to identify asymptomatic nocturnal hypoglycaemia. The diabetes nurse specialist occasionally visits the patient's place of work and teaches their colleagues and managers about hypoglycaemia.

Pregnant diabetic mothers are encouraged to eat every two hours to reduce the risk of pre-prandial hypoglycaemic episodes occurring during the day. Many are reluctant to eat regular snacks, particularly those whose weight increases considerably with advancing pregnancy. Insulin doses are reduced to pre-pregnancy levels immediately after the baby is born. Despite this, hypoglycaemia is still common in the early postnatal period, particularly in women who breastfeed. Lactation may require an additional 1000 kcal of energy daily, and has to be accommodated by an appropriate increase in dietary carbohydrate. Failure to do so, or to modify the insulin dose, may precipitate hypoglycaemia. Patients should be persuaded to continue to monitor their blood glucose for some days after delivery, although many often abandon frequent self-monitoring when pregnancy is over.

CONCLUSIONS

- Pregnancy is the one time when almost all women with type 1 diabetes are prepared to aim for blood glucose levels that are close to normal. As in other reports of intensive insulin therapy, this results in a marked increase in the frequency of hypoglycaemia, particularly during the first trimester.
- The risks are largely associated with the same factors that affect all patients who attempt to achieve strict blood glucose control in the non-pregnant state.
- There is some evidence suggesting that pregnancy itself may impair some of the physiological defences to hypoglycaemia and contribute to the development of impaired hypoglycaemia awareness.
- Despite some disconcerting evidence from animal studies, even severe hypoglycaemia does not appear to harm the developing human fetus, which is at far greater risk from a persistently elevated blood glucose.
- The ordeal of pregnancy for those with insulin-treated diabetes and the effect of repeated hypoglycaemia is perhaps best demonstrated by how few women choose to maintain their glycaemic control so strictly after pregnancy has ended.

REFERENCES

Björklund AO, Adamson UKC, Almström NHH et al (1996). Effects of hypoglycaemia on fetal heart activity and umbilical artery Doppler velocity waveforms in pregnant women with insulin-dependent diabetes mellitus. *Br J Obstet Gynaecol* **103**: 413–20.

Björklund A, Adamson U, Andreasson K et al (1998a). Hormonal counterregulation and subjective symptoms during induced hypoglycemia in insulin-depen-

dent diabetes mellitus patients during and after pregnancy. *Acta Obstet Gynecol Scand* **77**: 625–34.
Björklund AO, Adamson UKC, Carlström KAM et al (1998b). Placental hormones during induced hypoglycaemia in pregnant women with insulin-dependent diabetes mellitus: evidence of an active role for placenta in hormonal counter-regulation. *British J Obstet Gynaecol* **105**: 649–55.
Buchanan TA, Schemmer JK, Freinkel N (1986). Embryotoxic effects of brief maternal insulin-hypoglycemia during organogenesis in the rat. *J Clin Invest* **78**: 643–9.
Churchill JA, Berendes HW, Nemore J (1969). Neuropsychological deficits in children of diabetic mothers. *Am J Obstet Gynecol* **105**: 257–68.
Davis SN, Shavers C, Costa F, Mosqueda-Garcia R (1996). Role of cortisol in the pathogenesis of deficient counterregulation after antecedent hypoglycemia in normal humans. *J Clin Invest* **98**: 680–91.
Diamond MP, Reece EA, Caprio S et al (1992). Impairment of counterregulatory hormone responses to hypoglycemia in pregnant women with insulin-dependent diabetes mellitus. *Am J Obstet Gynecol* **166**: 70–7.
Ellington SK (1987). Development of rat embryos cultured in glucose-deficient media. *Diabetes* **36**: 1372–8.
Farquhar JW (1969). Prognosis for babies born to diabetic mothers in Edinburgh. *Arch Dis Child* **44**: 36–47.
Fuhrmann K, Reiker H. Semmler K, Glockner E (1969). Prevention of congenital malformation in infants of insulin dependent diabetic mothers. *Diabetes Care* **6**: 219–23.
Holden KP, Jovanovich L, Druzin ML, Petersen CM (1984). Increased fetal activity with low maternal blood glucose in pregnancies complicated by diabetes. *Am J Perinatol* **1**: 161–4.
Impastato DJ, Gabriel AR, Lardaro EH (1964). Electric and insulin shock therapy during pregnancy. *Dis Nerv Sys* **25**: 542–6.
Johnston DG, Beard RW, Chan SP et al (1995). Aspects of metabolism in normal and gestational diabetic pregnancy. *Biochem Soc Trans* **23**: 512–6.
Kimmerle R, Heinemann L, Delecki A, Berger M (1992). Severe hypoglycemia incidence and predisposing factors in 85 pregnancies of type 1 diabetic women. *Diabetes Care* **15**: 1034–7.
Kitzmiller JL, Gavin LA, Gin GD, Jovanovich-Peterson L, Main EK, Zingran WD (1991). Preconception care of diabetes. Glycemic control prevents congenital abnormalities. *J Am Med Assoc* **265**: 731–6.
Lankford HV, Bartholomew SP (1992). Severe hypoglycemia in diabetic pregnancy. *Virginia Med Q* **119**: 172–4.
Nisell H, Persson B, Hanson U et al (1994). Hormonal, metabolic, and circulatory responses to insulin-induced hypoglycemia in pregnant and nonpregnant women with insulin-dependent diabetes. *Am J Perinatol* **11**: 231–6.
Patrick J, Campbell K, Carmichael I, Richardson B (1982). Patterns of gross fetal body movements over 24–hour observation intervals during the last 10 weeks of pregnancy. *Am J Obstet Gynecol* **142**: 363–71.
Persson B, Hansson U (1993). Hypoglycaemia in pregnancy. *Bailliere's Clin Endocrinol Metab* **7**: 731–9.
Rayburn W, Piehl E, Jacober S, Schork, A Ploughman L (1986). Severe hypoglycemia during pregnancy: its frequency and predisposing factors in diabetic women. *Int J Obstet Gynaecol* **24**: 263–8.
Reece EA, Hagay Z, Roberts AB et al (1995). Fetal Doppler and behavioral

responses during hypoglycemia induced with the insulin clamp technique in pregnant diabetic women. *Am J Obstet Gynecol* **172**: 151–5.

Rizzo T, Metzger BE, Burns WJ, Burns K (1991). Correlations between antepartum maternal metabolism and intelligence of offspring. *N Eng J Med* **325**: 911–6.

Rosenn BM, Miodovnik M, Holcberg G, Khoury JC, Siddiqi TA (1995). Hypoglycemia: the price of intensive insulin therapy for pregnant women with insulin-dependent diabetes mellitus. *Obstet Gynecol* **85**: 417–22.

Rosenn BM, Miodovnik M, Khoury JC, Siddiqi TA (1996). Counterregulatory hormonal responses to hypoglycemia during pregnancy. *Obstet Gynecol* **87**: 568–74.

Rossi G, Lapaczewski P, Diamond MP. Jacob RJ, Shulman GI, Sherwin RS (1993). Inhibitory effect of pregnancy on counterregulatory hormone responses to hypoglycemia in awake rat. *Diabetes* **42**: 1440–5.

Smoak IW, Sadler TW (1990). Embryopathic effects of short-term exposure to hypoglycemia in mouse embryos in vitro. *Am J Obstet Gynecol* **63**: 619–24.

Stangenberg M, Persson B, Stange L, Carlström K (1983). Insulin induced hypoglycaemia in diabetics. Maternal and fetal cardiovascular reactions. *Acta Obstet Gynaecol Scand* **62**: 249–52.

Steel JM, Johnstone FD, Smith AF (1989). Pre-pregnancy preparation. In: Sutherland, HW, Stowers JM, Pearson DWM, eds. *Carbohydrate Metabolism in Pregnancy and the Newborn: IV*. Berlin: Springer-Verlag, 129–39.

Steel JM, Johnstone FD, Hepburn DA, Smith AF (1990). Can pre-pregnancy care of diabetic women reduce the risk of abnormal babies? *BMJ* **301**: 1070–4.

The Diabetes Control and Complications Trial Research Group (1996). Pregnancy outcomes in the Diabetes Control and Complications Trial. *Am J Obstet Gynecol* **174**: 1343–53.

Yssing M (1974). Oestriol excretion in pregnant diabetes related to long term prognosis of surviving children. *Acta Endocrinol* **182**: 95–104.

11

Living with Hypoglycaemia

BRIAN M. FRIER
Royal Infirmary of Edinburgh, Edinburgh

INTRODUCTION

Hypoglycaemia is recognised to be the single major limiting factor in achieving and maintaining good glycaemic control in people with insulin-treated diabetes. Because hypoglycaemia can occur at any time of day or night, is often unpredictable, affects intellectual and physical performance and disrupts the life of the affected individual and others, its effects can impinge on every aspect of everyday living. Irrespective of the causes and risk factors for hypoglycaemia, the effects on the affected individual are generally unpleasant, frightening and can have wide ramifications which include psychological sequelae (Box 11.1). Adverse experiences of severe hypoglycaemia can influence the subsequent behaviour of an individual in an attempt to avoid further events, and by the effect on their self-care of diabetes, may encourage poor glycaemic control.

PSYCHO-SOCIAL EFFECTS

Fear of Hypoglycaemia

In addition to the subjective experience of symptoms and physical changes induced by acute hypoglycaemia, the effects on cognitive and non-cognitive functions may be very disabling, leading to loss of control of events and reliance on others for assistance. The emotional consequences of living with the ever-present risk of hypoglycaemia can affect

Hypoglycaemia in Clinical Diabetes. Edited by B. M. Frier and B. M. Fisher.

Box 11.1 Psychological consequences of hypoglycaemia

Short-term
- Anxiety
- Transient cognitive dysfunction
- Aversion
- Depersonalisation
- Loss of control
- Guilt, frustration
- Embarassment
- Dependence on others
- Accidents

Long-term
- Stress
- Avoidance behaviour
- Obsessive self-monitoring
- Relationship conflicts
- Guilt, frustration
- Work/school problems
- Social isolation
- ? Permanent cognitive dysfunction

the personal lives of both the affected individual and other members of the family. It is not surprising that most individuals with recurrent exposure to severe hypoglycaemia develop an aversion to it. Many rate their fear of severe hypoglycaemia as equivalent to their concern about developing serious long-term complications of diabetes (Pramming et al, 1991) (Figure 11.1). In a group of 60 people with type 1 diabetes, 11 (18%) described severe hypoglycaemia as being the most frightening event in their lives (Sanders et al, 1975) and many associated this with feelings of insecurity, tension and depression.

People with insulin-treated diabetes who have experienced frequent severe hypoglycaemia, may show higher levels of psychological distress, including increased anxiety, depression, and fear of future hypoglycaemia (Wredling et al, 1992; Gold et al, 1994a). Fear of hypoglycaemia is also a common source of anxiety for relatives, and may strain marital and family relationships. The spouses of people with diabetes who have frequent severe hypoglycaemia, also have a greater fear of hypoglycaemia, and report having sleep disturbance through worrying about nocturnal hypoglycaemia compared with the spouses of people with diabetes who do not suffer severe hypoglycaemia (Gonder-Frederick et al, 1997). The negative consequences of hypoglycaemia not only affect spouses, but also the parents of children with diabetes (Clarke et al, 1998), the children of diabetic parents, and other family members. Two-thirds of a group of 60 spouses of people with diabetes said that the risk of severe hypoglycaemia was a major source of concern to them, and when their partner is late, one in five considered hypoglycaemia to be the principal cause (Stahl et al, 1998). About 10% felt that severe hypoglycaemia was "always" a burden. Similar worries may afflict a child who has previously discovered a

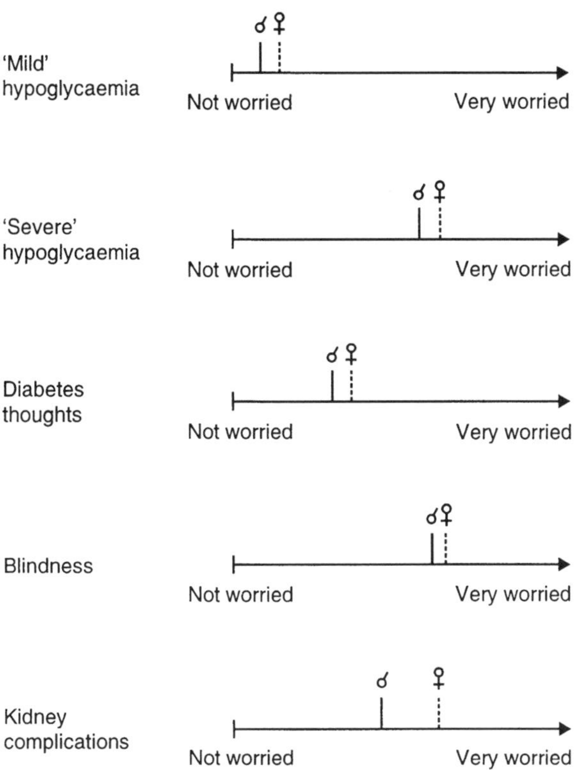

Figure 11.1 Attributes towards different aspects of diabetes indicated by 411 patients with type 1 diabetes on a visual analogue scale. Reproduced from Pramming et al (1991) with permission of *Diabetic Medicine*

comatose, hypoglycaemic diabetic parent. Whether episodic severe hypoglycaemia leads to increased marital breakdown and stress is not clear, although anecdotal evidence would suggest that this does occur.

Cox et al (1987) have devised a simple questionnaire, the Hypoglycaemia Fear Survey, which can assess an individual's fear of hypoglycaemia. In addition to measuring fear, it is possible to assess the way that people worry about hypoglycaemia and the behavioural responses which they take to avoid it. In some patients, hypoglycaemia may profoundly influence both the impact of diabetes on their daily life, and their approach to self-management. The consequences of evasion and subsequent fear of hypoglycaemia may promote a phobia and so encourage behavioural changes that maintain a high blood glucose to avoid future hypoglycaemia. Although the psychological consequences rarely produce frank psychiatric illness, the long-term effect of hypoglycaemia on subsequent behaviour may be much greater in many patients than is recognised by clinicians. This may partly explain the resistance shown by some individuals to therapeutic recommendations to improve their glycaemic control. Fear of hypoglycaemia was cited as the main reason why many young patients with type 1 diabetes were not enthusiastic about attaining strict glycaemic control despite the findings of the Diabetes Control and Complications Trial (DCCT) (Thompson et al, 1996). The non-cognitive effects of acute hypoglycaemia on mood and behaviour (Box 11.2) have been reviewed by Gold et al (1997) and are described in Chapter 2.

The disruption to domestic life caused by an episode of severe hypoglycaemia, the feeling of helplessness to prevent further episodes, and the increased tension and anxiety that are engendered by hypoglycaemia, both in the person with diabetes and in their relatives, are not conducive to a relaxed home environment. The psycho-social implications and consequences of hypoglycaemia on the family and on home life are little understood by many health professionals, who do not empathise with the domestic problems presented by hypoglycaemia.

NOCTURNAL HYPOGLYCAEMIA

Nocturnal hypoglycaemia is common in people with insulin-treated diabetes and often is not identified. The frequency of nocturnal hypogly-

Box 11.2 Effects of hypoglycaemia on non-cognitive psychological function

Mood
- Tense – tiredness
- Unhappiness; anger
- Pessimism about life expectations

Fear
- Related to frequency and severity of hypoglycaemia
- Affects personality traits
- Promotes anxiety (phobia)
- ? Behavioural modification

Behaviour
- Irritability; emotional lability
- Hostility; aggression (adults)
- Naughtiness (children)

caemia and its likely time of development with different insulin regimens are discussed in Chapter 3. Most people do not experience symptoms of hypoglycaemia while asleep, and are seldom awakened by a low blood glucose; this is a true physiological cause of impaired awareness of hypoglycaemia. Catecholamine responses to hypoglycaemia are diminished during sleep, indicative of a general reduction in sympatho-adrenal activity during deep sleep (Jones et al, 1998). Apart from the unknown long-term effect which recurrent exposure to protracted nocturnal hypoglycaemia may have on cognitive function, untreated episodic hypoglycaemia may contribute to the development of diminished symptomatic awareness and counterregulatory deficiency (Veneman et al, 1993). When these abnormalities are acquired, they potentially increase the vulnerability of people with insulin-treated diabetes to a fall in blood glucose during the night, so creating a vicious circle.

Features of Nocturnal Hypoglycaemia

Clues that a low blood glucose is occurring during the night may be subtle (Box 11. 3). Suspicion should be raised by a history of vivid dreams or nightmares, poor quality of sleep, morning headache, feeling "hungover" (without having taken alcohol) and feeling tired on awakening. A study of 10 subjects with type 1 diabetes, who were exposed to one hour of experimentally induced hypoglycaemia during the night, confirmed that their subjective well-being was affected the following day, with greater fatigue being experienced during exercise (King et al, 1998). However, tests of cognitive function were unaffected both in this (King et al, 1998) and other (Bendtson et al, 1992) studies on the morning after nocturnal hypoglycaemia. Nocturnal convulsions are particularly disturbing and have occasionally been associated with bone fractures and

Box 11.3 Clinical manifestations of nocturnal hypoglycaemia

- Vivid dreams; nightmares
- Morning headache; feeling "hungover"
- Poor-quality sleep
- Chronic fatigue; lethargy
- Depression
- Restless behaviour during sleep; disturbed or damp bedclothes
- Night sweats
- Nocturnal convulsions
- Enuresis (children)

soft tissue injuries. Nocturnal hypoglycaemia has also been implicated as the cause of the "dead in bed" syndrome (see Chapter 7).

The spouses or partners of people with insulin-treated diabetes who share the same bed, often become very sensitive to the features of nocturnal neuroglycopenia in their partner, are usually awakened by these cues, and can intervene to provide effective treatment. They report that their partner becomes very restless in bed, sweats profusely while asleep, and may be difficult to rouse. The person with hypoglycaemia may then be uncooperative, refusing to do blood glucose testing or to take oral carbohydrate. However, most children and teenagers, and many adults (particularly elderly people) sleep alone, highlighting the pressing need for a reliable and sensitive alarm device to detect a low blood glucose during sleep.

Blood Glucose Tests and Insulin Regimens

Conventional Insulin Regimens

The measurement of blood glucose at bedtime should be routine. If patients are reluctant to do regular testing, this is the single most important time of the day to estimate blood glucose, and its prophylactic value should be emphasised. Several studies have demonstrated that a blood glucose below 6.0 mmol/l at bedtime is associated with an increased risk of nocturnal hypoglycaemia when using conventional, twice-daily, soluble and isophane insulin regimens. The time when blood glucose is most likely to be low during the night is between 02.00 and 04.00 hours. This may be avoided by delaying the injection of the evening dose of isophane insulin, which should be administered as late as possible before retiring to bed, and certainly after 23.00 hours. People who retire to bed early and so inject their bedtime isophane insulin earlier in the evening, are at risk of developing hypoglycaemia in the later part of the night. The use of a continuous subcutaneous insulin infusion (CSII) overnight, in place of bedtime isophane insulin, has been shown to reduce the frequency of nocturnal hypoglycaemia (Kanc et al, 1998). However, few patients would regard this as a practical option.

Many people now eat their evening meal between 19.30 to 21.30 hours, which is much later than the traditional British "tea time" of 17.00 to 18.30 hours and is akin to the later timing of the evening meal prevalent in many Mediterranean countries. In this situation, a bedtime snack is redundant. Because of the relatively long duration of action (up to six hours) of soluble insulin, its administration in the mid to late evening risks inducing nocturnal hypoglycaemia at around 01.00 to 02.00 hours. The use of a rapid-acting insulin analogue, such as insulin lispro, injected immediately before a late evening meal, may then be preferable, as its hypoglycaemic action has usually waned before the individual retires to bed. In some patients this may increase the risk of early hypoglycaemia *after* the evening meal, and a late supper then promotes hyperglycaemia during the night (Mohn et al, 1999). Redistribution of the amount of carbohydrate consumed during the evening may prevent these problems.

Basal-bolus Insulin Regimens

The use of a short-acting insulin before meals and an intermediate-acting insulin at bedtime, rarely causes nocturnal hypoglycaemia between 02.00 and 04.00 hours, which is the traditional time that is recommended to patients to test blood glucose for the detection of nocturnal hypoglycaemia. Nocturnal hypoglycaemia associated with multiple injection regimens occurs with two peaks of frequency: "early night" hypoglycaemia occurring between 23.00 and 01.00 hours, and "early morning" hypoglycaemia between 04.00 and 07.30 hours (Figure 11.2) (Vervoort et al, 1996). Bedtime blood glucose values predict "early night" hypoglycaemia, which is absent when bedtime blood glucose is over 7.5 mmol/l. Fasting blood glucose values below 5.5 indicate preceding "early morning" hypoglycaemia. If a target pre-breakfast value above this level can be achieved, the frequency of nocturnal hypoglycaemia should be reduced.

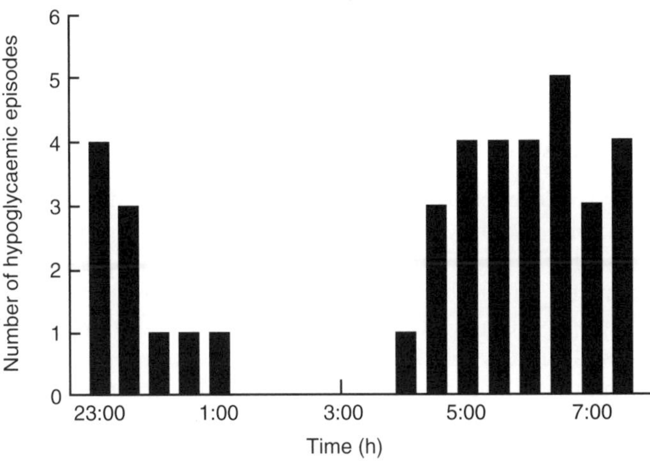

Figure 11.2 Time-related frequency of nocturnal hypoglycaemia in 31 patients with type 1 diabetes treated with a basal-bolus insulin regimen (short-acting soluble insulin before meals and intermediate-acting isophane insulin at bedtime). Reproduced from Vervoort et al (1996) with permission of *Diabetic Medicine*

For people on basal-bolus insulin regimens, daily monitoring of fasting and bedtime blood glucose concentrations should help to prevent hypoglycaemia during the night. These times of testing are clearly more valuable than periodic testing of blood glucose at 03.00 hours.

Availability of Carbohydrate

It is prudent for people treated with insulin to keep a supply of rapid-acting carbohydrate accessible by the bedside, either as dextrose tablets, a glucose drink or a snack such as biscuits. One young woman who attends my clinic, was sleeping alone in her own bedroom and awakened with florid symptoms of hypoglycaemia, but was unable to rise out of bed or call to other family members for help. Patients occasionally describe wakening with transient hemiplegia induced by nocturnal hypoglycaemia. The immediate availability of a supply of glucose would allow immediate self-treatment of this frightening situation. Some means of attracting attention (like a handbell) may also be of benefit, and for people who live alone, a telephone by the bedside is desirable so that emergency assistance can be summoned. This assumes that the hypoglycaemic individual is still able to use the telephone. While none of these measures will prevent hypoglycaemia occurring during the night, the prospect of lying incapacitated and stranded in bed, while the means of retrieving the situation is elsewhere in the house, causes understandable anxiety in many people treated with insulin. Measures to anticipate and treat this, often unpredictable, metabolic problem are essential, even if nocturnal hypoglycaemia is uncommon.

Prophylactic Measures to Avoid Nocturnal Hypoglycaemia

In addition to routine testing of blood glucose at bedtime, a fundamental measure to avoid hypoglycaemia occurring during the night is the ingestion of a suitable late supper or bedtime snack. In people with good glycaemic control, short-acting carbohydrate is ineffective in preventing nocturnal hypoglycaemia. Although transient hyperglycaemia may be achieved, this is rapidly dissipated and fails to counteract the nocturnal hyperinsulinaemia which is associated with many insulin regimens. The bedtime snack should contain slowly digested, long-acting carbohydrate. Preliminary studies using corn starch at bedtime have indicated a reduced frequency of nocturnal hypoglycaemia in children and adults with type 1 diabetes, although palatability may be a problem. Possible alternative foods which have a high content of starch and fibre, and therefore act as a "lente" carbohydrate, are breakfast cereals or porridge with milk, bread as a sandwich or toast, cereal bars or biscuits with a high content of fibre or a constituent such as oats. The composition of the evening meal may also be important. The consumption of a high-protein, low-fat meal at 19.00 hours has been shown to be more effective than an isocaloric low-protein, high-fat meal at maintaining blood glucose overnight in diabetic patients infused with a fixed dose of insulin (Winiger et al, 1995).

The conventional bedtime snack may not necessarily prevent the development of nocturnal hypoglycaemia but simply delay it to later in the night. In a study of 15 patients with type 1 diabetes, a bedtime snack (200 kcal) consisting of milk and a slice of toast, maintained the blood glucose for two to three hours, but thereafter was ineffective in preventing a decline into the hypoglycaemic range (Saleh and Cryer, 1997). By contrast, a bedtime dose of 40 g of alanine which promotes the release of endogenous glucagon, or the oral ingestion of 5 mg of the beta-2-adrenoceptor agonist, terbutaline, which stimulates the secretion of adrenaline, were more effective in preventing nocturnal hypoglycaemia. While the practicality of administering these particular agents is dubious, this is a promising approach to the prevention of nocturnal hypoglycaemia. Practical measures to avoid nocturnal hypoglycaemia are listed in Box 11.4.

The early detection (and rapid treatment) of nocturnal hypoglycaemia awaits the development of a non-invasive glucose sensor for the continuous measurement of blood glucose. An alarm system could then be triggered at a pre-determined blood glucose concentration, so awakening the patient and enabling the ingestion of oral glucose before progression to disabling neuroglycopenia. Devices that depend on changes in sweating and skin temperature have been shown to be unreliable, and are not

Box 11.4 Avoidance of nocturnal hypoglycaemia: possible measures and advice to patients

- Measure blood glucose at bedtime
- Keep rapid-acting carbohydrate beside bed for emergency treatment
- Take suitable bedtime snack containing long-acting carbohydrate
- Do an occasional blood glucose measurement during night
- Take care with timing of evening meals and timing of insulin administration
- Possible use of rapid-acting insulin analogue before evening meal (especially if late)
- Take care with consumption of alcohol and strenuous exercise during evening before bed.

specific to a low blood glucose (Clarke et al, 1988), although it has been claimed that a sensor for sweat detection may be useful (Davies and Evans, 1995).

The Somogyi Effect

The existence of the so-called "Somogyi effect", i.e. fasting hyperglycaemia promoted by the counterregulation associated with nocturnal hypoglycaemia, is disputed. Although asymptomatic nocturnal hypoglycaemia was shown by one research group to correlate with moderate fasting hyperglycaemia and higher plasma concentrations of counterregulatory hormones in 10 patients with type 1 diabetes (Perriello et al, 1998), this observation has not been confirmed by others (Hirsch et al, 1990), and in clinical practice the frequency and magnitude of the Somogyi effect are thought to be insignificant (Havlin and Cryer, 1987). The principal cause of fasting hyperglycaemia after nocturnal hypoglycaemia is thought to be the excessive ingestion of carbohydrate to treat the low blood glucose. Thus, the rebound hyperglycaemia may occur as a result of over-treatment, but this remains controversial.

EXERCISE

Regular exercise is particularly valuable for people with insulin-treated diabetes (Wassermann and Zinman, 1994). Exercise increases insulin sensitivity, helps to avoid weight gain and is beneficial for several metabolic parameters, including lipids and cardiovascular risk factors (Lehmann et al, 1997). However, exercise may not improve overall glycaemic control unless it is very frequent and intense (as pursued by many athletes).

In the non-diabetic individual, exercise promotes the release of counterregulatory hormones, especially adrenaline, and inhibits insulin secretion. This stimulates the hepatic output of glucose, initially through hepatic glycogenolysis, but if exercise is sustained, gluconeogenesis is also promoted. Glucose is utilised by skeletal muscle, so blood glucose concentration does not alter. In people with insulin-treated diabetes, the prevailing plasma concentration of insulin is independent of, and cannot be suppressed by, exercise, and this determines the metabolic consequences of exercise (Wasserman and Zinman, 1994). If plasma insulin is low, the peripheral uptake of glucose by muscle is reduced and hyperglycaemia results from exercise. If plasma insulin is high, hepatic output of glucose is inhibited, peripheral utilisation by muscle is stimulated, and the blood glucose falls, resulting in hypoglycaemia (see Chapter 3).

The temporal relationship between the time of exercise, the time of administration of insulin, and its time-action profile, are therefore major determinants of the metabolic outcome with respect to the blood glucose response. Other factors of relevance include the time of the ingestion of food, the nature of the food consumed, the intensity and duration of the exercise, and the site of insulin injection. Exercise of a limb into which insulin has recently been injected, will increase the rate of absorption by muscle action (Box 11.5). The risk of hypoglycaemia is increased if intramuscular injection is made inadvertently (Frid et al, 1990).

Prevention of Hypoglycaemia Following Exercise

The potential risk of associated hypoglycaemia requires the adoption of differing strategies to prevent an undesirable fall in blood glucose. The individual can either ingest additional short-acting carbohydrate, in liquid or solid form, or reduce the dose of insulin in anticipation of a period of physical activity. Both measures may be necessary and may be determined by the duration and the intensity of the exercise intended. Strenuous exercise as a short burst of activity, such as a game of squash or an aerobics class, may require prophylactic consumption of short-acting carbohydrate in advance of the exercise. Protracted physical activity lasting for several hours, such as hill walking, requires a substantial reduction in total insulin dose, in addition to an increase in consumption of carbohydrate. It is difficult to advocate specific measures for individuals or for particular events, as the response to exercise can be idiosyncratic and depends partly on the overall quality of glycaemic control. The risk of inducing hypoglycaemia with exercise is obviously heightened in individuals who have strict glycaemic control and who have a lower blood glucose at the start of exercise, than those with moderate hyperglycaemia. Some degree of trial and error may be neces-

Box 11.5 Factors influencing blood glucose response to exercise in people with insulin-treated diabetes

- Time of previous insulin administration
- Type of insulin used; insulin regimen
- Site of insulin injection
- Time of previous meal or snack
- Nature and quality of food consumed before exercise
- Duration and nature (intensity) of exercise
- Time of day of exercise

sary to assess the effect of specific activities on blood glucose in individuals.

A fall in blood glucose may not occur during, or immediately following physical exertion, but may be delayed for several hours, sometimes occurring up to 15 hours later (MacDonald, 1987). If the exercise is taken in the late afternoon or early evening, hypoglycaemia may occur during the night or even the following day. The response obviously depends on factors such as the efficiency of mobilisation of glucose from glycogen stores, how effectively these are replenished after exercise, the magnitude of the co-existing hormonal response and sympatho-adrenal activation, and the prevailing plasma insulin concentration during and after exercise.

For some patients one of the safest times of day to exercise is in the fasting state (before breakfast) and before the administration of morning insulin as at this time of day plasma insulin is relatively low (Ruegemer et al, 1990). In the fasting state the fall in blood glucose during moderate exercise is small or absent in subjects with insulin-treated diabetes, the prophylactic ingestion of carbohydrate may cause an unwanted rise in blood glucose, and may not therefore be necessary (Soo et al, 1996). The use of continuous subcutaneous insulin infusion (CSII) does not avoid the risk of exercise-induced hypoglycaemia, and interrupting the basal insulin infusion may be insufficient to prevent a fall in blood glucose after postprandial exercise if hyperinsulinaemia is present (Edelmann et al, 1986). In well controlled patients using CSII the insulin dose has to be reduced before, during, and after exercise to minimise the risk of acute and late hypoglycaemia (Sonnenberg et al, 1990). Measures to prevent hypoglycaemia occurring in relation to exercise are shown in Box 11.6.

Box 11.6 Measures to prevent hypoglycaemia induced by exercise

- Take extra carbohydrate (20–30 g short-acting) and possibly during exercise (if prolonged)
- Reduce insulin dose before exercise
- Monitor blood glucose frequently
- Avoid peak absorption and time of action of insulin for strenuous exercise (2–4 hours after soluble insulin)
- Use anterior abdominal wall for injection of insulin (avoid active limbs)
- Avoid exercise if blood glucose is high (> 17.0 mmol/l), especially if ketosis is present
- Learn the glycaemic response to different types of exercise
- Carry identification re insulin

Strenuous exercise may sometimes be unpremeditated, as in an emergency situation. In addition, it is very easy for individuals to become distracted during activities such as home decorating or gardening, during which they work much harder or longer than originally intended. It is therefore essential that all people with insulin-treated diabetes carry a supply of glucose tablets or an alternative source of quick-acting refined carbohydrate *at all times* to counter a sudden decline in blood glucose.

Sport

Some sports are inherently dangerous and may be inadvisable for an individual who is at risk of developing hypoglycaemia. Dangerous activities are those involving height, water, extremes of climate and exposure to inhospitable terrain. Activities such as hang-gliding and parachuting, subaqua-diving or unaccompanied rock climbing are usually proscribed for people treated with insulin. Apart from the risk to the individual, the safety of others must be considered, and they should not be put at risk by an individual experiencing acute hypoglycaemia. However, with adequate precautions and careful preparation, there are few sports that cannot be tackled safely by people with insulin-treated diabetes, and many diabetic athletes or professional sportsmen and women have achieved distinction at the highest levels of sporting prowess. For the average individual, for whom sport is simply a form of recreation and a means of obtaining regular exercise, measures to avoid hypoglycaemia are relatively straightforward, as described earlier.

Most team sports such as football and hockey, and competitive games such as squash or tennis usually have a predictable duration, but other activities such as swimming, cycling or running may be much more variable. Protracted and demanding physical activities require more elaborate planning. Long-distance running requires a considerable reduction in insulin dose. In 13 runners with diabetes who participated in the New York marathon the total insulin dose was reduced by a mean of 38% (Grimm and Muchnick, 1993). The frequent ingestion of beverages and snacks which are rich in carbohydrate is also necessary. A personal account of a marathon run (Kjeldby, 1997) emphasised the difficulty in determining how much intermediate-acting insulin to inject in the evening after the run, and the necessity to do frequent measurements of blood glucose over the next 24 to 48 hours to avoid delayed hypoglycaemia.

Outward Bound mountain courses and holidays for young people with type 1 diabetes that include rock climbing, canoeing, horse-riding, caving and mountain expeditions have been described by Hillson (1984; 1987) who has detailed the sort of measures necessary for participants to avoid and to treat hypoglycaemia (Box 11.7). Anticipation of potential hazards for people with diabetes at risk of hypoglycaemia must be considered for all activities, with consideration given to the timing of meals and administration of insulin, travelling time and how much energy is likely to be expended. It may be difficult to distinguish between physical exhaustion and hypoglycaemia, both of which may co-exist (Hillson, 1984), and hypothermia can be induced by hypoglycaemia as well as by cold and wet conditions. It may be necessary to reduce insulin dosage and increase carbohydrate intake at summer camps for children with diabetes (Braatvedt et al, 1997), as frequent hypoglycaemia is associated with the sudden increase in energetic activities when the children arrive at camp. In children, this policy may have to be applied to holidays in general (see Chapter 9).

RECREATION

Strenuous and protracted exercise may occur during recreational activities, such as prolonged and vigorous dancing, and these social events may also involve the consumption of alcohol, another potential cause of hypoglycaemia. Some "recreational" drugs such as amphetamines have

Box 11.7 Measures to prevent hypoglycaemia in outdoor activities and holidays (derived from Hillson, 1984; 1987)

- Reduce total insulin dose (by 10–15%)
- Ensure a good intake of high-fibre carbohydrate with plentiful quick-acting carbohydrate
- Increase carbohydrate at main meals and double the amount taken at snacks, or the number of snacks between main meals
- Consume glucose tablets or drinks immediately before climbing up or down anything high, or during water activities
- Carry glucose at all times and keep by the bed at night
- Monitor blood glucose four times daily and respond appropriately to the results. Aim for a blood glucose of 10.0 mmol/l. Blood glucose may be difficult to measure in cold or wet weather
- Take an hourly snack during prolonged exercise such as cycling or mountain walking
- Take a large pre-bedtime snack to avoid delayed hypoglycaemia

been associated with frenetic behaviour and increased metabolic rate that can induce hypoglycaemia in people treated with insulin (Jenks and Watkinson, 1998). Young people with type 1 diabetes who attend discos or parties often avoid the potential risk and embarrassment of hypoglycaemia by omitting the administration of insulin before the social event. While this may be a pragmatic approach, the problem with this strategy is that exercise may worsen the pre-existing hyperglycaemia, and could promote the development of ketoacidosis. A modest reduction of insulin dose, combined with appropriate high-carbohydrate snacks and the judicious consumption of alcohol should avoid hypoglycaemia, though this requires forward planning and is not conducive to the spontaneity of social activity desired by many young adults. Similarly, unpremeditated and energetic sexual intercourse can precipitate unexpected hypoglycaemia, depending on the related metabolic circumstances, and care should be taken to avoid this hazard if possible! It is easy to see why meticulous self-care of diabetes could inhibit the social activities of teenagers and young adults and interfere with late nights and parties. It is also clear why many do not strive for good glycaemic control in this situation. An episode of severe hypoglycaemia will ruin a social outing, but chronic hyperglycaemia is equally undesirable.

DRIVING

For people with diabetes who are treated with insulin, the potential risks of hypoglycaemia are always present and have therefore influenced the ways in which modern society regulates and restricts their activities. This principally affects driving licences and some forms of employment. While most of these restrictions are reasonable and important for public safety, much lay, and even medical, ignorance exists about hypoglycaemia and its effects, so that discriminatory practices still occur, particularly with regard to employment.

Effect of Hypoglycaemia on Driving

Driving is a common and everyday activity that demands complex psychomotor skills, including good visuo-spatial functions, rapid information processing, vigilance and satisfactory judgment. Because hypoglycaemia rapidly interferes with cognitive functions, even modest degrees of neuroglycopenia may affect driving skills, without necessarily provoking symptomatic awareness of hypoglycaemia. Cox et al (1993) used a sophisticated driving simulator to study the driving abilities of 25 drivers with type 1 diabetes at different blood glucose concentrations, maintained by a glucose clamp. Driving performance over a trial period of four minutes was significantly disrupted in nine patients (36%) at an arterialised blood glucose of 2.6 mmol/l, and mainly affected steering, with, in addition, increased swerving and spinning of the vehicle, poor road positioning and compensatory slowing. What was disconcerting was that around half of the affected drivers did not experience warning symptoms of hypoglycaemia and said they felt competent to drive while their blood glucose was low (Cox et al, 1993). Allowing for the artificial conditions of a driving simulator and the very short period of testing, there is little doubt that hypoglycaemia can adversely affect the ability to drive and in individual cases hypoglycaemia has been implicated as a precipitating cause of road traffic accidents, causing the occasional fatality. In a study of insulin-treated drivers in Northern Ireland, the number of hypoglycaemic episodes that occurred while driving in the preceding year was shown to be associated with the total number of accidents during the previous five years (Stevens et al, 1989), consistent with Scottish studies which showed a greater rate of accidents among diabetic drivers who experienced hypoglycaemia while driving (Frier et al, 1980; Eadington and Frier, 1989; MacLeod et al, 1993).

Hypoglycaemia can impair cognitive function and judgment as a direct effect of neuroglycopenia, without necessarily provoking warning symptoms or altering consciousness. Automatism may occur and irrational and compulsive behaviour during hypoglycaemia has been described by insulin-treated diabetic drivers (Frier et al, 1980). Diabetic drivers experiencing hypoglycaemia have occasionally been arrested by the police on the suspicion that inebriation was the cause of their altered behaviour and symptoms. Impaired awareness of hypoglycaemia, with its increased risk of severe hypoglycaemia, is clearly a hazard to safe driving, and is a common reason why the driving licence is revoked.

Risk of Accidents and Restriction of Driving Licences

It is difficult to quantitate how often hypoglycaemia occurs during driving and how often this precipitates an accident, particularly as fatal cases are not usually detected. Around a third of insulin-treated diabetic drivers have admitted experiencing hypoglycaemia while driving during the preceding six to 12 months (Frier et al, 1980; Stevens et al, 1989; Eadington and Frier, 1989). The rate of hypoglycaemia-induced accidents is extremely difficult to evaluate and is, of necessity, anecdotal. Studies in the UK have suggested that the accident rate of diabetic drivers is very similar to non-diabetic drivers (Stevens et al, 1989; Eadington and Frier, 1989), and this premise is supported by studies from Germany (Chantelau et al, 1990) and the USA (Songer et al, 1988) (Table 11.1). In an

Table 11.1 Hypoglycaemia-related road traffic accidents: rates per mileage driven

Reference	n	Time (years)	Hypo-related accidents	Total mileage ($\times 10^6$)	Hypo-related accidents per 10^6 miles
Eadington and Frier (1989)	166	8	9	10.5	0.90
Chantelau et al (1990)	241	2	10	5.7	1.76
Songer et al (1988)	127	1	2	1.5	1.30

assessment of medical factors causing road traffic accidents, a study in Iceland showed that disorders such as diabetes were not over-represented (Gislason et al, 1997). However, one American study has observed a "slight increase" in the risk of motor vehicle accidents in diabetic drivers (Hansotia and Broste, 1991), but considered this to be insufficient to "warrant further restrictions on driving privileges".

These studies have been criticised for being retrospective, excluding fatal accidents and being influenced by the removal of diabetic drivers who have ceased driving either by their own volition or through the efforts of the regulatory authorities. However, most licencing authorities issue ordinary driving licences to people with insulin-treated diabetes that are restricted in duration, and are subject to medical review. Other than visual impairment, the principal factors that commonly lead to an ordinary driving licence being revoked are impaired awareness of hypoglycaemia and recurrent severe hypoglycaemia during waking hours.

Vocational Driving Licences

A more stringent approach has been adopted by the European Community towards vocational licences, i.e. those for large goods vehicles (LGV) and passenger carrying vehicles (PCV), and for several years drivers treated with insulin have been disbarred from holding vocational driving licences in most European countries. However, there is a wide international variation in the policies of governments towards vocational licensing for diabetic drivers (DiaMond Project Group on Social Issues, 1993) and even between states in the USA (Gower et al, 1992). The Federal Highways Administration in North America have considered relaxation of the restrictive licensing for insulin-treated diabetic drivers who operate commercial trucks and drive between states. In a pilot study, strict medical qualifications, which includes freedom from severe hypoglycaemia in the preceding five years, are being applied and it is possible that individual case assessment may be introduced in the USA.

In Europe, following the issue of the second EC directive on driving, a further development has been the reclassification of vocational licences and the withdrawal of the rights of people treated with insulin to drive vehicles, such as vans or lorries, weighing 3.5 to 7.5 tonnes (3500 to 7500 kg) (C1 licence), and minibuses with 16 passengers (D1 licence). The governments of most European countries, including the UK, have now agreed to issue C1 licences to "exceptional cases", i.e. drivers with insulin-treated diabetes who drive such vehicles for their employment, subject to more stringent annual review of medical fitness to drive. In the UK, this concession does not include D1 licences. The main concern is the risk of hypoglycaemia affecting drivers of these larger vehicles. The need to safeguard public safety has to be balanced against the rights of the individual with diabetes, but this issue has aroused considerable controversy.

Advice for Diabetic Drivers

Although this chapter is primarily concerned with hypoglycaemia, there are various reasons why an individual driver who is taking insulin may be advised to cease driving, albeit temporarily (Box 11.8). Cox et al (1994) have claimed that blood glucose awareness training in a small number of people with impaired awareness of hypoglycaemia, led to fewer road traffic accidents in subsequent years, suggesting an indirect benefit of this approach to improving the recognition of blood glucose fluctuations (see Chapter 5). Prevention of hypoglycaemia while driving is essential (Box 11.9) and it is important for the driver to plan each journey (no matter

Box 11.8 Diabetic drivers – Reasons to cease driving

Hypoglycaemia

- People with newly diagnosed type 1 diabetes, or any patient commencing treatment with insulin, should cease driving until glycaemic control and vision are stable
- Recurrent hypoglycaemia (especially if severe)
- Impaired awareness of hypoglycaemia (if disabling)

Other

- Reduced (corrected) visual acuity for distance (worse than 6/12 on Snellen chart) in both eyes. Care after use of mydriatic for eye examination
- Sensorimotor peripheral neuropathy with loss of proprioception
- Severe peripheral vascular disease; amputation (hand controls and automatic transmission may be feasible)

Box 11.9 Advice for diabetic drivers regarding hypoglycaemia

- If hypoglycaemia occurs while driving stop the vehicle in a suitable location; leave the driver's seat.
- Always keep an emergency supply of readily accessible fast-acting carbohydrate (e.g. glucose tablets or sweets) *in the vehicle.*
- Check blood glucose before driving (even on short journeys) and estimate at regular intervals on long journeys.
- Take regular meals and snacks, and rest periods on long journeys; avoid alcohol.
- If hypoglycaemia is experienced, do not drive until 45 minutes after blood glucose is restored to normal (delayed recovery of cognitive function).
- Carry personal identification indicating "diabetes" in case of injury in a road traffic accident.

how short) in advance. Blood glucose monitoring is necessary before, and during, long journeys, and rest periods for snacks and meals should be taken. A supply of both quick-acting and more substantial carbohydrate should be kept permanently in the vehicle in case of unexpected delays or emergencies (traffic jams, breakdowns) or unpremeditated exercise such as changing a wheel. If hypoglycaemia occurs while driving, the driver should stop the vehicle, switch off the engine and leave the driver's seat, as in British law a charge of driving under the influence of a drug (insulin) can be made even if the car is stationary. It is also important that driving is not recommended immediately after normoglycaemia is restored. In this situation, blood glucose does not accurately reflect glucose in the brain, with the rise in intracerebral glucose lagging behind that in the peripheral blood. The recovery of cognitive function following hypoglycaemia takes at least 45 minutes after blood glucose has returned to normal.

Medico-legal Aspects

Physicians who specialise in diabetes are often required to provide medico-legal reports on road traffic accidents involving drivers with insulin-treated diabetes, in whom hypoglycaemia has been implicated as a possible cause. A detailed history of the circumstances should be taken from the diabetic driver to identify whether hypoglycaemia was likely at the time of the accident, as a contemporaneous blood glucose is seldom available. Occasionally, a blood glucose has been measured at the scene of the accident by paramedical ambulance staff or on subsequent admission to hospital. However, any significant delay before the blood glucose is estimated may obscure the glycaemic status at the time of the accident, through the effect of counterregulatory hormones released by the stress of the accident and/or hypoglycaemia *per se*, or as a result of treatment.

The presentation of a convincing story of hypoglycaemia preceding the accident has to be accompanied by a careful description of the potential effects of hypoglycaemia on cognitive function and behaviour, comprehensible to a lay person. Although this mitigating factor may not allow legal charges to be dismissed, in my experience the penalty may be substantially reduced if hypoglycaemia is accepted to be the principal problem that has affected the individual's driving ability and precipitated the accident. However, this must not be considered to be a foregone conclusion, as the legal view of hypoglycaemia occurring in a person treated with insulin (or an oral hypoglycaemic drug) is that this represents "careless" behaviour on their part and is therefore the "fault" of the individual, even though in clinical practice no cause can be determined for many episodes of hypoglycaemia. By contrast, spontaneous hypoglycaemia is an accepted defence, and one of my patients with insulin-treated diabetes had charges of dangerous driving dismissed when it was shown that at the time of the offence he had developed undiagnosed and untreated Addison's disease—a rare but recognised cause of increased and unpredictable severe hypoglycaemia in type 1 diabetes. Medico-legal aspects of hypoglycaemia and diabetes have been reviewed previously (Frier and Maher, 1988).

TRAVEL

Many of the measures recommended for longer car journeys (Box 11.9) are appropriate to long-distance travel, irrespective of the mode of transport used. Forward planning is essential to avoid hypoglycaemia, with emphasis on adjustment of insulin dose (or regimen) if necessary, carrying equipment for blood glucose monitoring and ensuring an adequate supply both of quick-acting carbohydrate and of non-perishable emergency rations in case suitable food is not available during travel. Standard airline meals are often low in unrefined carbohydrate. Advice for travel and holidays is available from various sources, but with respect to avoiding (and treating) hypoglycaemia, some practical points can be made.

- For long-distance air travel, crossing several time zones, frequent administration of short-acting (soluble) insulin is much simpler than attempting to modify the times of administration and dosage of intermediate-acting insulins. Disposable insulin pens are also very useful for this purpose. Rapid-acting insulin analogues have the advantage that their administration can be delayed until the food on offer is available and its palatability assessed, or can be taken after the meal, providing greater flexibility of dosage.

- Some blood glucose meters are inaccurate in the hypoglycaemic range and many do not give accurate readings at high altitude or at extremes of temperature. Visually read strips for blood glucose estimation may therefore be necessary in some situations. It is advisable to carry a spare blood glucose meter in case of equipment failure.
- A supply of quick-acting carbohydrate is essential, but should be stored appropriately. Dextrose tablets may disintegrate or become very hard in hot and humid climates unless wrapped in silver foil or stored in a suitable container, and obviously chocolate will melt if the temperature is high. At very cold temperatures, the wrapper may become welded to the chocolate. Cartons of orange juice can not be re-used once opened, so a plastic bottle with a screw top is preferable. Sealed packets of powdered glucose may be more suitable to carry in hot damp climates.
- Travelling companions should carry a supply of quick-acting carbohydrate (and glucagon) for emergency use.

The nature of the travel undertaken, how much energy is expended, the quality and nature of food and the risk of intermittent illness (such as travel sickness or gastroenteritis) are all potential factors that can influence blood glucose and potentially induce hypoglycaemia. While many situations are predictable, the most important measure is frequent monitoring of blood glucose so that sensible adjustments in insulin therapy and ingestion of food can be made.

EMPLOYMENT

The risk of developing acute hypoglycaemia and its consequences (mainly in people with insulin-treated diabetes) is one of the reasons why some forms of employment are not available to individuals who require insulin therapy. Employment prospects are often restricted where the threat of hypoglycaemia poses a risk to the diabetic worker, to his or her colleagues, or to the general public. With some occupations, such as a train or bus driver, or a commercial airline pilot, any risk of hypoglycaemia is unacceptable. In other areas the potential risks of hypoglycaemia may be less well defined, and restrictions to employment have been established by individual industries or firms, rather than by legislation. While medical advice has usually been sought, this has not always been well informed, and may not have involved physicians with expertise in diabetes. Some restrictions have been challenged successfully, with one example in the UK being the reinstatement of several active firefighters, based on individual medical assessment.

People with insulin-treated diabetes are not usually permitted to work alone in isolated or dangerous areas nor at unprotected heights. They are also disbarred from serving in the armed forces. This is presumably on the grounds that all service personnel (including non-combatants) could be involved in a conflict at short notice, and maintaining provision of insulin and appropriate dietary requirements could present difficulties in a wartime situation. Employment is not usually permitted in emergency teams, civil aviation, work in the off-shore oil industry and in many forms of commercial driving (Waclawski, 1989). A list of jobs with which the employment of people with insulin-treated diabetes (both types 1 and 2) is restricted is shown in Table 11.2.

The civil aviation authority in the UK does not permit diabetic indivi-

Table 11.2 Employment restrictions placed on diabetic workers treated with insulin in UK (adapted from Waclawski, 1989)

Vocational driving	Large goods vehicles (LGV licences) Passenger carrying vehicles (PCV licences) Locomotives and underground trains Professional drivers (chauffeurs) Taxi drivers (variable; depends on local authority)
Civil aviation	Commercial pilots; flight engineers Aircrew Air-traffic controllers
National and emergency services	Armed forces (Army, Navy, Air Force) Police force Fire brigade or Rescue services Prison and Security services
Dangerous areas for work	Offshore oil-rig work Moving machinery Incinerator loading Hot-metal areas Work on railway tracks Coal mining
Work at heights	Overhead linesmen Crane driving Scaffolding/high ladders or platforms

duals who are treated either with insulin or with sulphonylureas to fly commercial aircraft, or to work as air-traffic controllers, although in the USA an air-traffic controller has appealed successfully against dismissal on grounds of discrimination. In the European Community, discussions are proceeding to produce common air-worthiness regulations for pilots with medical disorders, including diabetes.

Hypoglycaemia at Work

Although anecdotal accounts exist of severe hypoglycaemia affecting individuals with insulin-treated diabetes while they are at work, no evidence is available to suggest that this is a widespread problem. While isolated episodes of severe hypoglycaemia occurring in the work place are inevitable, it appears that most hypoglycaemia is mild, quickly self-treated and does not cause disruption. The times of day at which hypoglycaemia is most common were observed in a prospective study of 60 patients with type 1 diabetes, half of whom had impaired awareness of hypoglycaemia (Gold et al, 1994b). Most episodes of severe hypoglycaemia occurred during the evening or night, or in the early morning before the subjects went to work (Figure 11.3). The reason for the higher frequency of severe hypoglycaemia in the evening or during the night was not attributable to the insulin regimens being used. People treated with insulin may be more vigilant while at work to try to avoid develop-

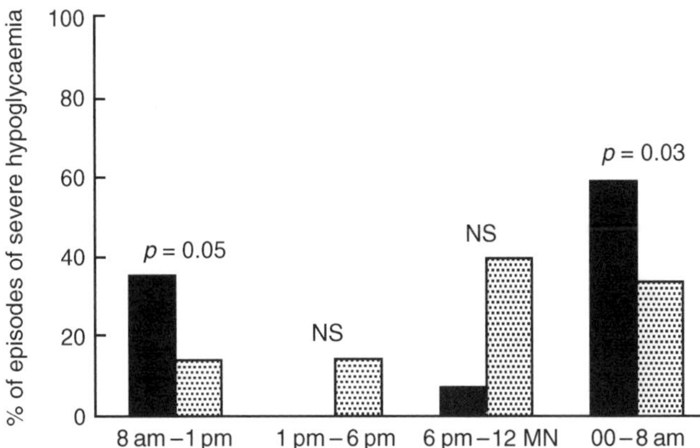

Figure 11.3 Percentages of total number of episodes of severe hypoglycaemia occurring at different times of day in patients with type 1 diabetes with normal (solid bars) and impaired (hatched bars) awareness of hypoglycaemia. Reproduced from Gold et al (1994b) with permission of the American Diabetes Association

ing a low blood glucose, working activities may be more regular than at home or at weekends, or they self-treat a low blood glucose promptly, so avoiding significant neuroglycopenia. A pilot study of 40 people with insulin-treated diabetes in full-time employment in Edinburgh, conducted over three months, indicated that the frequency of severe hypoglycaemia was very low during working hours, although hypoglycaemia was recorded at home and at other times (Beck et al, 1997).

Shift work is generally not a contraindication to the employment of people with type 1 diabetes. However, occasionally a frequent change of shift rota can cause difficulties with glycaemic control, although this usually causes a deterioration in control rather than hypoglycaemia (Poole et al, 1992). Measures to avoid and/or treat hypoglycaemia at work are no different from any other time or circumstance, although in some jobs, blood glucose monitoring may not be feasible while at work, and break times for snacks and meals may be variable. It is essential that workmates or colleagues are familiar with the emergency treatment of diabetes and that a supply of quick-acting carbohydrate is available in the work place. It is advisable that the individual's employer is aware that he or she has type 1 diabetes, although some people conceal this fact, fearing dismissal or discrimination. Legislation to avoid this is in place in many Western countries, but widespread ignorance remains about the nature of diabetes, its treatment and the possible side-effects, and this has to be confronted by those with specialist expertise.

Similar arrangements for emergency treatment should be in place in schools (see Chapter 9), colleges and other venues of tertiary education, including university accommodation. In one tragic, fatal case (Strachan et al, 1998), a young student with type 1 diabetes was left lying unconscious for two days on the floor of his room in the hall of residence, despite being observed by the domestic staff who thought he was asleep, or inebriated. Although the warden knew that the student had diabetes, the domestic staff were not aware of this information, and in this case hypoglycaemic coma was followed by the development of fatal diabetic ketoacidosis. At the subsequent fatal accident enquiry, the dichotomy between maintaining the privacy and confidentiality of the individual, and the duty of care owed to young people living in university accommodation was discussed by the Sheriff. As a result of his report and recommendations, the residential management of students with type 1 diabetes was modified in practice in most Scottish universities. However, this case highlights the importance of disclosure of diabetes, and its potential metabolic problems, (especially hypoglycaemia) to the appropriate authorities and those who may potentially be required to render emergency assistance.

Specialist Medical Reports

Physicians specialising in diabetes are often required to provide medical reports for employers, either related to the suitability of specific types of work for a person with type 1 diabetes, or to their capability of performing the job. It is often necessary to advocate on the behalf of patients when a problem at work is specifically related to some aspect of their diabetic management, such as hypoglycaemia. The introduction of insulin therapy sometimes has to be delayed because of the impact which this will have on the individual's employment. By strict dietary measures, one of my patients who was an oil tanker driver (holding a LGV licence), and who had longstanding type 2 diabetes, managed to maintain satisfactory glycaemic control on the maximum dose of combined oral hypoglycaemic therapy for nearly two years, delaying conversion to insulin. He was anxious to protect his pension rights until his retirement, at which point insulin was commenced. However, procrastination with starting insulin therapy is usually not advisable, particularly in patients presenting with type 1 diabetes, and sympathetic medical counselling may be necessary to recommend an alternative occupation. This is often necessary in people who hold vocational driving licences.

PRISON AND POLICE CUSTODY

Police Custody and Hypoglycaemia

Many features of acute hypoglycaemia simulate those of alcoholic inebriation, so that people with insulin-treated diabetes have occasionally been arrested by the police under the mistaken impression that they are drunk or under the influence of drugs. The danger of this situation is often compounded by their detention at a police station, with confinement in a cell, instead of their urgent transfer to hospital. Unfortunately, the consumption of alcohol can promote hypoglycaemia in people treated with insulin, and may be a contributory factor to inducing the low blood glucose, so causing further difficulty with identification of the underlying metabolic problem. This emphasises the importance of an individual with insulin-treated diabetes carrying some form of identification to indicate that they are taking insulin and may be at risk of developing hypoglycaemia-induced coma. In addition to the risk of being arrested during an episode of hypoglycaemia because of aggressive or abnormal behaviour, a low blood glucose may develop while in custody. The police may have limited comprehension of the needs of a person with diabetes and the risks of hypoglycaemia. The young male patient with undiagnosed Addison's disease, described earlier, who was arrested on a driving charge, was profoundly neuroglycopenic when taken into custody. He was detained without treatment for two hours until his father arrived at the police station. He recognised immediately that his son was severely hypoglycaemic and needed emergency treatment with dextrose. This type of situation is clearly alarming, and potentially could have a fatal outcome.

Management of Diabetes in Prison

The general problems of managing diabetes in prison have been examined in two British studies (Gill and MacFarlane, 1989; MacFarlane et al, 1992) and recommendations have been made to improve the care of people with diabetes in prison, by the American Diabetes Association (Eichold, 1989) and the British Diabetic Association (Gill et al, 1992).

Imprisonment causes particular problems for the management of diabetes, which are conducive to the development of hypoglycaemia. These include:

- an inadequate or inappropriate prison diet
- long "lock-up" periods necessitated by prison routine
- solitary confinement for individual prisoners
- restrictions in the time and place of insulin administration
- the use of some insulin regimens (e.g. basal-bolus and/or injection of bedtime isophane insulin) are precluded by prison routine
- a long time interval between the evening meal and breakfast the following morning (sometimes over 12 hours)
- no blood glucose monitoring facilities being allowed in cells
- lack of medical knowledge among most prison officers, with few personnel having any medical training.

Many of these problems predispose to a risk of nocturnal hypoglycaemia, and actively discourage any attempt at achieving strict glycaemic control. Various measures can be suggested to try to prevent hypoglycaemia in prisoners with insulin-treated diabetes. These include:

- availability of dextrose tablets (or an alternative source of carbohydrate, e.g. biscuits) in cells
- provision of a late evening snack
- avoidance of solitary confinement if possible
- sharing cells with prisoner(s) who can recognise hypoglycaemia
- arranging access to specialist advice on management of diabetes.

CONCLUSIONS

- Fear of hypoglycaemia is common and may influence self-management of blood glucose by individual patients. Worries about hypoglycaemia extend to relatives, spouses and partners of the person with diabetes and recurrent hypoglycaemia can disrupt family life.
- The lack of symptomatic awareness during sleep contributes to the potential severity of nocturnal hypoglycaemia. The time of occurrence of low blood glucose during the night depends on the insulin regimen used. Measures to prevent nocturnal hypoglycaemia include blood glucose testing at bedtime, use of a rapid-acting insulin analogue before the evening meal, and a suitable bedtime snack that is high in unrefined, slowly digested, carbohydrate.
- The risk of hypoglycaemia occurring during exercise depends on the prevailing plasma concentrations of insulin and glucose. Strategies to avoid a fall in blood glucose include the ingestion of additional carbohydrate and a reduction in insulin dose. The contributory effect of alcohol may be important. Sport, recreational activities and travel all require forward planning and preventative measures. Some dangerous activities are not advisable.
- Although the risk of hypoglycaemia-related driving accidents is difficult to quantitate, hypoglycaemia is a potential hazard when driving, and impaired awareness of hypoglycaemia may cause revocation of the driving licence. The diabetic driver must carry a supply of glucose in the vehicle and take suitable precautions on all journeys.
- Hypoglycaemia at work is uncommon but the potential risk disbars insulin-treated people from certain occupations. Discrimination by employers against people with type 1 diabetes may occur occasionally.
- The problems of managing diabetes in prison include inadequate facilities for preventing hypoglycaemia, especially overnight. Retention of diabetic individuals in police custody may cause difficulties by failure of the custodians to recognise hypoglycaemia, and its similarity to the features of inebriation.

REFERENCES

Beck J, Miller BG, Frier BM, Grant J, Waclawski ER (1997). A pilot study of the frequency of hypoglycaemic episodes in people with insulin-treated diabetes and the relationship of hypoglycaemia to employment.Technical memorandum. Institute of Occupational Medicine, Edinburgh: 1997.

Bendtson I, Gade J, Theilgaard A, Binder C (1992). Cognitive function in type 1 (insulin-dependent) diabetic patients after nocturnal hypoglycaemia. *Diabetologia* **35**: 898–903.

Braatvedt GD, Mildenhall L, Patten C, Harris G (1997). Insulin requirements and metabolic control in children with diabetes mellitus attending a summer camp. *Diabet Med* **14**: 258–61.

Chantelau E, Dannbeck S, Kimmerle R, Ross D (1990). Zur verkehrstüchtigkeit insulin-behandelter diabetiker. *Münch Med Wschr.* **132**: 468–71.

Clarke WL, Carter WR, Moll M, Cox DJ, Gonder-Frederick LA, Cryer PE (1988). Metabolic and cutaneous events associated with hypoglycemia detected by Sleep-Sentry. *Diabetes Care* **11**: 630–5.

Clarke WL, Gonder-Frederick LA, Miller S, Richardson T, Snyder A (1998). Maternal fear of hypoglycemia in their children with insulin-dependent diabetes mellitus. *J Pediatr Endocrinol Metab* **4**: 189–94

Cox DJ, Irvine A, Gonder-Frederick L, Nowacek G, Butterfield J (1987). Fear of hypoglycemia: quantification, validation and utilization. *Diabetes Care* **10**: 617–21.

Cox DJ, Gonder-Frederick L, Clarke W (1993). Driving decrements in type 1 diabetes during moderate hypoglycemia *Diabetes* **42**: 239–43

Cox DJ, Gonder-Frederick L, Julian DM, Clarke W (1994). Long-term follow-up evaluation of blood glucose awareness training. *Diabetes Care* **17**: 1–5.

Davies AG, Evans S (1995). Sweat detection as an indicator of nocturnal hypoglycaemia. *Lancet* **346**: 772 (letter).

DiaMond Project Group on Social Issues (1993). Global regulations on diabetics treated with insulin and their operation of commercial motor vehicles. *BMJ* **307**: 250–3.

Eadington DW, Frier BM (1989). type 1 diabetes and driving experience: an eight-year cohort study. *Diabet Med* **6**: 137-41

Edelmann E, Staudner V, Bachmann W, Walter H, Haas W, Mehnert H (1986). Exercise-induced hypoglycaemia and subcutaneous insulin infusion. *Diabet Med* **3**: 526–31.

Eichold S (1989). Diabetes in correctional institutions. *Diabetes Care* **12**: 509–10.

Frid A, Östman J, Linde B (1990). Hypoglycemia risk during exercise after intramuscular injection of insulin in thigh in IDDM. *Diabetes Care* **13**: 473–7.

Frier BM, Maher G (1988). Diabetes and hypoglycaemia: medico-legal aspects of criminal responsibility. *Diabet Med* **5**: 521–6.

Frier BM, Matthews DM, Steel JM, Duncan LJP (1980). Driving and insulin-dependent diabetes. *Lancet* **315**: 1232–4

Gill GV, MacFarlane IA (1989). Problems of diabetics in prison. *BMJ* **298**: 221–3.

Gill GV, MacFarlane IA, Tucker NH (1992). Diabetes care in British prisons: existing problems and potential solutions. *Diabet Med* **9**: 109–13.

Gislason T, Tomasson K, Reynisdottir H, Björnsson JK, Kristbjarnarson H (1997). Medical risk factors amongst drivers in single-car accidents. *J Intern Med* **241**: 213–9.

Gold AE, Deary IJ, Jones RW, O'Hare JP, Reckless JPD, Frier BM (1994a). Severe deterioration in cognitive function and personality in five patients with long-standing diabetes: a complication of diabetes or a consequence of treatment? *Diabetic Medicine* **11**: 499–505.

Gold AE, MacLeod KM, Frier BM (1994b). Frequency of severe hypoglycemia in patients with type 1 diabetes with impaired awareness of hypoglycemia. *Diabetes Care* **17**: 697–703.

Gold AE, Deary IJ, Frier BM (1997). Hypoglycaemia and non-cognitive aspects of psychological function in insulin-dependent (type 1) diabetes mellitus (IDDM). *Diabet Med* **14**: 111–8.

Gonder-Frederick L, Cox D, Kovatchev B, Julian D, Clarke W (1997). The psychosocial impact of severe hypoglycemic episodes on spouses of patients with IDDM. *Diabetes Care* **20**: 1543–6.

Gower IF, Songer TJ, Hylton H, et al (1992). Epidemiology of insulin-using commercial motor vehicle drivers. *Diabetes Care* **15**: 1464–7.

Grimm J-J, Muchnick S (1993). Type 1 diabetes and marathon running. *Diabetes Care* **16**: 1624 (letter).

Hansotia P, Broste SK (1991). The effect of epilepsy or diabetes mellitus on the risk of automobile accidents. *N Eng J Med* **324**: 22–6.

Havlin CE, Cryer PE (1987). Nocturnal hypoglycemia does not commonly result in major morning hyperglycemia in patients with diabetes mellitus. *Diabetes Care* **10**: 141–7.

Hillson RM (1984). Diabetes Outward Bound mountain course, Eskdale, Cumbria. *Diabet Med* **1**: 59–63.

Hillson RM (1987). British Diabetic Association activities for young people – safety while adventuring. *Pract Diabet* **4**: 233–4.

Hirsch IB, Smith LJ, Havlin CE, Shah SD, Clutter WE, Cryer PE (1990). Failure of nocturnal hypoglycemia to cause daytime hyperglycemia in patients with IDDM. *Diabetes Care* **13**: 133–42.

Jenks J, Watkinson M (1998). Minimising the risks of amphetamine use for young adults with diabetes. *J Diabet Nursing* **2**: 179–82.

Jones TW, Porter P, Sherwin RS, et al (1998). Decreased epinephrine responses to hypoglycemia during sleep.*N Eng J Med* **338**: 1657–62.

Kanc K, Janssen MMJ, Keulen ETP, Jacobs MAJM, Popp-Snijders C, Snoek FJ, Heine RJ (1998). Substitution of night-time continuous subcutaneous insulin infusion therapy for bedtime NPH insulin in a multiple injection regimen improves counterregulatory hormonal responses and warning symptoms of hypoglycaemia in IDDM. *Diabetologia* **41**: 322–9.

King P, Kong M-F, Parkin H, Macdonald IA, Tattersall RB (1998). Well-being, cerebral function, and physical fatigue after nocturnal hypoglycemia in IDDM. *Diabetes Care* **21**: 341–5.

Kjeldby B (1997). Running the New York marathon with diabetes. *BMJ* **314**: 1053–4.

Lehmann R, Kaplan V, Bingisser R, Bloch KE, Spinas GA (1997). Impact of physical activity on cardiovascular risk factors in IDDM. *Diabetes Care* **20**: 1603–11.

MacDonald MJ (1987). Postexercise late-onset hypoglycemia in insulin-dependent diabetic patients. *Diabetes Care* **10**: 584–8.

MacFarlane IA, Gill GV, Masson E, Tucker NH (1992). Diabetics in prison: can good diabetic care be achieved? *BMJ* **304**: 152–5.

MacLeod KM, Hepburn DA, Frier BM (1993). Frequency and morbidity of severe hypoglycaemia in insulin-treated diabetic patients. *Diabet Med* **10**: 238–45.

Mohn A, Matyka KA, Harris DA, Ross KM, Edge JA, Dunger DB (1999). Lispro or regular insulin for multiple injection therapy in adolesence. Differences in free insulin insulin and glucose levels overnight. *Diabetes Care* **22**: 27–32.

Perriello G, De Feo P, Torlone E, et al (1998). The effect of asymptomatic nocturnal hypoglycemia on glycemic control in diabetes mellitus. *N Eng J Med* **319**: 1233–9.

Poole C, Wright A, Nattrass M (1992). Control of diabetes mellitus in shift workers. *Br J Ind Med* **49**: 513–5.

Pramming S, Thorsteinsson B, Bendtson I, Binder C (1991). Symptomatic hypoglycaemia in 411 type 1 diabetic patients. *Diabet Med* **8**: 217–22.

Ruegemer JJ, Squires RW, March HM, et al (1990). Differences between prebreakfast and late afternoon glycemic responses to exercise in IDDM patients. *Diabetes Care* **13**: 104–10.

Saleh TY, Cryer PE (1997). Alanine and terbutaline in the prevention of nocturnal hypoglycemia in IDDM. *Diabetes Care* **20**: 1231-6.

Sanders K, Mills J, Martin FIR, Horne DJD (1975). Emotional attitudes in adult insulin-dependent diabetics. *J Psychosom Res.* **19**: 241–6.

Songer TJ, LaPorte RE, Dorman JS, et al (1988). Motor vehicle accidents and IDDM. *Diabetes Care* **11**: 701–7.

Sonnenberg GE, Kemmer FW, Berger M (1990). Exercise in type 1 (insulin-dependent) diabetic patients treated with continuous subcutaneous insulin infusion. Prevention of exercise induced hypoglycaemia. *Diabetologia* **33**: 696–703.

Soo K, Furler SM, Samaras K, Jenkins AB, Campbell LV, Chisholm DJ (1996). Glycemic responses to exercise in IDDM after simple and complex carbohydrate supplementation. *Diabetes Care* **19**: 575–9.

Stahl M, Berger W, Schaechinger H, Cox DJ (1998). Spouse's worries concerning diabetic partner's possible hypoglycaemia. *Diabet Med* **15**: 619–20 (letter).

Stevens AB, Roberts M, McKane R, Atkinson AB, Bell PM, Hayes JR (1989). Motor vehicle driving among diabetics taking insulin and non-diabetics. *BMJ* **299**: 591-5.

Strachan MWJ, Lammie GA, Fineron PW, Perros P, MacCuish AC, Frier BM (1998). A fatal case of diabetic ketoacidosis (DKA): precipitated by preceding severe hypoglycaemia? *Diabet Med* **15** (suppl 1): S47 (abstract).

Thompson CJ, Cummings JFR, Chalmers J, Gould C, Newton RW (1996). How have patients reacted to the implications of the DCCT? *Diabetes Care* **19**: 876–8.

Veneman T, Mitrakou A, Mokan M, Cryer P, Gerich J (1993). Induction of hypoglycemia unawareness by asymptomatic nocturnal hypoglycemia. *Diabetes* **42**: 1233–7.

Vervoort G, Goldschmidt HMG, van Doorn LG (1996). Nocturnal blood glucose profiles in patients with type 1 diabetes mellitus on multiple (> 4) daily insulin injection regimens. *Diabet Med* **13**: 794–9.

Waclawski ER (1989). Employment and diabetes: a survey of the prevalence of diabetic workers known by occupation physicians, and the restrictions placed on diabetic workers in employment. *Diabet Med* **6**: 16–9.

Wasserman DH, Zinman B (1994). Exercise in individuals with IDDM. *Diabetes Care* **17**: 924–37.

Winiger G, Keller U, Laager R, Girard J, Berger W (1995). Protein content of the evening meal and nocturnal plasma glucose regulation in type 1 diabetic subjects. *Hormone Res* **44**: 101–4.

Wredling RAM, Theorell PGT, Roll HM, Lins PES, Adamson UKC (1992). Psychosocial state of patients with IDDM prone to recurrent episodes of severe hypoglycemia. *Diabetes Care* **15**: 518–21.

Index

Note: page references in **bold** are to figures, those in *italics* are to tables.

Index compiled by Liz Granger